Quality of Life

Guest Editors

BRAD E. DICIANNO, MD
RORY A. COOPER, PhD

PHYSICAL MEDICINE AND REHABILITATION CLINICS OF NORTH AMERICA

www.pmr.theclinics.com

Consulting Editor
GEORGE H. KRAFT, MD, MS

February 2010 • Volume 21 • Number 1

SAUNDERS an imprint of ELSEVIER, Inc.

W.B. SAUNDERS COMPANY
A Division of Elsevier Inc.

1600 John F. Kennedy Boulevard • Suite 1800 • Philadelphia, Pennsylvania 19103

http://www.theclinics.com

PHYSICAL MEDICINE AND REHABILITATION CLINICS OF NORTH AMERICA Volume 21, Number 1
February 2010 ISSN 1047-9651, ISBN-13: 978-1-4377-1859-1

Editor: Debora Dellapena

Reprints. For copies of 100 or more of articles in this publication, please contact the Commercial Reprints Department, Elsevier Inc., 360 Park Avenue South, New York, NY 10010-1710. Tel.: 212-633-3812; Fax: 212-462-1935; E-mail: reprints@elsevier.com.

Physical Medicine and Rehabilitation Clinics of North America (ISSN 1047-9651) is published quarterly by Elsevier Inc., 360 Park Avenue South, New York, NY 10010-1710. Months of issue are February, May, August, and November. Business and Editorial Offices: 1600 John F. Kennedy Blvd., Suite 1800, Philadelphia, PA 19103-2899. Customer Service Office: 3251 Riverport Lane, Maryland Heights, MO 63043. Periodicals postage paid at New York, NY and additional mailing offices. Subscription price per year is $230.00 (US individuals), $376.00 (US institutions), $116.00 (US students), $280.00 (Canadian individuals), $491.00 (Canadian institutions), $167.00 (Canadian students), $345.00 (foreign individuals), $491.00 (foreign institutions), and $167.00 (foreign students). Foreign air speed delivery is included in all *Clinics* subscription prices. All prices are subject to change without notice. **POSTMASTER:** Send address changes to *Physical Medicine and Rehabilitation Clinics of North America*, Customer Service Office: Elsevier Health Sciences Division, Subscription Customer Service, 3251 Riverport Lane, Maryland Heights, MO 63043. **Customer Service: 1-800-654-2452 (US). From outside of the United States, call 314-447-8871. Fax: 314-447-8029. E-mail: JournalsCustomerService-usa@elsevier.com (for print support); JournalsOnlineSupport-usa@elsevier.com (for online support).**

Physical Medicine and Rehabilitation Clinics of North America is indexed in *Excerpta Medica, MEDLINE/ PubMed (Index Medicus), Cinahl,* and *Cumulative Index to Nursing and Allied Health Literature.*

Printed and bound by CPI Group (UK) Ltd, Croydon, CR0 4YY

Transferred to Digital Print 2011

Contributors

CONSULTING EDITOR

GEORGE H. KRAFT, MD, MS
Alvord Professor of Multiple Sclerosis Research; Professor, Department of Rehabilitation Medicine, and Adjunct Professor, Department of Neurology, University of Washington School of Medicine, Seattle, Washington

GUEST EDITORS

BRAD E. DICIANNO, MD
Assistant Professor, Departments of Physical Medicine and Rehabilitation, and Rehabilitation Science and Technology, University of Pittsburgh Medical Center; Medical Director, University of Pittsburgh Medical Center, Center for Assistive Technology; Associate Medical Director, Department of Veterans Affairs, Human Engineering Research Laboratories, Veterans Affairs Pittsburgh Healthcare System, Pittsburgh, Pennsylvania

RORY A. COOPER, PhD
Director, Department of Veterans Affairs, Human Engineering Research Laboratories, Pittsburgh Veterans Affairs Rehabilitation Research and Development Center, Veterans Affairs Pittsburgh Healthcare System; Distinguished Professor and FISA Foundation–Paralyzed Veterans of America Chair, Departments of Rehabilitation Science and Technology, Bioengineering, and Physical Medicine and Rehabilitation, University of Pittsburgh, Pittsburgh, Pennsylvania

AUTHORS

SONYA ALLIN, PhD
Adjunct Research Scientist, Toronto Rehabilitation Institute, Toronto, Postdoctoral Researcher, Natural Sciences and Engineering Research Council of Canada, Department of Occupational Science and Occupational Therapy, Intelligent Assistive Technology and Systems Lab, University of Toronto, Toronto, Canada

VICTORIA C. ANDERSON-BARNES, BA
Center for Neuroscience and Regenerative Medicine, Uniformed Services University, Bethesda, Maryland

NAHOM M. BEYENE, MS
Human Engineering Research Laboratories, Department of Veterans Affairs, Veterans Affairs Pittsburgh Healthcare System; University of Pittsburgh, Pittsburgh, Pennsylvania

NIELS BIRBAUMER, PhD
Professor, Institute of Medical Psychology and Behavioral Neurobiology, University of Tuebingen, Tuebingen, Germany

MICHAEL L. BONINGER, MD
Chair and Professor, Departments of Physical Medicine and Rehabilitation and Bioengineering, University of Pittsburgh; Medical Director, Human Engineering Research Laboratories, Veterans Affairs Pittsburgh Healthcare System, Pittsburgh, Pennsylvania

BAMBI R. BREWER, PhD
Assistant Professor, Department of Rehabilitation Science and Technology, University of Pittsburgh, Pittsburgh, Pennsylvania

STEVEN W. BROSE, DO
Spinal Cord Injury Medicine Fellow, Department of Physical Medicine and Rehabilitation, University of Pittsburgh, Pittsburgh, Pennsylvania

LEONARDO G. COHEN, MD
Senior Investigator, Human Cortical Physiology Section and Stroke Neurorehabilitation Section, National Institute of Neurological Disorders and Stroke, National Institutes of Health, Bethesda, Maryland

JENNIFER L. COLLINGER, PhD
Research Bioengineer, Department of Physical Medicine and Rehabilitation, University of Pittsburgh; Human Engineering Research Laboratories, Veterans Affairs Pittsburgh Healthcare System, Pittsburgh, Pennsylvania

JOHN COLTELLARO, MS, ATP
Rehabilitation Engineer, University of Pittsburgh Medical Center, Center for Assistive Technology, Pittsburgh, Pennsylvania

RORY A. COOPER, PhD
Director, Human Engineering Research Laboratories, Department of Veterans Affairs, Pittsburgh Veterans Affairs Rehabilitation Research and Development Center, Veterans Affairs Pittsburgh Healthcare System; Distinguished Professor and FISA Foundation–Paralyzed Veterans of America Chair, Departments of Rehabilitation Science and Technology, Bioengineering, and Physical Medicine and Rehabilitation, University of Pittsburgh, Pittsburgh, Pennsylvania

ROSEMARIE COOPER, MPT, ATP
Assistant Professor, Human Engineering Research Laboratories, Pittsburgh Veterans Affairs Rehabilitation Research and Development Center, Veterans Affairs Pittsburgh Healthcare System; Assistant Professor, Department of Rehabilitation Science and Technology, University of Pittsburgh; Center for Assistive Technology, Pittsburgh, Pennsylvania

BEATRIZ CRESPO-RUIZ
Sport Science, National Hospital for Spinal Cord Injury, The Healthcare Service of Castilla–La Mancha (SESCAM), Toledo, Spain

S. DE GROOT, PhD
Centre for Human Movement Sciences, University Medical Centre Groningen, University of Groningen; Duyvensz-Nagel Research Laboratory, Rehabilitation Centre Amsterdam, The Netherlands

ANTONIO DEL AMA-ESPINOSA
Engineer, National Hospital for Spinal Cord Injury, The Healthcare Service of Castilla–La Mancha (SESCAM), Toledo, Spain

BRAD E. DICIANNO, MD
Assistant Professor, Departments of Physical Medicine and Rehabilitation, and Rehabilitation Science and Technology, University of Pittsburgh Medical Center; Medical Director, University of Pittsburgh Medical Center, Center for Assistive Technology; Associate Medical Director, Department of Veterans Affairs, Human Engineering Research Laboratories, Veterans Affairs Pittsburgh Healthcare System, Pittsburgh, Pennsylvania

DAN DING, PhD
Assistant Professor, Department of Rehabilitation Science and Technology, University of Pittsburgh; Human Engineering Research Laboratories, Department of Veterans Affairs, Veterans Affairs Pittsburgh Healthcare System, Pittsburgh, Pennsylvania

EMILY ECKEL, MS, OTR/L
Assistant Professor, Master of Occupational Therapy Program, Chatham University, Pittsburgh, Pennsylvania

ANDREA FAIRMAN, OTR/L, CPRP
Graduate Student Researcher, School of Health and Rehabilitation Science, Department of Rehabilitation Science and Technology, University of Pittsburgh, Pittsburgh, Pennsylvania

ROBERT GAILEY, PhD, PT
Director, Functional Outcomes Research and Evaluation Center, Veterans Affairs Miami Health Care System; Associate Professor, Department of Physical Therapy, University of Miami Miller School of Medicine, Miami, Florida

ANGEL GIL-AGUDO, MD
Coordinator, Departments of Physical Medicine and Rehabilitation and Department of Biomechanics and Technical Aids, National Hospital for Spinal Cord Injury, The Healthcare Service of Castilla–La Mancha (SESCAM), Toledo, Spain

JEFFREY S. GIUGGIO, MArch
Human Engineering Research Laboratories, Department of Veterans Affairs, Rehabilitation Research and Development Service; Department of Rehabilitation Science and Technology, University of Pittsburgh, Pittsburgh, Pennsylvania

W. GROEN, MSc
Faculty of Human Movement Sciences, Research Institute MOVE, Vrije Universiteit, Amsterdam, The Netherlands

F.J. HETTINGA, PhD
Centre for Human Movement Sciences, University Medical Centre Groningen, University of Groningen, Groningen, The Netherlands

KATYA HILL, PhD, CCC-SLP
Associate Professor, Communication Science and Disorders, School of Health and Rehabilitation Sciences, University of Pittsburgh; Executive Director, Augmentative and Alternative Communication (AAC) Institute, Pittsburgh, Pennsylvania

HEIDI HORSTMANN KOESTER, PhD
Koester Performance Research, Ann Arbor, Michigan

ALEXANDRA N. JEFFERDS, BS
Human Engineering Research Laboratories, Department of Veterans Affairs, Veterans Affairs Pittsburgh Healthcare System; University of Pittsburgh, Pittsburgh, Pennsylvania

JUSTIN Z. LAFERRIER, MSPT, OCS, SCS, ATP, CSCS
Human Engineering Research Laboratories, Veterans Affairs Rehabilitation Research and Development Service, Veterans Affairs Pittsburgh Healthcare System; Department of Rehabilitation Science and Technology, University of Pittsburgh, Pittsburgh, Pennsylvania

ROGER LITTLE, MS
Department of Rehabilitation Science and Technology, School of Health and
Rehabilitation Sciences, University of Pittsburgh, Pittsburgh, Pennsylvania

HSIN-YI LIU, MS
Student, Department of Rehabilitation Science and Technology, University of
Pittsburgh; Human Engineering Research Laboratories, Department of Veterans Affairs,
Veterans Affairs Pittsburgh Healthcare System, Pittsburgh, Pennsylvania

EDMUND LoPRESTI, PhD
Koester Performance Research, Ann Arbor, Michigan; AT Sciences, Pittsburgh,
Pennsylvania

HEATHER MARKHAM, MS
Doctoral Student Researcher, Department of Rehabilitation Science and Technology,
University of Pittsburgh, Pittsburgh, Pennsylvania

MICHAEL MCCUE, PhD
Associate Professor and Vice-Chair of Rehabilitation Science and Technology, Director
of the Rehabilitation Counseling Program and Co-Director of the Rehabilitation
Engineering Research Center on Telerehabilitation, Department of Rehabilitation Science
and Technology, School of Health and Rehabilitation Science, University of Pittsburgh,
Pittsburgh, Pennsylvania

GREGORY J. PAQUIN, BSc
Rehabilitation Engineer, California Department of Rehabilitation, Santa Fe Springs,
California

LAVINIA FICI PASQUINA, MArch
Associate Professor, School of Architecture and Planning, The Catholic University
of America, Washington, District of Columbia

PAUL F. PASQUINA, MD
Chairman, Department of Orthopaedics and Rehabilitation, Walter Reed Army Medical
Center, Bethesda, Maryland

JONATHAN L. PEARLMAN, PhD
Human Engineering Research Laboratories, Department of Veterans Affairs, Veterans
Affairs Pittsburgh Healthcare System; University of Pittsburgh, Pittsburgh, Pennsylvania

MONICA A. PEREZ, PhD, PT
Assistant Professor, Department of Physical Medicine and Rehabilitation, University
of Pittsburgh, Pittsburgh, Pennsylvania

MICHAEL PRAMUKA, PhD, CRC
Assistant Professor, School of Health and Rehabilitation Science, Department of
Rehabilitation Science and Technology, University of Pittsburgh, Pittsburgh, Pennsylvania

ANDREW B. SCHWARTZ, PhD
Professor, Departments of Bioengineering and Neurobiology, University of Pittsburgh,
Pittsburgh, Pennsylvania

PUNEET SHOKER, BPT
Indian Spinal Injuries Centre, New Delhi, India

DAN SIEWIOREK, PhD
Buhl University Professor of Computer Science, Electrical and Computer Engineering, School of Computer Science, Carnegie Mellon University, Pittsburgh, Pennsylvania

RICHARD SIMPSON, PhD, ATP
Associate Professor, Departments of Veterans Affairs and Rehabilitation Science and Technology, Human Engineering Research Labs, University of Pittsburgh, Pittsburgh, Pennsylvania

ASIM SMAILAGIC, PhD
Research Professor, School of Computer Science, Institute for Complex Engineered Systems, Carnegie Mellon University, Pittsburgh, Pennsylvania

AARON M. STEINFELD, PhD
Systems Scientist, Robotics Institute, Carnegie Mellon University, Pittsburgh, Pennsylvania

ELIZABETH C. TYLER-KABARA, MD, PhD
Assistant Professor, Departments of Bioengineering and Neurological Surgery, University of Pittsburgh, Pittsburgh, Pennsylvania

NEKRAM UPADHYAY, MS
Indian Spinal Injuries Centre, New Delhi, India

L. VALENT, PhD
Heliomare Rehabilitation Research and Development, Wijk aan Zee, The Netherlands

L.H.V. VAN DER WOUDE, PhD
Centre for Human Movement Sciences, University Medical Centre Groningen, University of Groningen, Groningen, The Netherlands

S. VAN DRONGELEN, PhD
Swiss Paraplegic Research, Nottwil, Switzerland

LINDA VAN ROOSMALEN, PhD
Visiting Assistant Professor, Department of Rehabilitation Science and Technology, University of Pittsburgh, Pittsburgh, Pennsylvania

WEI WANG, MD, PhD
Assistant Professor, Departments of Physical Medicine and Rehabilitation and Bioengineering, University of Pittsburgh; Quality of Life Technology Engineering Research Center, Pittsburgh, Pennsylvania

DOUGLAS J. WEBER, PhD
Assistant Professor, Departments of Physical Medicine and Rehabilitation and Bioengineering, University of Pittsburgh; Quality of Life Technology Engineering Research Center, Pittsburgh, Pennsylvania

JOY WEE, MSc, MD, FRCPC
Providence Care, St. Mary's of the Lake Hospital, Queen's University, Kingston, Ontario, Canada

Contents

> Technology plays a critical role in promoting well-being, activity, and participation for individuals with spinal cord injury (SCI). As technology has improved, so has the realm of possibilities open to people with SCI. School, work, travel, and leisure activities are all facilitated by technology. Advances in materials have made wheelchairs lighter, and developments in design have made wheelchairs that fit individual needs. Software has made computer interfaces adaptive and in some case intelligent, through learning the user's behavior and optimizing its structure. As participatory action design and aware systems take greater hold, transformational change is likely to take place in the technology available to people with SCI.

> Computer access technology (CAT) allows people who have trouble using a standard computer keyboard, mouse, or monitor to access a computer. CAT is critical for enhancing the educational and vocational opportunities of people with disabilities. Choosing the most appropriate CAT is a collaborative decision-making process involving the consumer, clinician(s), and third party payers. The challenges involved and potential technological solutions are discussed.

> Electronic aids to daily living (EADLs) are devices that facilitate the operation of electrical appliances in a given environment for a person with a severe physical disability. These specialized devices can provide tremendous psychological and functional benefits to someone with a severe disability, their family members and caregivers. This article provides an overview of the utility, functionality, access, acquisition, and evaluation of EADLs. It also highlights challenges in obtaining and measuring the benefits of these devices.

Augmentative and alternative communication (AAC) technology is recommended for individuals with significant communication disorders, who may have motor limitations and other challenges that impact quality of life (QOL). The goal of AAC treatment is to optimize communication. This article presents innovations to the primary, secondary, and tertiary AAC components that are considered by rehabilitation clinicians when matching people with technology (MPT). Language considerations are paramount to the MPT process, and innovations are discussed on how features may enhance language performance. AAC technology has made performance and outcome gains contributing to the QOL of people who cannot speak.

This review explores recent trends in the development and evaluation of assistive robotic arms, both prosthetic and externally mounted. Evaluations have been organized according to the CATOR taxonomy of assistive device outcomes, which takes into consideration device effectiveness, social significance, and impact on subjective well-being. Questions that have informed the review include: (1) Are robotic arms being comprehensively evaluated along axes of the CATOR taxonomy? (2) Are definitions of effectiveness in accordance with the priorities of users? (3) What gaps in robotic arm evaluation exist, and how might these best be addressed? (4) What further advances can be expected in the next 15 years? Results highlight the need for increased standardization of evaluation methods, increased emphasis on the social significance (i.e., social cost) of devices, and increased emphasis on device impact on quality of life. Several open areas for future research, in terms of both device evaluation and device development, are also discussed.

Recent advancements in control interface technology have made the use of end devices such as power wheelchairs easier for individuals with disabilities, especially persons with movement disorders. In this article, we discuss the current state of control interface technology and the devices available clinically for power wheelchair control. We also discuss our research on novel hardware and software approaches that are revolutionizing joystick interface technology and allowing more customizability for individual users with special needs and abilities. Finally, we discuss the future of control interfaces and what research gaps remain.

> The boundaries once faced by individuals with amputations are quickly being overcome through biotechnology. Although there are currently no prosthetics capable of replicating anatomic function, there have been radical advancements in prosthetic technology, medical science, and rehabilitation in the past 30 years, vastly improving functional mobility and quality of life for individuals with lower-limb amputations. What once seemed impossible is rapidly becoming reality. The future seems limitless, and the replication of anatomic function now seems possible.

> Motor vehicles are a technology that has been embedded in the built environment since the early 1900s. Personal transportation is important for the quality of life of individuals who have disabilities because it gives a feeling of freedom and enables individuals who have mobility impairments to participate in the community. This article describes the evaluation of individuals and their cognitive, sensory, and physical abilities that are important for (safe) driving. A case is made for independent mobility for individuals who have disabilities and elderly individuals by first giving an overview of the functional, cognitive, and sensory abilities that are critical for driving. Second, the types of vehicle modifications and state-of-the-art controls that are available and on the horizon are described and the way in which these technologies are selected to meet driver needs is explained. Requirements for driver safety systems for drivers who remain in their wheelchairs are then discussed. Finally, emerging and innovative driving enhancement systems, such as obstacle avoidance and navigation, are discussed, as are their benefits in helping drivers who have disabilities and elderly drivers to experience safe and independent driving.

> By studying exercise and performance in hand-cycling in both activities of daily living and in Paralympic sport settings, new insights can be gained for rehabilitation practice, adapted physical activity, and sports. This review looks into the pros and cons of hand-cycling in both rehabilitation and optimal sports performance settings as suggested from the current—but still limited—scientific literature and experimentation. Despite the limited evidence-base and the diversity of study approaches and methodologies, this study suggests an important role for hand-cycling during and after rehabilitation, and in wheeled mobility recreation and sports. An approach that combines biomechanical, physiological, and psychosocial elements may

lead to a better understanding of the benefits of hand-cycling and of the fundamentals of exercise in rehabilitation, activities of daily living, and sports.

Classification systems are one of the key elements in sports for people with disability, including wheelchair basketball. Further scientific studies to validate classification systems are needed. This article describes the most relevant research, with emphasis on biomechanics.

This article reviews neural interface technology and its relationship with neuroplasticity. Two types of neural interface technology are reviewed, highlighting specific technologies that the authors directly work with: (1) neural interface technology for neural recording, such as the micro-ECoG BCI system for hand prosthesis control, and the comprehensive rehabilitation paradigm combining MEG-BCI, action observation, and motor imagery training; (2) neural interface technology for functional neural stimulation, such as somatosensory neural stimulation for restoring somatosensation, and non-invasive cortical stimulation using rTMS and tDCS for modulating cortical excitability and stroke rehabilitation. The close interaction between neural interface devices and neuroplasticity leads to increased efficacy of neural interface devices and improved functional recovery of the nervous system. This symbiotic relationship between neural interface technology and the nervous system is expected to maximize functional gain for individuals with various sensory, motor, and cognitive impairments, eventually leading to better quality of life.

"Virtual Coach" refers to a coaching program or device aiming to guide users through tasks for the purpose of prompting positive behavior or assisting with learning new skills. This article reviews virtual coach interventions with the purpose of guiding rehabilitation professionals to comprehend more effectively the essential components of such interventions, the underlying technologies and their integration, and example applications. A design space of virtual coach interventions including self-monitoring, context awareness, interface modality, and coaching strategies were identified and discussed to address when, how, and what coaching messages to deliver in an automated and intelligent way. Example applications that address various health-related issues also are provided to illustrate how a virtual coach intervention is developed and evaluated. Finally, the article provides some insight into addressing key challenges and opportunities in designing and implementing virtual coach interventions. It is expected that more virtual coach interventions will be developed in the field of rehabilitation to support self-care and prevent secondary conditions in individuals with disabilities.

Michael McCue, Andrea Fairman, and Michael Pramuka

Telerehabilitation is an emerging method of delivering rehabilitation services that uses technology to serve clients, clinicians, and systems by minimizing the barriers of distance, time, and cost. The driving force for telerehabilitation has been as an alternative to face-to-face rehabilitation approaches to reduce costs, increase geographic accessibility, or act as a mechanism to extend limited resources. A rationale for telerehabilitation is the potential to enhance outcomes beyond what may result from face-to-face interventions by enabling naturalistic, in vivo interventions. There is considerable support for the value of interventions delivered in the natural environment, ranging from addressing efficacy concerns by addressing problems of generalization, to increasing patient participation, including environmental context in rehabilitation, and increasing patient satisfaction. Further clinical and research exploration should explore telerehabilitation as a tool for the delivery of rehabilitation services in vivo.

Paul F. Pasquina, Lavinia Fici Pasquina, Victoria C. Anderson-Barnes, Jeffrey S. Giuggio, and Rory A. Cooper

Today, injured service members are surviving wounds that would have been fatal in previous wars. A recent RAND report estimates that approximately 320,000 service members may have experienced a traumatic brain injury (TBI) during deployment, and it is not uncommon for a soldier to sustain multiple associated injuries such as limb loss, paralysis, sensory loss, and psychological damage. As a result, many military service members and their families face significant challenges returning to a high quality of independent life. The architectural concepts of universal design (UD) and evidence-based design (EBD) are gaining interest as an integral part of the rehabilitation process of veterans with TBI. This article examines the possibilities presented by UD and EBD in accordance with the Americans with Disabilities Act of 1990, in terms of high-end building and interior design quality, and possible technological options for individuals with disabilities.

Alexandra N. Jefferds, Nahom M. Beyene, Nekram Upadhyay,
Puneet Shoker, Jonathan L. Pearlman, Rory A. Cooper, and Joy Wee

This article reviews mobility technology in less-resourced countries, with reference to people with disabilities in several locations, and describes technology provision to date. It also discusses a recent collaborative study between a United States University and an Indian spinal injuries hospital of Indian wheelchair users' community participation, satisfaction, and wheelchair skills. The data suggest that individuals who received technology from the hospital's assistive technology department experienced increased community participation and improved wheelchair skills. This evidence may have already enabled the hospital to improve Indian governmental policies toward people with disabilities, and it is hoped that future research will benefit other people similarly.

THE CLINICS ARE NOW AVAILABLE ONLINE!

Access your subscription at:
www.theclinics.com

Foreword

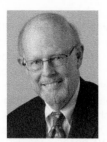

George H. Kraft, MD, MS
Consulting Editor

I am indebted to Drs. Rory Cooper and Brad Dicianno for preparing this issue on quality of life (QOL) and trust that the readers of the *Physical Medicine and Rehabilitation Clinics of North America* also are. QOL research is currently a "hot" topic in rehabilitation, and these guest editors have gathered together several qualified experts on a wide variety of relevant QOL topics.

This is the first issue in many years to come from the remarkably successful Department of Physical Medicine and Rehabilitation at the University of Pittsburgh. Perhaps this is an appropriate time for this publication, as Pittsburgh is in the news with the meeting in that city of the Group of Twenty Finance Ministers and Central Bank Governors (G-20). Rory Cooper, PhD, and physiatrist, Brad Dicianno, MD, at the University of Pittsburgh's Center for Assistive Technology have incorporated a phenomenally broad array of important topics. How can the medical field of rehabilitation, which at its core manages chronically disabling conditions, improve function? The answer is assistive technology—the thrust of this issue.

Technology can improve QOL. Examples are use of environmental controls, robotics, improved joystick technology, augmentative and alternative communication, personal transportation, and virtual coach technology to improve self-care. Can neural interface technology enhance neuroplasticity? This question is addressed.

Avocational activities and their contribution to QOL are not ignored; hand cycling and wheelchair basketball are discussed. Specific disease states are covered: spinal cord injuries, lower limb amputations and prosthetics, and military-acquired traumatic brain injury. Finally, can health care be improved using computer assessment and telerehabilitation? Finally, what is the status of mobility technology in countries with fewer resources?

Phys Med Rehabil Clin N Am 21 (2010) xvii–xviii
doi:10.1016/j.pmr.2009.09.002
1047-9651/09/$ – see front matter © 2010 Elsevier Inc. All rights reserved.

pmr.theclinics.com

These are important questions, and this is an important issue. I hope that this issue of the *Clinics* will serve as a resource on technology and QOL. As it is now indexed in PubMed, this information will be useful for years to come.

George H. Kraft, MD, MS
Alvord Professor of Multiple Sclerosis
Research Professor
Department of
Rehabilitation Medicine
Adjunct Professor Department of Neurology
University of Washington, Box 356490
1959 NE Pacific Street
Seattle, WA 98195-6490, USA

E-mail address:
ghkraft@uw.edu (G.H. Kraft)

Preface

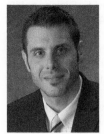 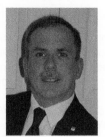

Brad E. Dicianno, MD   Rory A. Cooper, PhD
Guest Editors

Quality-of-life technology is of paramount importance to allowing the elderly and those with disabilities to function independently in their homes and communities. Such technology will become increasingly important in the upcoming decades, as twice as many individuals older than 65 years will be alive in the United States in 2025 than in 1997 and as the number of individuals with disabilities continues to skyrocket.

In this collection of work from some of the top investigators in the field of quality-of-life technology, research in key areas where strides are being made to meet the technology needs of future generations is discussed. Independence in carrying out daily activities and employment is enhanced by new technology in computer access devices, environmental control, augmentative communication, and robotics. New mobility technology—from control interfaces for wheelchairs to prosthetic limbs—has exploded, with new options for customizing devices for each user's individual needs. Social participation is enhanced by technology that makes transportation safe and efficient. Individuals are able to exercise and participate in sports because of advancements made in adaptive equipment, such as hand cycles and sports wheelchairs.

This issue also discusses how the future of rehabilitation technology is already upon us. It presents present a glimpse of the ways sophisticated algorithms, human–systems interfaces, and brain–computer interfaces can give individuals with severe motor impairments the ability to control a host of end devices. Work on virtual coaching, which can allow users to reap even more benefits from the technology they use, is discussed. Discoveries in telerehabilitation allow multidisciplinary teams to collaborate and provide remote service delivery to users in need who have never before been connected to rehabilitation professionals. A picture is painted of universal design of contemporary, comfortable, and aesthetically pleasing spaces for living and work that everyone can soon enjoy. Finally, how those in areas of the world with fewer resources are challenged to meet the needs of their own growing populations with unique and fascinating approaches to implementing technology relevant to their communities is discussed.

Phys Med Rehabil Clin N Am 21 (2010) xix–xx
doi:10.1016/j.pmr.2009.08.002
1047-9651/09/$ – see front matter © 2010 Elsevier Inc. All rights reserved.

pmr.theclinics.com

We hope that readers not only feel challenged by the obstacles that they face today but also are inspired by the possibilities that quality-of-life technology affords.

Brad E. Dicianno, MD
Assistant Professor
Department of Physical Medicine and Rehabilitation
Department of Rehabilitation Science and Technology
University of Pittsburgh Medical Center, Kaufmann Medical Building
Suite 202, 3471 5th Avenue, Pittsburgh, PA 15213, USA

Medical Director of UPMC Center for Assistive Technology
Associate Medical Director for Department of Veterans Affairs
Human Engineering Research Laboratories
7180 Highland Drive, 151R-1, Pittsburgh, PA 15206, USA

Rory A. Cooper, PhD
Director
Department of Veterans Affairs
Human Engineering Research Laboratories
Pittsburgh VA Rehabilitation Research and Development Center
VA Pittsburgh Healthcare System
7180 Highland Drive, 151R-1, Pittsburgh, PA 15206, USA

Distinguished Professor
FISA Foundation–Paralyzed Veterans of America Chair
Department of Rehabilitation Science and Technology
Departments of Bioengineering and
Physical Medicine and Rehabilitation
University of Pittsburgh, 3471 5th Avenue, Pittsburgh, PA 15213, USA

E-mail addresses:
dicianno@pitt.edu (B.E. Dicianno)
rcooper@pitt.edu (R.A. Cooper)

Quality-of-Life Technology for People with Spinal Cord Injuries

Rory A. Cooper, PhD[a,b,c,d],*, Rosemarie Cooper, MPT, ATP[a]

KEYWORDS
- Rehabilitation • Spinal cord injury • Wheelchair • Seating
- Computer access • Adaptive recreation

Technology plays a critical role in promoting well-being, activity, and participation for individuals with spinal cord injury (SCI). It is one of the few things that can be provided to people with SCI where one can see an immediate and profound benefit. As technology has improved, so has the realm of possibilities open to people with SCI. The range of activities in which people with SCI participate is impressive and yet still growing. School, work, travel, and leisure activities are all facilitated by technology.[1,2] Advances in materials have made wheelchairs lighter, and developments in design have made wheelchairs that fit individual needs. Software has made computer interfaces adaptive and in some case intelligent, through learning the user's behavior and optimizing its structure. The trend is certainly taking us in two exciting directions: (1) personalized design where the technology matches and adapts to the user's needs; (2) and aware systems that learn from the user's behavior, the context, and the environment to support the end-user. As participatory action design and aware systems take greater hold, transformational change is likely to take place in the technology available to people with SCI.

Universal design is likely superseded in many areas of assistive technology in favor of adaptive and smart design. The basic premise of universal design is that products,

[a] Human Engineering Research Laboratories, Pittsburgh VA Rehabilitation Research & Development Center, VA Pittsburgh Healthcare System, 7180 Highland Drive, Pittsburgh, PA 15206, USA
[b] Department of Rehabilitation Science & Technology, University of Pittsburgh, Pittsburgh, PA 15206, USA
[c] Department of Bioengineering, University of Pittsburgh, Pittsburgh, PA 15206, USA
[d] Department of Physical Medicine & Rehabilitation, University of Pittsburgh, Pittsburgh, PA 15206, USA
* Corresponding author. Human Engineering Research Laboratories, Pittsburgh VA Rehabilitation Research & Development Center, VA Pittsburgh Healthcare System, 7180 Highland Drive, Pittsburgh, PA 15206.
E-mail address: rcooper@pitt.edu (R.A. Cooper).

Phys Med Rehabil Clin N Am 21 (2010) 1–13
doi:10.1016/j.pmr.2009.07.004
1047-9651/09/$ – see front matter. Published by Elsevier Inc.

pmr.theclinics.com

buildings, and entire systems be created that accommodate the maximum possible range of people. This is a noble goal, but it often leads to unsatisfactory results for large sectors of people; although, architecture and city planning are notable exceptions where universal design has been successful and has been a stimulus for creative thinking. Of course, there are other examples as well. Adaptive design is already making inroads, especially in devices and even systems that are programmable. For example an ubiquitous cellular telephone can be adapted in many ways. The cell phone software allows for personalization (eg, ring tone, address book), and limited learning (eg, recording numbers called and received). The appearance of some cell phones can be changed by changing the snap-on plastic cover. Another entirely different approach is used in the eyeglass business that allows people to try various colors of a fixed frame style at no risk; this is feasible because most of the cost is in the lenses, which are transferred between frames. This latter approach can be seen as smart design, where the needs of various customers are anticipated in advance and incorporated into the range of products and options made available. Rapid prototyping and flexible manufacturing are already making their impact on smart design. Rapid prototyping in a classical sense uses computer-aided engineering, design, and manufacturing to make products or components using more or less standard manufacturing processes. This removes much of the human labor and specialized tooling from the product pathways. State-of-the-art rapid prototyping uses constructive processes, such as 3-dimensioal printing, to assemble devices from basic materials. Flexible manufacturing is making change to the way products are designed and manufactured; as factories became more automated to reduce costs and increase flexibility, the concept grew to include making multiple products for different companies within the same factory. Flexible manufacturing allows the machines and product flow to change to meet an individual customer's needs. Personal computers are an example of flexible manufacturing that most people may be familiar with. Quite readily, one can order a computer through the Internet or via telephone that is manufactured for them from a wide selection of options and features that they choose from. These technological changes are impacting assistive technology and will continue to do so for some time to come.

THE TEAM APPROACH

Like other areas of rehabilitation, the delivery of assistive technology (AT) services are best provided using a team approach.[1,2] The individual with SCI and the family members are critical members of the team, and they should set the goals. Ideally, an AT team would include a physician, therapist, AT supplier, and a rehabilitation engineer. Each has a unique but complementary role, and in cooperation with the end-user provides a comprehensive view of the AT needs. Physiatrists make ideal physicians on AT teams with their residency training and the opportunities that AT provides to benefit people with disabilities. The increasing complexity of AT selection, justification, fitting, tuning, and training requires specialized knowledge. The Rehabilitation Engineering and Assistive Technology Society of North America (RESNA) recognized the need for consumers and insurers to be able to distinguish individuals with relevant experience and specialized knowledge.[3] Over the following 10 years, RESNA created three credentials that each year continue to grow throughout the United States and appears to be slowly becoming a model for several other countries. The Assistive Technology Supplier (ATS) credential is intended for distributors and manufacturer representatives of AT. The ATS is the most important of the credentials offered by RESNA, as it has started to bring order to an area of AT that was largely unregulated. Before the ATS there was no reliable credential for a supplier or manufacturer representative to demonstrate competency and for consumers to readily identify qualified suppliers. The Assistive Technology Provider (ATP) credential is geared toward therapists (physical, occupational, speech/language, counselors, and special educators). The ATP provides recognition for qualified clinicians who wish to be recognized for their specialized knowledge and expertise. For decades, rehabilitation engineers provided clinical services without formal recognition of their expertise and in many cases their services were not reimbursed by some insurance agencies. The Rehabilitation Engineering Technology (RET) credential addresses the needs of rehabilitation engineers and provides other professionals and consumers a clear way to recognize clinical rehabilitation engineers. In order to obtain the RET, the engineer must also have obtained the ATP credential. All of the RESNA credentials require proof of relevant experience and a passing score on a comprehensive examination. It is too early to tell, but the signs indicate that the credentials have improved the quality of services available. Although there remain some significant challenges ahead. It is difficult for comprehensive AT clinics to survive from reimbursement for their services. Therefore, most AT clinics are associated with a university, not-for-profit organization (eg, Easter Seals, United Cerebral Palsy), or a rehabilitation center; whereas other sources can assist in underwriting the costs.

WHEELCHAIRS

There are four basic classes of wheelchair: (a) manual wheelchair, (b) power-assisted wheelchair, (c) electric-powered wheelchair, and (d) robotic wheelchair. We will discuss the benefits, applications, and likely advances for each of these categories. There are a large variety of manual wheelchair makes and models available; however, the ultralight manual wheelchair clearly shines brighter than the others.[4,5] And even the ultralight wheelchair itself is being redefined as newer materials and design techniques are bringing down the mass and improving ergonomics. Let's start with the decades old questions: what is more important, weight or fit? The short answer to this question appears simple, both, but a more effective way to determine the answer is to ask a related question. Which wheelchair and features are most functional and will cause the least harm. Weight is certainly important in preventing repetitive strain injuries, for ease of loading in a car, and for making it easier to propel up slopes or curbs. Ergonomics affect all of these properties and in addition affect seated comfort (or prevention of discomfort), propulsion over all terrain, and control over the wheelchair (eg, wheelies).[6,7] Fortunately, weight and ergonomics often go together because designing a very light (less then 10 kg) manual wheelchair requires both good design and ergonomics. To keep the weight low, designers must carefully choose those features that will be fixed and those that will be adjustable. This also forces the clinician-consumer team to take equal care in selecting the wheelchair. Some options may make the chair slightly heavier such as ergonomic pushrims or solid backrests, but frequently they are worth the weight.

Research tells us that there are several guidelines that can be followed to choose and set up a properly fitting and functioning manual wheelchair.[8–10] The seat width should be about 25 mm or less wider than the distance between the trochantors while seated. This keeps the chair narrow for negotiating doorways, aisles, and hallways. More importantly, it brings the wheels in so that the shoulders remain in a more neutral position close to the body while propelling. The seat depth should be about 50 mm less then the seated distance between the back and the popliteal area behind the knees. This will allow some repositioning within the seat, and provide a large surface area for the cushion. The seat back height should be such that the person can move freely for activities performed in the chair: eating, reaching, dressing, slouching, sitting, propelling. Too high a back height can be restrictive, and too low can lead to discomfort and reduced trunk stability. The seat height should be such that users while sitting upright in the chair can reach the axles comfortably with their hands extended at their sides. Seat inclination (dump) is more of an individual decision. About 5 degrees is common, but higher angles can help to hold the pelvis against the backrest increasing trunk stability; however, this often makes transfer from the chair more difficult. Positioning of the rear wheels is one of the most critical dimensions. Placing the axles forward of the backrest and nearer to the center of mass of the user and chair together reduces rolling resistance, decreases the downhill turning moment on side slopes, and allows the user to grasp the pushrims over a wide arc. All of these are positive attributes, but one negative result is that the wheelchair becomes less stable in the rearward direction. Therefore, it is wise to have the clinician-consumer team work on wheelie skills and balance to determine the best rear axle position.

When starting to use a wheelchair it is best to select one that provides the ability to adjust many of its seating and wheel positions. Typically people who first have a SCI go through a series of physical and functional changes, and the chair will need to be adjusted as these changes take place. Once the end-users have become more skilled at using a wheelchair and their function has stabilized, a change to a chair with more fixed features is likely warranted. Throughout a person's life it is important to keep pace with improvements in wheelchair technology, as many times the advances can increase function, reduce discomfort, and protect against injury. Ultralight manual wheelchairs should be recommended for almost all individuals with paraplegia and for individuals with lower tetraplegia, unless there is a secondary condition or diagnosis to suggest otherwise.

The power-assisted wheelchair has become more popular within the past decade because of the availability of the pushrim-activated power-assist wheelchair (PAPAW). The PAPAW uses small motors that react to the torque applied to the pushrims. The motors are powered by a high-density battery (eg, NiMH, NiCd, Lithium).[11] The PAPAW serves two important purposes: (1) it reduces the physical and physiologic strain on the user; and (2) it provides lightweight (about 20 kg) power-assisted mobility and transportability.[12–14] A PAPAW can be a custom-designed wheelchair or it can be an ultralight manual wheelchair adapted to accept power-assist wheels. Fitting individuals for a PAPAW is much like fitting them for an ultralight manual wheelchair, with two notable exceptions: (1) the axle position should be more rearward for added stability; and (2) the power-assist wheels need to be tuned for the user. Key factors with the electronics of a PAPAW to pay attention to are: can the end-user safely operate at the maximum assisted speed; does the device provide adequate braking assistance and control on slopes; is the chair easy to maneuver in close quarters. A PAPAW is effectively a heavy manual wheelchair if the batteries lose their charge; therefore, regular charging is important.

There has been a virtual explosion in electric-powered wheelchair (EPW) designs. This has provided people with many more choices, but not all of them are appropriate for people with SCI.[15,16] The taxonomy of EPW can be described based on function, drive wheel position, intended environment, and seating functions. A number of EPWs really do not need to be considered for people with SCI. Our goal should be to maximize functional mobility within the home and community at large. Therefore, activity duty EPWs are most appropriate. Although controversial, there is growing evidence to support the recommendation of powered seating functions for individuals with

SCI. Powered seat elevation may be the most helpful to aide in transfers either assisted or unassisted. Seat height is also critical for extending the functional work space. Powered tilt and/or powered recline are also very important seating functions. Tilt and recline facilitates weight shift to increase comfort, reduce risk of soft tissue breakdown, decrease discomfort, and improve circulation in the lower extremities. The controversy stems basically from cost; powered seat functions increase the cost of the EPW, and therefore some will argue that they are unnecessary if the individual can perform an independent weight shift or transfer. The flaw in this logic is that performing an independent weight shift or transfer or even a few is not enough to determine what a person's abilities and risks are in their home and community. The needs of people change from day to day and week to week; powered seating functions allow the end-user to adapt to these changes.

The location of the drive wheels of an EPW affect the driving behavior. Rear-wheel-drive EPWs hold their direction the best when rolling forward down a path. When steering, they turn about a point behind the driver, requiring the person to plan when turning into a doorway, for example. They were most popular before digital controls, although are still popular today. Mid-wheel-drive EPWs place the powered wheels near the center of mass of the user. This provides for turning about the center of the chair, which makes them maneuverable and easier for most end-users to judge turns. Mid-wheel-drive EPWs require six wheels, two front outriggers and two rear outriggers to remain stable. Setting the tension on the outrigger suspension is important to provide mobility and control; too soft and the chair rocks, and too hard and the chair cannot climb obstacles. Front-wheel-drive EPWs are popular among some individuals for their obstacle climbing ability. By having the powered wheels encounter the obstacle first, they can often climb over them. When turning a front-wheel-drive EPW, the rear end sweeps, which requires the driver to plan where it will move through the turn.

The controls of EPWs have been gradually improving, but have a long way toward achieving their full potential. Most EPWs allow for adjusting the maximum speed, rate of turning, and braking distance, which have made it possible to accommodate a larger population of end-users. Some systems allow for filter adjustments to compensate for tremor. The use of advanced control algorithms, such as robust control, has yet to be widely applied. A significant barrier to the use of advanced controls is that most wheelchair controllers come from only a few sources, and that EPWs are essentially assembled with existing commercial controllers. This barrier may be partially reduced through open-source software that manufacturers could ask controller suppliers to adopt so as to improve their products.

The operation of an EPW requires an effective and reliable user interface.[17,18] The most common user interface is the motion joystick, which produces a speed and direction signal proportional to the position of the stick. Signal processing can be used to condition the joystick output to make it easier to control the EPW. Essentially, any reliable and sufficiently rapid source of information can be used to create a user interface. Switches (eg, hand, head, or tongue), gyroscopes and accelerometers (eg, head position), pressure sensors (eg, sip and puff), and isometric joysticks (a.k.a. force-sensing joysticks) are all used to control EPWs. The greatest challenges are in selecting the most effective user interface and tuning it to the user. Selection is typically based on a process of elimination starting with continuous interfaces (eg, joystick) and if necessary transitioning to switch control. The ability to produce continuous input signals most often results in more rapid and smoother control over the EPW. Switch control usually results in slower control dictated by a series of discrete commands. Research and development is active in creating more effective signal-processing algorithms and eventually aware algorithms to intuit the user's intent and generate control signals.

Driving an EPW is not a simple activity; it requires judgment, vigilance, and adequate vision to effectively navigate in a community environment.[19,20] When driving down a street, the driver must pay attention to pedestrians, look out for obstacles or cracks in the sidewalk, and align the chair with the curb-cut when crossing the street, as well as watch for traffic. Imagine trying to talk to a friend, talking on the phone, or carrying something on your lap during the circumstances described in the preceding sentence. Robotic mobility systems may offer a solution. Advances in robotics suggest that it may be possible to create mobility devices that are more aware of the environment and that can work in partnership with the user.[21] For example, a fully robotic device could potentially transport an individual from one location to another simply by indicating the desired destination. One could envision current EPWs as the other end of a spectrum that would transverse through reliance solely on commands generated continuously by the driver and commands automatically generated by the robotic device based on broad commands provided by the user. Work is in progress toward the creation of robotic mobility devices. Presently the focal point is obstacle detection, obstacle avoidance, and route navigation. Currently, none of these mobility devices have become commercially available, primarily because they are not yet reliable enough to use in real-world situations. Thus far only simple stationary obstacles, commonly cardboard boxes, can be reliably detected. Advances in imaging processing, image tracking, multisensor integration, and aware systems need to be made before practical robotic mobility devices will be available; however, their deployment could be transformational. There has been limited commercial success in robotic mobility devices with such devices like the IBOT4000 that uses robotics technology to provide unprecedented mobility. The IBOT4000 demonstrates that a multilink design rather than a chassis (like classical EPW) allows the structure to change form to match the desired driving task. For examples, in standard function the links connecting the wheel clusters, base, and seat are at acute angles with respect to one another, whereas in standing function that links open to obtuse angles with respect to one another resulting in an extended height. Furthermore, the IBOT4000 detects the center of mass of the payload (user plus items being carried) and adjusts its response.

There is one unbreakable principle when selecting or recommending a wheelchair and that is to never recommend any wheelchair that has not been tested to and found to be in compliance with the RESNA or International Standards Organization (ISO) standards.[22–24] The RESNA and ISO standards are intended to ensure minimal quality. Best results are often obtained through independent testing conducted within a reputable testing laboratory.

SEATING

Wheelchair users, especially those users who have limited ability to reposition and have a loss of sensation in the areas where weight is being supported, are at high risk for developing pressure ulcers[25–27]; however, high pressure alone usually is insufficient for the development of a pressure ulcer. Research has demonstrated that the damaging effects of pressure are related to both its magnitude and duration. The support surface characteristics, pressure distribution, shear, temperature control, and moisture control all contribute to pressure ulcer prevention.[28] These relationships are related to seat cushions made from elastic, viscoelastic, fluid-filled, low-air-loss, air-fluidized, and alternating pressure support surfaces. The magnitude of shear and friction forces and the additive effects of temperature and moisture can be affected by the characteristics of the support surface chosen for a given individual. Although extrinsic factors such as temperature, moisture, and mechanical characteristics are critical to the development of pressure ulcers, factors intrinsic to the person's skin and its supporting structures, vasculature, or lymphatic also play a significant role in susceptibility to these factors.[29-31] The wide variance in tissue tolerance between people means that scientists have been unable to pinpoint a general pressure threshold below which pressure ulcers will not develop. The often-quoted safe pressure threshold of 32 mm Hg is unsubstantiated. Many experts suggest that interface pressure measurement is better for identifying inappropriate support surfaces than for determining appropriate ones, ie, clinicians should use pressure measurement to exclude certain interventions attributable to high loading, but should not use it as a singular assessment measure. To choose an appropriate support surface, you must consider more than normal pressure. When choosing a wheelchair cushion, for example, also consider its effect on transfers, posture, propulsion, comfort, and stability.

An elastic material deforms in proportion to the applied load. Greater loads result in predictably greater alterations in the shape of the material. Support surfaces that are made from resilient foam exhibit this type of elastic response. Foam is limited in its ability to immerse and envelop by its stiffness and thickness. Soft foams will envelop better than stiffer foams, but will necessarily be thicker to avoid bottoming out. Foam seat cushions are frequently contoured to improve their performance. Precontouring the seat cushion to provide a better match between the buttocks and the cushion increases the contact area, thus reducing average pressure. Precontouring also increases immersion and envelopment properties, thus decreasing pressure peaks. Foam tends to increase skin temperature because foam materials and the air they entrap are generally poor conductors of heat. If time is also a factor in the load versus deformation characteristic, then the response is considered to be viscoelastic.

Viscoelastic foam acts like a self-contouring surface because the elastic response diminishes over time, even after the foam is compressed. The disadvantage of the temperature and time-sensitive response is that the desirable effects may not be realized when the ambient temperature is too low. Solid gel products are also viscoelastic in nature.

Fluid-filled products may consist of small or large chambers filled with air, water, or other viscous fluid materials such as silicon elastomer, silicon, or polyvinyl. The fluid flow from chamber to chamber or within a single chamber is passive in response to movement and requires no supplemental power. Given the large variety of materials used as covers for products in the fluid-filled category, it is difficult to generalize on moisture control characteristics; however, the insulating effects of rubber and plastic used in some fluid-filled products have been shown to increase the relative humidity attributable to perspiration.

Alternating pressure describes a support surface feature in which the pressure distribution is periodically altered. Most surfaces using this feature contain air-filled chambers or cylinders arranged lengthwise, interdigitated, or in various other patterns. Air is pumped into the chambers at periodic intervals to inflate and deflate the chambers in opposite phases, thereby changing the location of the contact pressure. Pulsating pressure differs from alternating therapy in that the duration of peak inflation is shorter and the cycling time is more frequent. The latter appears to have a dramatic effect on increasing lymphatic flow.

Although support surface technologies have been designed to reduce mechanical (pressure, shear, friction) and additive (moisture, temperature) factors implicated in pressure ulcer formation, most support surface comparisons have relied solely on interface pressure measurement, a limited and highly variable method.

TRANSPORTATION

Transportation is a key component to full integration into the community.[32,33] Matching the appropriate transportation to the user is essential. Accessible public transportation is necessary to provide persons with disabilities the same opportunities as others: employment, education, religious worship, and recreation. In the United States, the Individuals with Disabilities Education Act and the Americans with Disabilities Act of 1990 (ADA) have provided the opportunity for access to school and public transportation by people with disabilities.[32,33] The ADA transportation requirements mandate accessible fixed-route vehicles, as well as complementary paratransit services for those unable to use the fixed-route service. In addition, advances in technology for adapting vehicles have made personal vehicle transportation available to many people with disabilities, either as a passenger or a driver.

A subset of wheelchair users may not be able to transfer to a vehicle seat and might, therefore, remain seated in the wheelchair. When selecting a wheelchair and vehicle, it is critical to ensure that the two devices are compatible. A common mistake is to choose the wheelchair and motor vehicle in isolation, which frequently leads to incompatibility that can be difficult and costly to address. A reasonable goal is that the wheelchair user has the same level of safety afforded to passengers sitting in vehicle seats that must meet federal safety standards.[34–36] The reality is that the wheelchair-seated passenger is at an increased risk of injury in event of a vehicle collision, and even an emergency maneuver. Despite the existence of voluntary safety standards that address the design and performance of devices used to safely transport the wheelchair-seated passenger, devices that comply with these standards, particularly ISO 7176-19 wheelchairs, are not widely used.[37,38] In addition, widely used 4-pt tie-down systems are not user friendly, resulting is disuse or misuse. This results in continued problems with unsafe and inadequate wheelchairs and wheelchair securement.

COMPUTER ACCESS

The most familiar pointing devices are the mouse and the trackpad.[39] Other frequently seen pointing devices include the trackball and the trackpoint.[39] Pointing devices that are more commonly associated with individuals with SCI include touch screens, head-mounted mouse emulators, and mouse keys. People can have problems generating mouse clicks for several reasons. Some people have trouble activating a switch. Others are accustomed to a pointing device that does not have a mouse button. People who use a head-mounted mouse emulator may not want to be tethered to the computer by a cord attached to a mouse button. An alternative to a physical mouse button (or buttons) is mouse click emulation software.

Virtual keyboards consist of text entry methods that are not operated by directly selecting from a collection of buttons. Virtual keyboards include (1) software-based on-screen keyboards that can be operated by a pointing device or switch and (2) Morse code systems. The advantage of on-screen keyboards is their extreme flexibility. Their size and layout can be changed readily. The primary disadvantage of an on-screen keyboard is that it consumes screen space that could otherwise be used by an application.

A quality microphone is critical for good performance with voice recognition. The preferred type of microphone is the headset, which positions the microphone within an inch of the user's mouth. A disadvantage of a headset is the need to put the headset on and take the headset off, which some individuals are unable to do independently. Boom microphones and array microphones eliminate the need to wear anything, but equivalent sound quality from a boom or array microphone is more costly than for a headset. Voice recognition users are often disappointed to learn that speaking to a computer is not at all like speaking to a person. Voice recognition software is based almost entirely on signal-processing algorithms, and does not consider context, syntax, or semantics when interpreting what a user says. Voice recognition software relies on a voice model that must be trained for each individual user, and the quality of the voice model determines the accuracy of the voice recognition software.

Scanning systems allow a user to select from a set of items (eg, letters, numbers, words) using one or two switches. There are a variety of switches available, distinguished by their size, sensitivity, and the type of motion to which they respond. The type of switch used, and its location, depends on what motion(s) the client can perform both consistently and reliably. The simplest form of scanning is one-switch linear scanning, in which each item is highlighted in turn and the user presses the switch when the desired item is highlighted. A more common form of one-switch scanning is row-column scanning. A common implementation of row-column scanning with one switch requires three switch hits to make one selection from a 2-dimensional matrix of items. The first switch hit initiates a scan through the rows of the matrix. Each row of the matrix, beginning with the first, is highlighted in turn until the second switch hit is made to select a row. Each column of the row is then highlighted in turn until the target is highlighted, when the third switch hit is made to select the target. Persons with disabilities have varying needs when it comes to computing technologies. Technology solutions can be used on the client side to aid users in making the electronic information accessible.[40] Changes in design approaches, technological advances in computer access methods, and cutting edge research have played important roles in making electronic information more accessible.[41]

SPORTS AND RECREATION

Sports and recreation are important modalities of rehabilitation and reintegration of people with SCI.[42,43] Experiencing success and simply having fun again play important roles in achieving rehabilitation goals. In addition, developing long-term healthy habits is critical to achieving a successful life. Human occupational functioning theory cites the importance of the "volitional elements of the personality" as critical factors in a person's motivation for the rehabilitation process.[44] Volitional elements support an individual's sense of personal ability and effectiveness and judgment of what is important and meaningful. Sports and recreation represent an engagement in a valued form of daily life activity. Healthy competition with self and others through sports and recreation creates an arena for continuing the gains of medical rehabilitation, challenging personally held ideas about disability and handicap learned, and provides opportunities to develop a new self-concept that hopefully includes acceptance of disability.[45,46]

Although there are regular opportunities for people with SCI to participate in sports and recreation activities, there are too few integrated local facilities. There are excellent programs like the National Veterans Wheelchair Games (NVWG) and the National Disabled Veterans Winter Sports Clinic (NDVWSC). The NVWG is held in a different city each year in the United States, and is open to all armed services veterans with a disability that necessitates the use of a wheelchair for the participation in sport. There are approximately 600 participants each year from throughout the United States, Puerto Rico, and England. The NVWG promotes sport as a tool for building confidence, camaraderie, and fitness. A wide variety of sports are included, as well as dual track classification—novice/open/master and impairment level. The variety of sports allows participants to find the activities that they enjoy. There are clearly two highlights that illustrate the keys to the success of the NVWG. The slalom is a timed obstacle course for wheelchair users. Colorful obstacles that reflect real-world challenges are negotiated by the participants. Curbs, ramps, ladders, ropes, sand traps, doors, and narrow passages all await slalom participants. The success of this event is in making the course challenging but passable by all of the participants. The top competitors are invited to compete in the "Super-G," which is a longer course consisting of even more difficult tasks—balance beam, paintball shooting, teeter-totter, and log-run. The slalom is interesting for competitors and spectators, and does not require the competitor to bring any special equipment. The NVWG uses a very interesting model for team sports. To integrate novice athletes, and to make the competitions balanced, the teams are assembled by the event organizers (basketball, softball, rugby). Each team is assigned an experienced athlete to serve as the coach. Players are then distributed among the teams based on the classification and their skill. The goal is to keep all of the teams competitive. The coaches are also charged with developing the talents of the novice athletes. During games, every player must get a minimum amount of game time. Therefore, every player participates in every game. This makes nearly every game competitive and exciting for both players and spectators.

The NDVWSC is the world's largest winter sports clinic for people with disabilities. Approximately 350 veterans with a wide variety of disabilities participate and are instructed by over 600 trainers and coaches. Because it is a clinic, the participants may try a plethora of winter sports and recreation activities with equipment available from the NDVWSC. Individuals with SCI may learn downhill skiing, cross-country skiing, scuba diving, rock climbing, shooting, sledge hockey, and fencing. Participants are divided into teams and given tasks to help them get to know each other. There are also numerous social activities that create a sense of camaraderie. Both the NVWG and the NDVWSC are free for the participants; naturally they must pay for their travel costs and lodging. The popularity and the surveys from participants in the NVWG and NDVWSC indicate that these events provide invaluable opportunities. Logically, they should be copied by other organizations to create opportunities for people with disabilities who are not veterans.

DIRECTIONS FOR FUTURE TECHNOLOGIES

Technology is and is likely to remain critical for rehabilitation and supporting community reintegration. The trends point toward smarter more adaptable technologies, greater flexibility in manufacturing, and further translation of research findings into improved products and services.[47] Transformational technologies for people with SCI are likely to involve aware systems that augment the body and the mind. Model-rich technologies that learn from functional activities, context, previous experience, human and social behaviors, physiology, physical capacity, and cognition are possible with focused effort. Future technologies will need to be aware: by understanding and adapting to the intent of the person, the context, and the attributes of the environment. It is critical that new smart, aware technologies are safe, reliable, and provide timely, gracious assistance. These technologies will aide with assessment, training, and increase capabilities of end-users.

SUMMARY

Despite the significant advances in assistive technology for people with spinal cord injuries there remains much to be done. There seem to be a few critical areas for further clinical evidence. There is little evidence to construct the optimal AT service delivery team and practice guidelines. Credentialing has certainly helped to raise standards, and there is evidence that a team approach is better than an isolated clinician model. Comprehensive AT teams can assist in matching the person's needs with the technology and ensuring that the pieces all fit together.

There is strong evidence in support of ultralight manual wheelchairs that are fitted to the user. There is need for evidence for manual wheelchair training techniques and for understanding the mechanisms, time course, and treatment of upper limb injuries among manual wheelchair users. More research is needed into the ergonomics of both manual and electric-powered wheelchairs. Little is know about usage, user training, impairment compensation, and control of EPWs. It seems clear the EPWs need to incorporate smarter interfaces (seating and control) and to become more "aware."

There has been significant investigation into wheelchair seating for decades, yet the knowledge of pressure sore development has still only scratched the surface. It remains elusive why some people are more susceptible than others, and it is as yet unknown a priori as to how pressure ulcers can be prevented. Advances in sensor technologies that yield new assessment tools should help.

Transportation is critical to maintaining health, participating in the community, and employment. Legislative mandates have made improvements, but technology deployment and adoption has not kept pace. Transportation remains accessible on only select areas, and is not simple to use for many people whether public or personal. Computer access technology is crucial for some individuals to participate in the exchange of electronic information and for employment.

There have been a number of hardware and software devices developed to facilitate computer access. Technologies are needed to make computer access systems become more contextually aware, adaptive, and able to increase communication rate.

Sports and recreation are important to the successful reintegration of people with SCI into the community; however, there are too few opportunities for exercise, especially in public facilities. Accessible sports and exercise equipment technologies need to be developed, as well as validated exercise programs.

ACKNOWLEDGMENT

This work was supported in part by the US Department of Education, National Institute on Disability and Rehabilitation (H133N000019), and the US Department of Veterans Affairs, Rehabilitation Research and Development Service (B3142C).

REFERENCES

1. Chavez E, Boninger ML, Cooper R, et al. Application of a participation system to assess the influence of assistive technology on the lives of people with spinal cord injury. Arch Phys Med Rehabil 2004;85(11):1854–8.
2. Hunt PC, Boninger ML, Cooper RA, et al. Factors associated with wheelchair type and quality among individuals with traumatic spinal cord injury. Arch Phys Med Rehabil 2004;85(11):1859–64.
3. Available at: www.resna.org. Accessed January 5, 2007.
4. Fitzgerald SG, Collins DM, Cooper RA, et al. Issues in the maintenance and repairs of wheelchairs: a pilot study. J Rehabil Rev Dev 2005;42(6):853–62.
5. Fitzgerald SG, Cooper RA, Boninger ML, et al. Comparison of fatigue life for three types of manual wheelchairs. Arch Phys Med Rehabil 2001;82(10):1484–8.

6. DiGiovine MM, Cooper RA, Boninger ML, et al. User assessment of manual wheelchair ride comfort and ergonomics. Arch Phys Med Rehabil 2000;81(4):490–4.

7. Crane BA, Holm MB, Hobson DA, et al. Test-retsest reliability, internal item consistency, and concurrent validity of the wheelchair seating discomfort assessment tool. Assist Technol 2005;17(2):98–107.

8. Boninger ML, Koontz AM, Sisto SA, et al. Pushrim biomechanics and injury prevention in spinal cord injury: recommendations based on CULP-SCI investigations. J Rehabil Res Dev 2005;42(3):9–20.

9. Boninger ML, Impink B, Cooper RA, et al. Relationship between median and ulnar nerve function and wrist kinematics during wheelchair propulsion. Arch Phys Med Rehabil 2004;85(7):1141–5.

10. Boninger ML, Baldwin M, Cooper RA, et al. Manual wheelchair pushrim biomechanics and axle position. Arch Phys Med Rehabil 2000;81(5):608–13.

11. Cooper RA, Fitzgerald SG, Boninger ML, et al. Evaluation of a pushrim activated power assisted wheelchair. Arch Phys Med Rehabil 2001;82(5):702–8.

12. Algood SD, Cooper RA, Fitzgerald SG, et al. Effect of a pushrim activated power assist wheelchair on the functional capabilities of individuals with tetraplegia. Arch Phys Med Rehabil 2005;86(3):380–6.

13. Algood SD, Cooper RA, Boninger ML, et al. Impact of a pushrim activated power assist wheelchair on the metabolic demands, stroke frequency, and range of motion among individuals with tetraplegia. Arch Phys Med Rehabil 2004; 85(11):1865–71.

14. Corfman TA, Cooper RA, Boninger ML, et al. Range of motion and stroke frequency differences between manual wheelchair propulsion and pushrim activated power assisted wheelchair propulsion. J Spinal Cord Med 2003;26(2): 135–40.

15. Cooper RA, Cooper R, Tolerico M, et al. Advances in electric powered wheelchairs. Top Spinal Cord Inj Rehabil 2006;11(4):15–29.

16. Cooper RA, Thorman T, Cooper R, et al. Driving characteristics of electric powered wheelchair users: how far, fast, and often do people drive? Arch Phys Med Rehabil 2002;83(2):250–5.

17. Ding D, Cooper RA, Kaminski BA, et al. Integrated control of assistive technology. Assist Technol 2003;15(2):89–96.

18. Dicianno BE, Spaeth DM, Cooper RA, et al. Advancements in power wheelchair joystick technology: effects of isometric joysticks and signal conditioning on driving performance. Am J Phys Med Rehabil 2006;85(8):631–9.

19. Cooper RA. Intelligent control of power wheelchairs. IEEE Eng Med Biol Mag 1995;15(4):423–31.

20. Dan D, Cooper RA. Review of control technology and algorithms for electric powered wheelchairs. IEEE Controls Syst Mag N Y 2005;25(2):22–34.

21. Simpson R, LoPresti E, Hayashi S, et al. Smart power assistance module for manual wheelchairs: preliminary results. J Neuroeng Rehabil 2005;2(30):1–11.

22. Pearlman JL, Cooper RA, Karnawat J, et al. Evaluation of the safety and durability of low-cost electric powered wheelchairs. Arch Phys Med Rehabil 2005;86(12): 2361–70.

23. Fass MV, Cooper RA, Fitzgerald SG, et al. Durability, value, and reliability of selected electric powered wheelchairs. Arch Phys Med Rehabil 2004;85(5): 805–14.

24. Rentschler AJ, Cooper RA, Fitzgerald SG, et al. Evaluation of selected electric powered wheelchairs using the ANSI/RESNA standards. Arch Phys Med Rehabil 2004;85(4):611–9.

25. Yarkony G. Pressure ulcers: a review. Arch Phys Med Rehabil 1994;75:908–17.
26. Sprigle SH, Chung K-C, Brubaker CE. Reduction of sitting pressures with custom contoured cushions. J Rehabil Res Dev 1990;27:135–40.
27. Bennett L, Kavner D, Lee BY, et al. Skin stress and blood flow in sitting paraplegic patients. Arch Phys Med Rehabil 1984;65:189–90.
28. Holzapfel S. Support surfaces and their use in the prevention and treatment of pressure ulcers. J ET Nurs 1993;20:251–60.
29. Levine SP, Kett RL, Brooks SV, et al. Electrical muscle stimulation for pressure sore prevention: tissue shape variation. Arch Phys Med Rehabil 1990;71:210–5.
30. Mak AF, Huang L, Wang Q. A biphasic poroelastic analysis of the flow dependent subcutaneous tissue pressure and compaction due to epidermal loadings: issues in pressure sores. J Biomech Eng 1994;116:421–9.
31. Nicholson GP, Scales JT, Clark RP, et al. A method for determining the heat transfer and water vapor permeability of patient support systems. Med Eng Phys 1999;21:701–12.
32. IDEA-97 Individuals with Disabilities Education Act of 1997, (PL105–17) 34CFR.300 Federal Register March 12, Volume 64, Number 48.
33. ADA 1990- Americans with Disabilities Act of 1990(PL101-336), 49CFR37: Transportation Services for Individuals with Disabilities (Act). Washington, DC: Federal Register.
34. MDA DB2001(03)- device bulletin: guidance on the safe transportation of wheelchairs. Medical Devices Agency. Washington, DC: Department of Health; 2001.
35. Shaw G, Gillispie T. Appropriate protection for wheelchair riders on public transit buses. J Rehabil Res Dev 2003;40(4):309–20.
36. Sprigle S, Morris B, Nowacek G, et al. Assessment of adaptive transportation technology: a survey of users and equipment vendors. Assist Technol 1994;6:111–9.
37. van Roosmalen L, Reed M, Bertocci GE, et al. Wheelchair occupant restraint usability issues. Assist Technol 2005;17:23–36.
38. Bertocci GE, Digges K, Hobson DA, et al. Shoulder belt anchor location influences on wheelchair occupant crash protection. J Rehabil Res Dev 1996;33(3):279–89.
39. Burgstahler SE. Disabled students gain independence through adaptive technology services. EDUCOM Review 1992;27(2):45–6.
40. Waddell CD. The growing digital divide in access for people with disabilities: overcoming barriers to participation in the digital economy. Available at: http://www.icdri.org/CynthiaW/the_digital_divide.htm. 1999. Accessed August 7, 2009.
41. Shneiderman B, Hochheiser H. Universal usability as a stimulus to advanced interface design. Behav Inf Technol 2001;20(5):367–76.
42. Heath GW, Fentem PH. Physical activity among persons with disabilities—a public health perspective. Exerc Sport Sci Rev 1997;25:195–234.
43. Rimmer JH, Braddock D, Pitteti KH, et al. Research on physical activity and disability: an emerging national priority. Med Sci Sports Exerc 1996;28:1366–72.
44. Kielhofner G. A model of human occupation: theory and application. Baltimore (MD): William & Wilkins; 1985.
45. Scruton J. Stoke Mandeville road to the paralympics. Aylesbury (UK): The Peterhouse Press; 1998.
46. Steardward RD, Peterson C. Paralympics: where heroes come. In: Peterson B, editor. One shot. Edmonton, Alberta (CA): Holdings Publishing Division; 1999.
47. Cooper RA, Dan D, Simpson R, et al. Virtual reality applied to wheeled mobility: an overview of work in Pittsburgh. Assist Technol 2005;17(2):159–70.

Research in Computer Access Assessment and Intervention

Richard Simpson, PhD, ATP[a,b,*], Heidi Horstmann Koester, PhD[c],
Edmund LoPresti, PhD[c,d]

KEYWORDS

- Computer access • Assistive technology
- Automatic adaptation • Telerehabilitation • Assessment

IMPORTANCE OF COMPUTER ACCESS TECHNOLOGY

Computer access technology (CAT) allows people who have trouble using a standard computer keyboard, mouse, or monitor to access a computer. CAT includes inexpensive devices, such as trackballs and small-footprint keyboards, and sophisticated technologies, such as automatic speech recognition, eyegaze tracking, and brain-computer interfaces. CAT services are provided by a range of rehabilitation professionals, including rehabilitation engineers, occupational therapists, speech-language pathologists, special educators, and vocational rehabilitation counselors.

CAT is critical for enhancing the educational and vocational opportunities of people with disabilities.[1,2] In addition, CAT has been shown to contribute to improved health status by providing access to health information and interaction with clinicians and peers.[3] CAT can reduce social isolation by eliminating physical barriers, facilitating communication, and providing a forum for the exchange of information.[4] Individuals with disabilities often appreciate the anonymity of the Internet, where they can be evaluated for the strength of their contributions rather than their physical appearance or disability.[5,6] The Internet also provides protection against self-consciousness and social anxiety, and active participation can lead to greater levels of self-acceptance and decreased feelings of isolation.[7,8]

This work was supported by the National Science Foundation (#0540865) and the National Institutes of Health (#2R44HD045015-03).

[a] Department of Veterans Affairs, Human Engineering Research Labs, University of Pittsburgh, Forbes Tower, Suite 5044, 3600 Forbes Avenue at Atwood Street, Pittsburgh, PA 15260, USA
[b] Department of Rehabilitation Science and Technology, University of Pittsburgh, Forbes Tower, Suite 5044, 3600 Forbes Avenue at Atwood Street, Pittsburgh, PA 15260, USA
[c] Koester Performance Research, 2408 Antietam, Ann Arbor, MI 48105, USA
[d] AT Sciences, 160 N. Craig Street Suite 117, Pittsburgh, PA 15213, USA
* Corresponding author. Department of Rehabilitation Science and Technology, University of Pittsburgh, Forbes Tower, Suite 5044, 3600 Forbes Avenue at Atwood Street, Pittsburgh, PA 15260, USA.
E-mail address: ris20@pitt.edu (R. Simpson).

Phys Med Rehabil Clin N Am 21 (2010) 15–32
doi:10.1016/j.pmr.2009.07.006
1047-9651/09/$ – see front matter © 2010 Elsevier Inc. All rights reserved.

Fifty-seven percent (74.2 million) of working-age (between 18 and 64 years of age) computer users are likely or very likely to benefit from the use of CAT[9]:

- 17% (21.9 million) of working-age computer users have a mild visual difficulty or impairment, and 9% (11.1 million) have a severe visual difficulty or impairment.[9]
- 19% (24.4 million) of working-age computer users have a mild dexterity difficulty or impairment, and 5% (6.8 million) have a severe dexterity difficulty or impairment.[9]
- 18% (24.0 million) of working-age computer users have a mild hearing difficulty or impairment, and 2% (2.5 million) have a severe hearing difficulty or impairment.[9]

Choosing the most appropriate CAT is a collaborative decision-making process involving the consumer, clinician(s), and third-party payers. The challenges involved in a successful computer access intervention include

1. Evaluating and documenting client abilities and specific difficulties with the standard computer interface[10]
2. Choosing the most appropriate assistive technology to address these difficulties
3. Configuring the technology to the user's needs
4. Training the user in appropriate use of their system[11–13] and
5. Providing continuous follow-up to ensure that the interface remains well suited to the user[13–17]

The consequences of failing to successfully meet any 1 of these challenges include wasted human and material resources spent in the intervention process, unnecessary obstacles placed in the individual's path toward their goals, technology abandonment,[14,18] and a lack of computer use amongst individuals with disabilities.[3,19] By all reported measures, we are largely failing to meet these challenges.

People with disabilities do not use computers at the same rate as people without disabilities. Whereas 85% of working-age adults without disabilities use computers, computer usage among those who have mild impairments is 80%, and 63% among individuals who have severe disabilities and are likely to benefit from the use of CAT.[9]

Many people with disabilities who do own computers do not take advantage of CAT. One study found that only 24% of working-age computer users with severe disabilities use CAT.[20] A significant barrier to obtaining CAT is cost. Twenty-eight percent of working-age computer users with mild difficulties/impairments and 32% with severe disabilities report there is a CAT that they do not own but would purchase if it became more affordable.[20]

A second obstacle is awareness. Of computer users with mild or severe disabilities, 20% were not aware that CAT appropriate for them existed.[20] Awareness of the free, built-in accessibility settings offered by the Windows and Mac operating systems is even lower. Of computer users with mild or severe disabilities, 36% were unaware of the available adjustments for the mouse and 35% were unaware of the available keyboard adjustment options.[20]

Amongst computer users who do own and use CAT, there is ample evidence that it is not configured correctly. For example, Trewin and Pain reported target acquisition error rates of greater than 10% for 14 of 20 users with physical disabilities, and observed that 55% of the dragging tasks made by these users were unsuccessful.[21] An average of 28% of clicks in this study included a mouse movement, which is a potential source of error, and 40% of multiple click attempts were unsuccessful.[21]

Worst of all, approximately a third of computer users who do receive CAT eventually abandon it. A study of 115 individuals with disabilities who received 136 assistive technology devices in a 5–year period, including computers, communication devices. and adapted software, reported a total abandonment rate of 32.4%. The abandonment rate within the study for computer access and communication devices was 30.8%.[22]

CHALLENGES TO COMPUTER ACCESS SERVICE DELIVERY
The Cost of CAT and Clinical Services

A significant obstacle to obtaining the most appropriate CAT is cost. CAT (for working-age adults) is often funded through vocational rehabilitation agencies, which have small budgets relative to the demand for their services. Funds spent on clinician time and CAT for 1 client are unavailable to other clients, so maximizing each dollar spent is critical. Consumers who are retired, or not seeking employment, are equally cost sensitive as they may have to purchase their own equipment. As the population ages, an increasing number of older computer users will potentially benefit from CAT[20] but are unlikely to be candidates for vocational rehabilitation and are thus likely to be using their own funds.

The Variety of Devices Available

Another challenge for computer access is the simple fact that there are too many options for any consumer to reasonably compare. There is a nearly limitless variety of alternatives to the traditional computer keyboard and mouse. Within each of these categories of devices there are multiple products, and each product has its own unique set of configuration options.

Given this variety of options, a consumer could spend weeks or months comparing devices, but a decision is often needed after 1 or 2 clinical sessions. In particular, consumers who need to obtain CAT to return to work or school often need to make decisions quickly to meet other deadlines. Beyond that, most consumers lack the patience or funding for multiple clinical visits. It is therefore critical to make optimal use of the time that client and clinician spend together in the clinic.

Consumer Needs Change Over Time

Even if a consumer who needs CAT receives a successful technology intervention, it is unlikely that the solution will remain effective indefinitely. Indeed, a consumer's needs can change long before he or she has the opportunity to be reevaluated by a clinician. Regular follow-up evaluations are critically important,[11–13] but often do not occur because of various barriers, such as the time and travel required and a lack of funding.

In addition, a single configuration may not be appropriate for a user at all times. A user's needs may change as a result of changes in his or her abilities, which may happen over the course of a day (eg, fatigue) or longer (eg, because of progression of the disability, recovery of function, or other factors). The user's needs may also change based on the user's desired tasks (eg, some computer activities may require greater precision than others). Even if a clinician is available to recommend an initial configuration, he or she may not be available every time adjustments to the configuration are desirable. If a user is responsible for his or her own adjustments, he or she may not notice, or know how to respond to, a gradual decline in performance.

POTENTIAL TECHNOLOGY SOLUTIONS

The problems with the computer access assessment process will not be solved through technology alone. The assessment process should be based on each client's individual priorities, taking into account preferences, physical and functional needs, social environments, and related issues,[23] which makes the involvement of a trained clinician crucial. A clinician will always be needed to work with the consumer and other stakeholders to choose the most appropriate technology. Similarly, a clinician or other caregiver is essential for training in many circumstances. Funding and reimbursement issues are public policy problems rather than technology problems.

In other areas, however, technology can play a prominent supporting (or even leading) role. These include computer access assessment tools that clinicians can use to evaluate and document a client's abilities, utilities to automatically configure technology for each client's individual needs, and technology to provide follow-up services through remote client-clinician interaction. Research in each of these areas is discussed in this review.

Assessment Tools

Many different methods are currently employed in assessments for computer access. Informal clinical observation is the oldest method and is characterized by brief trials with candidate systems in a clinic setting and qualitative judgments of client performance during these trials. The lack of an explicit objective framework in this approach makes it likely that appropriate candidate systems may not be considered, that criteria for selecting candidate systems may not be clearly defined, and that objective data to guide the ultimate selection may not be available, particularly when evaluations are performed by inexperienced clinicians.

The need for a systematic approach to delivering assistive technology services has long been recognized.[24,25] The systems and approaches developed to date are diverse and can be categorized on the following dimensions

1. types of information gathered (qualitative vs quantitative)
2. method of data collection and management (manual vs computerized)
3. focus of approach (assessment of ability vs prescription of "best" device)

Several conceptual models for the "ideal" assistive technology assessment process have been developed. These conceptual models are designed to structure the evaluation to ensure that important considerations are not overlooked. Forms and worksheets are often provided to help guide the evaluator's activities and lead to a recommendation of the most appropriate device. A weakness in this approach is that little or no support is provided for measuring specific aspects of client performance, such as speed and accuracy. The procurement and management of objective quantitative data are left to the evaluator, who may or may not perform this task in a consistent or valid way.

Generalized qualitative assessment models (applying to all aspects of assistive technology) include:

- **The Student, Environment, Tasks, Tools (SETT) model.**[26] A general framework (rather than an actual protocol) for evaluating a person, environment, and goals to identify the most appropriate assistive technology.
- **Matching persons with technology (MPT).**[13,23,27,28] A validated measure that evaluates how individuals judge their own functional and health status. The MPT measures quality of life and predisposition toward assistive technology (AT) use, and has been shown to successfully predict satisfaction with AT 1 month after discharge.[28]
- **Considering AT.**[29] A flowchart to guide professionals through consideration of AT by asking a series of questions.

- **Assessing students' needs for AT**.[30] A protocol for evaluating a child's assistive technology needs in the context of an individual education plan (IEP).
- **Education Tech Points**.[31] Assessment forms and a manual documenting the components of effective AT service delivery.

As shown in **Table 1**, several assessment tools have been developed specifically for computer access. Qualitative assessment methods designed specifically for computer access include:

Table 1
Computer access assessment models and products

Tool	Recommends Assessment Protocol	Computerized Skill Evaluation	Automatic Report Generation	Recommends Devices	Skills Evaluated
Compass	N	Y	Y	N	Use of text entry pointing devices; sensory abilities; cognitive abilities
REACH interface author	N	Y	Y	N	Use of text entry and pointing devices; switch skills
Alternative computer access: a guide to selection	Y	N	N	N	Use of text entry and pointing devices; sensory abilities; cognitive abilities
Control of computer-based technology for people with disabilities	Y	N	N	N	Background; environment; text entry, pointing, and switch skills
Lifespace	Y	N	Y	N	Physical, cognitive, emotional, support resources, and environmental characteristics
Assessment of computer task performance	Y	N	N	N	Text entry and pointing skills
EvaluWare	N	Y	Y	N	Looking, listening, pointing, switch, some text entry skills
VOCAselect	Y	N	Y	Y	Criteria for an appropriate AAC device
Computer access selector	Y	N	Y	Y	Criteria for an appropriate computer access device

Abbreviation: AAC, augmentative and alternative communication.

- **Alternative computer access: a guide to selection.**[1] A decision tree that guides clinicians through the assessment process. Decision points prompt the clinician to evaluate the client's motor, sensory, and cognitive skills. The leaves of the tree are suggestions of appropriate types of computer access devices.
- **Control of computer-based technology for people with physical disabilities: an assessment manual.**[32] A manual with data collection instruments, procedures for client observations, testing procedures for various computer access methods, and guidelines for matching client needs and device characteristics.
- **Assessment of computer task performance.**[33] A series of tests and measurement criteria for assessing computer skills. No software is provided to support testing. Instead, the tests are administered using icons present on the computer desktop and standard word processing software. A series of transparencies are provided, which can be placed on the computer monitor to support the tests (eg, indicating a path that the client should follow with the cursor).
- **Lifespace access profile.**[34] A team-based assessment tool that uses worksheets to measure physical, perceptual, cognitive and emotional skills, support resources, and environmental considerations. The worksheets are computerized, but data consist of subjective ratings from each team member.
- **EvaluWare**. A software package that presents evaluation exercises for a range of computer access skills. Despite the use of computerized tests, EvaluWare does not automatically record performance data.

Several computerized systems attempt to support the evaluator through all stages of the assessment process, producing a recommendation for the most appropriate assistive device. Examples of these systems include:

- **Computer access selector.**[35] Uses device criteria chosen from a series of prompts by a clinician to identify the most appropriate device from a list of known devices.
- **Assistive technology expert system.**[36,37] Presents a series of questions to the clinician based on rules in an expert system. Answers to each question determine subsequent questions, until a device is identified.

Systems with a primary focus on device prescription generally use assessment data only as a means to that end, which tends to limit the main use for these systems to one-time major evaluations lasting several hours or more. They are not easily applicable to assessments that take place in a single therapy session and are not designed to track performance across multiple assessments. Furthermore, the systems developed to date are limited to recommending a single device at a time, and are unable to coordinate a multifaceted approach to computer access.

What most models, protocols, guidelines, and tools uniformly lack is a means of collecting detailed quantitative performance data for use in decision making. As a result, computer access assessments primarily consist of brief trials with candidate systems resulting in qualitative judgments of client performance. Some clinicians collect quantitative data with a stopwatch, typing test software, or video games, but these approaches do not necessarily produce valid comparisons between devices.

The Compass software system,[38–41] which measures users' skills in various kinds of computer interaction, is designed to help clinical and educational professionals perform computer access evaluations with their clients by providing them with a clear picture of a client's strengths and limitations. Compass tests the skill families of text entry, pointing, and switch use through a hierarchy of tests that tap into successively more complex aspects of each skill. A hierarchy of complexity helps accommodate differing client abilities. For example, matching single letters of the alphabet may be a more appropriate assessment of keyboarding skill in a young student than transcription of full sentences. The hierarchy also provides a way to isolate the physical component of the test from its perceptual and cognitive aspects. As one moves up the hierarchy, tests incorporate more perceptual and cognitive skills. Performance on higher level tests may be compared with performance at the lower level of the hierarchy to reveal how perceptual and cognitive issues affect keyboarding and pointing for a particular client.

Automatically Adapting Device Configuration

The behavior of most computer input devices, such as keyboards and mice, is adjustable. Because each person's disability is unique, tuning these devices to a user's strengths and limitations is critical for success in many cases. Ideally, configuration is performed in consultation with a clinician who has expertise in computer access for people with disabilities. However, a trained clinician may not be available, and even when one is available, proper tuning of a device to the needs of a particular user can be a difficult and time-consuming task. The challenge is magnified because the user's needs and abilities may change over time, whether in the short term caused by factors such as fatigue or in the long term because of factors such as changes in the individual's underlying impairment. For these reasons, input devices are often not appropriately configured to meet users' needs, with consequent negative effects on user productivity and comfort.

A user's system is typically configured in 1 or more of 3 ways. The first, and perhaps the most common, is to use the default values for the device. Moderately inappropriate values may result in multiple keyboarding errors and/or difficulty selecting targets with the mouse, decreasing user performance and satisfaction. In a more extreme case, the system may be virtually unusable at the default values.

A second scenario is when the user makes his or her own adjustments. This requires that the user knows what parameters are available and how to adjust them. This is a complex task. Performing all possible adjustments for keyboard and mouse within Windows XP requires accessing 3 separate Control Panel applications with 12 tabbed panels; making objects larger for easier selection would require accessing several additional Control Panel applications. Terminology can be ambiguous; for example, to invoke BounceKeys, the user chooses to "ignore repeated keystrokes," whereas to adjust the repeat settings, the user must select "ignore quick keystrokes." Another potential source of confusion is that the repeat settings can be adjusted in 2 different control panels, with the accessibility settings overriding the keyboard control panel settings. Even if the user can successfully navigate the options, knowing the most appropriate values for all applicable settings may be even more difficult. Users may not understand how the parameter settings relate to the interface problems they are having, or if they do, the best choice of specific values may be unclear. Recent versions of the Windows operating system include an accessory program called the Accessibility Wizard, which does provide some help in reducing the complexity of configuration for keyboards, pointers, and the visual display. However, it does not include all available settings (eg, the key repeat settings are not available), and does not give specific suggestions about how to appropriately set parameter values based on user performance.

A third scenario occurs when a clinician or teacher is available to assist with the configuration process, using clinical observations and knowledge of the possible accommodations as a guide. However, most users with physical disabilities do not have a qualified clinician available to them. Trewin and Pain[42] found that only 35%

of 30 computer users with physical disabilities had a computer teacher. Further, not all clinicians have the skills to assist effectively. Even when a clinician or other advisor with relevant expertise is available, input device configuration often requires considerable trial and error.

Under each of these 3 approaches, it may be difficult to define appropriate settings for a user's initial configuration. It is equally difficult, if not more so, to address changes in the user's abilities over time, which may happen over the course of a day, a month, or a year, depending on the nature of the user's disability. Current methods may lead to appropriate input device configurations in some cases, but it does take special knowledge, additional time, and continued maintenance to do it right.[1] As a result, input devices are often not appropriately configured to meet users' needs, with consequent negative effects on user productivity and comfort.

An automated agent on the user's computer could help ensure that input devices are properly configured for the individual, and reconfigured as the user's needs change. Such an agent would need a means to observe the user's performance and predict appropriate input device configuration settings based on that performance. Several groups have been working toward configuration agents that would support this process.[43–48] A configuration agent models a user's strengths and limitations, and based on the model, helps configure the user's input devices appropriately.

Automatically configuring keyboards

Tuning a keyboard to a user's strengths and limitations may yield significant performance and comfort benefits. Conversely, the potential consequences of inappropriate settings are many. (Desktop sharing refers to the ability of 1 computer user to remotely operate another computer while seeing the windows and icons on the remote computer's desktop). For example, for someone who types with a mouthstick, not having StickyKeys active makes it cumbersome to type capital letters and impossible to use other key combinations such as Ctrl-C.

Trewin and colleagues have been developing a configuration agent for keyboard settings.[21,42,49–53] The agent creates a user model based on free typing and determines settings for a range of parameters such as StickyKeys, Repeat Delay, and BounceKeys (**Table 2**). The agent's recommendations were evaluated with 20 keyboard users who have physical disabilities. For StickyKeys, the agent's recommendation correlated significantly with users' opinions on how useful StickyKeys would be for them. However, the discrimination of the agent was imperfect, as 9 users felt that StickyKeys was useful for them, even though the agent did not recommend it for them. For repeat delay, use of the agent-recommended settings significantly reduced key repeat errors (from 2610 to 151 errors).[54] The agent accurately recommended use of BounceKeys for 5 of 7 subjects who made bounce errors. Effects on productivity measures, such as typing speed, were not measured.

One of the challenges in Trewin's approach is that it makes inferences based on unconstrained typing tasks. The agent accurately detected only 55% of inadvertent keypress errors illustrating the difficulty of this approach.[42] The use of unconstrained typing tasks allows for continuous monitoring, which is less obtrusive to the user, but may compromise the success of the agent's suggestions.

Koester and colleagues[55] are developing a software system called IDA (Input Device Agent) with the goal of optimally configuring input devices for people with physical impairments. In a study of 12 typists with physical impairments, IDA recommended 3 keyboard parameters in response to measurements of typing performance: repeat rate, repeat delay, and use of StickyKeys. For 2 participants with significant problems with inadvertent key repeats, use of the IDA-recommended repeat settings reduced

Table 2
Keyboard configuration parameters

Parameter	Description
Repeat delay	How long a key must be held down before it begins to repeat
Repeat rate	Once the keyboard begins to repeat a character, the rate at which it repeats
SlowKeys	How long a key must be held down before it is accepted
BounceKeys	Tells the operating system to ignore keystrokes that are depressed within x seconds of the previous key release
StickyKeys	When StickyKeys are activated, the typist can enter key combinations (eg, Shift-A to type a capital A) by pressing the modifier key (eg, Shift) and other keys (eg, "A") in series, rather than holding down multiple keys simultaneously
ToggleKeys	Gives an auditory signal when locking keys, such as Caps Lock, are depressed

the number of repeated characters by 96% and significantly improved text entry rate and typing accuracy. IDA recommended StickyKeys for 6 participants, which eliminated their modifier-related errors and significantly improved their typing speed. IDA did not recommend StickyKeys for the 6 participants who demonstrated no need for it.

Automatically configuring pointing devices
Pointing devices include the standard mouse, trackballs, laptop trackpads, head-controlled pointers, and many other devices. Typical parameters for pointing device configuration include those shown in **Table 3**. Other settings may be available, depending on the specific device and device driver being used. For example, Logitech trackballs (Logitech, Fremont, CA) allow the user to program the buttons to perform different functions. The trackpads common on laptop computers include settings related to cursor speed and whether the user can click by pressing on the trackpad or whether the buttons must be used.

Table 3
Typical configuration options for pointing devices

Parameter	Description
Button-handedness	Controls the functions assigned to the left and right mouse buttons
Click method	Whether the user performs a single or double click to select icons
Double-click speed	Controls the allowable time between 2 clicks in a double-click
Pointer speed (gain)	How quickly the cursor moves across the screen in response to mouse movements
Enhanced pointer precision	The enhance pointer precision (EPP) setting enables a complex algorithm controlling the velocity and acceleration of the mouse cursor
Snap-to-default	If this option is active, when a dialog box appears on the screen, the cursor will immediately move to the default button (eg, "OK")
Object size	It is possible to change the size (in pixels) of icons, menu bars, and other objects in the user interface. Increasing the size of these objects may make them easier to select, at the cost of reduced space on the screen. There may be many separate settings that could be adjusted to make different classes of objects larger

Proper adjustment of these settings can be critical to efficient use of the pointing device for people with disabilities.[1] For someone with impaired motor control, the default pointer speed on the pointing device may cause the cursor to move much too quickly, making it difficult or impossible to select small targets such as toolbar buttons. Other difficult tasks include dragging the pointer with the mouse button depressed and clicking and double-clicking the mouse button while keeping the pointer still.

If a relationship can be found between an individual's movement patterns and his or her optimal configuration settings, a software agent could customize the settings in response to the user's needs. This concept has been explored with a force-sensing joystick that adapts to hand tremor using measurements of the user's tracking ability and tremor.[45] A preliminary study with 3 subjects who had Friedrich's ataxia indicated that the adaptive joystick provided some improvement in performance for tracking tasks.

Tracey and Winters developed a system to configure mouse settings in the Windows operating system based on subject performance on computer tracking exercises and questions directed to an assistive technology clinician who had observed the user.[12] The principle limitation of this system is its assumption of the presence of an assistive technology expert when, in some cases, users may need or want to configure their systems independently.

LoPresti developed and evaluated a system that automatically adjusted the gain for users of head-controlled pointing devices.[17] For 16 subjects with physical disabilities, the system was able to select settings that were appropriate for most subjects and provided a modest but significant improvement in performance ($P<.05$). IDA recommends a setting for the computer's control-display gain based on observations of a user's performance in a target selection task.[56] In a study involving 12 participants with motor impairments, the IDA-selected gain was not associated with significant improvements in selection time or error-free performance compared with the operating system's default gain. However, 2 participants did have notable and consistent improvement in selection time and error-free performance using the IDA-selected gain.[56]

Switches

Individuals who cannot use adapted keyboards or pointing devices may use switch-based input techniques. One example is single-switch scanning, in which the system presents choices sequentially to the user. A common implementation of single-switch scanning requires 3 switch hits to make 1 selection from a row-column matrix of letters, numbers, symbols, words, or phrases. The first switch hit initiates a scan through the rows of the matrix. Each row of the matrix is highlighted in turn until a second switch hit is made to select a row. Each column of the row is then highlighted in turn until the target is highlighted, when the third switch hit is made to select the target. Depending on the scanning system used, there may be 3 or more adjustable parameters (**Table 4**), with the scan rate being most important. Switch-based parameters are incorporated into the switch system used and are not a feature of the operating system. The scan rate and other configuration parameters determine the minimum letter selection time that is possible for a user. If the scan rate in single-switch scanning is too fast, the user will make a lot of errors or may be unable to use the system. A scan rate that is too slow will unnecessarily slow down performance in a process that is already inherently very slow.[1]

One-switch row-column scanning can be tiring to use and is generally a slow method of communication. An able-bodied individual using an optimally designed

Table 4	
Typical configuration options for single-switch scanning	
Parameter	**Description**
Scan period	The amount of time an item remains highlighted for the user to make a selection
Initial scan delay	Additional delay applied to the first row or column
Column scans	Maximum number of times the columns within a row are scanned
Layout	Arrangement of targets within the scanning matrix

matrix of 26 letters and a space can produce between 6 and 8 words per minute using this method.[57,58] Despite its limitations, however, row-column scanning fills an important niche within access techniques by providing an affordable and reliable option for many individuals with limited movement and limited vocal abilities. Hence, despite increasing interest in speech recognition, eye-tracking, and direct-brain interfaces for accessing assistive technology, there remain valid reasons for seeking to enhance performance using row-column scanning.

Three research groups have worked on methods of automatically adapting the scan period of a single-switch row-column scanning system. Cronk and Schubert[59] developed an expert system for the adaptation of scan period, but it was never integrated into any commercial systems. Lesher and colleagues[60,61] developed a rule-based method of scan period adjustment based on user errors and the time required for the user to make a selection relative to the available time. Their primary goal was to provide a means of scan period adjustment for empiric studies comparing different scanning displays, and their system performed well enough to meet this goal with able-bodied subjects.[61]

Simpson and Koester[46] developed and evaluated a single-switch scanning system that used a Bayesian network to adjust the user's scan period in real time. Two studies, involving a total of 16 subjects without disabilities, demonstrated that the system could make reasonable adaptation decisions, with no human intervention, for a system with a single scan delay. Subjects' text entry performance and subjective opinion was no different with the automatic system compared with a manual adjustment protocol, in which able-bodied subjects could change the scan period at will with a single keypress. A major limitation is that the work was not validated with users with disabilities.

IDA's ability to make recommendations for scan period in a row-column scanning system was evaluate with 2 groups of individuals (8 people who were either able-bodied or had spinal cord injuries and 6 individuals with severe physical disability secondary to cerebral palsy).[62] Participants' speed, accuracy, and subjective ratings when using the IDA-recommended scan rate suggest that IDA can recommend an appropriate scan rate. Participants' performance was at least as good for the IDA-selected scan period as for the self-selected scan period.[62]

Monitoring and Telerehabilitation

The Institute of Medicine defines *telemedicine* as "the use of electronic information and communications technologies to provide and support health care when distance separates the participants."[63] The Shepherd Center has further defined *telerehabilitation* as "the use of telecommunications technology to provide rehabilitation and long-term support to people with disabilities."[64] Telerehabilitation technology can either be used *interactively* or in a *store-and-forward* mode. Interactive telerehabilitation sessions involve the client and clinician participating in the session at the same time, typically using audio- and videoconferencing technology. Store-and-forward telerehabilitation sessions, on the other hand, allow the clinician to collect data from the client without the need for simultaneous interaction.

Telerehabilitation technology can allow a clinician to collect performance data during a "loan period" to evaluate how well a potential computer access solution meets the consumer's needs. Often, the sole measurable outcome of a loan period is the consumer's subjective impression of the AT. Although the consumer's impression is important, there is typically no record of how often the device was used during the loan period, how well the consumer performed when using the device, or how the device was configured, all of which are important for making informed comparisons between multiple potential solutions. In addition, self-reports can be unreliable. Studies[65–67] have shown that "estimates of concordance of client self-reports and proxy-reports with performance-based measures range from a low of 63% to a high of 94% depending on the specific daily living task."[68]

Telerehabilitation can also be a cost-effective solution to providing follow-up to consumers after a device has been purchased. Receiving a device is no guarantee that the device will be installed and configured correctly, particularly if funding for an in-person visit from a clinician is not available. Telerehabilitation may reduce the cost of a clinician's involvement in the installation and configuration process to the point where this service can be provided with each piece of equipment received. Follow-up assistance may take several forms, including

- Interactive desktop sharing, videoconferencing, or text messaging to allow the clinician to guide (or control) the installation/configuration process
- Interactive or store-and-forward use of skill tests, which allow the clinician to compare performance obtained in the clinic with results on the consumer's home or work computer

Several clinical teams have documented the use of telerehabilitation to enhance the provision of computer access and augmentative communication services, although these publications have thus far been limited to case studies with little or no statistical analysis. In the United States, the Shepherd Center of Georgia has perhaps the most experience using telerehabilitation technology for computer access. They have described 1 instance in which a videophone was used to evaluate how well a computer access system was configured for a client,[64] and have also described using telerehabilitation technology for training a client to use speech-recognition software for computer access.[69]

Another American researcher, Elliot Cole, has described a computer-based cognitive rehabilitation intervention that made use of telecommunications technology.[70] Cole developed computer software that assisted a client with communication and information storage and retrieval. The client was trained to use the software using videoconferencing technology and desktop sharing software. This is the only reported instance we could identify in which telerehabilitation was used as a means of conducting follow-up evaluations. Specifically, Cole modified the system based on data automatically collected by the system during regular use.

In Europe, the Oxford Aiding Communication in Education (ACE) Center has made extensive use of telerehabilitation technology to support computer access and augmentative communication interventions. The TELENET[71] and CATCHNET[16] projects evaluated the effectiveness of low-cost videoconferencing and online software sharing in providing computer access assessment, training and support. Both projects used an integrative services digital network (ISDN) line to connect clinicians at the ACE Center with clinicians and clients in remote clinical sites, and reported general client and clinician satisfaction with the approach.

The Telesupport for Loan Equipment project[10] compared in-person support for computer access teams with remote support. The ACE runs a technology loan library and has observed a need for "good quality, on-going training while a piece of equipment is borrowed."[10] Results indicated that telerehabilitation interventions provided the following benefits to users and aides[10]:

- Clients could interact in real time with clinicians.
- Trained clinicians could configure devices remotely.
- Training and support via videoconferencing technology was perceived to be of higher quality than more conventional communication methods (eg, phone, email).

In Europe, the Remote Service of Rehabilitation Technology (RESORT) project[72-74] developed telerehabilitation technology that allows a clinician to establish a communication channel with a client for transmitting audio and visual data and for desktop sharing. A clinician can use RESORT to interact with a client, monitor (but not collect data on) the client's computer use, and adjust the configuration of the software. The RESORT team also developed an application programming interface (API) that allows an application on the client's computer to be synchronized with the clinician's computer. This API is different from other application-sharing technologies (eg, Microsoft NetMeeting) in that it supports real-time synchronization.

DISCUSSION

Quantitative evaluation tools such as Compass provide the means for clinicians to collect evidence in a rigorous manner. The underlying technology, however, can be advanced in several directions. One opportunity for potential improvement is the integration of additional performance measures, many of which were developed by the human-computer interaction (HCI) community. For example, MacKenzie and colleagues[75] have developed error measures that compare the cursor's actual path of travel to the "ideal" path of travel. Keates and Hwang[76-80] extended this work by developing error measures that incorporated the "instantaneous" optimal cursor path, referred to as the instantaneous task axis (ITA). These measures can provide the client and clinician with a great deal of additional information, but it is likely that a distinct subset of measures will be of greatest interest for each client, device, and task. Hence, a means of flexibly integrating user- and device-specific errors would also be useful.

Clinical assessment tools would also benefit from adoption of protocols originally developed for HCI research. For example, investigators within the field of human factors have recently begun employing "unconstrained" text entry protocols[81-85] in which the user is allowed to make errors and to decide whether or not to correct the errors that occur. The primary advantage of this approach is that it allows users to enter text under more natural, realistic conditions.[81-85] This approach also allows investigators to analyze the entire input stream, including errors and error corrections,[85] thus providing a more detailed picture of text entry.

Wobbrock has recently demonstrated how the text input stream can be categorized into[85]

- Non-errors: correct keystrokes (ie, the correct key pressed at the correct time)
- Substitutions: incorrect keystrokes in which 1 character is entered instead of another
- Insertions: incorrect keystrokes in which additional characters are entered
- Omissions: errors in which a character that should appear in the input stream does not
- Fixes: keystrokes used to remove characters or reposition the cursor (eg, back-space, delete, arrow keys)

The algorithms developed by Wobbrock, however, make certain assumptions that are not necessarily valid for individuals with disabilities or for text entry methods such as word completion and abbreviation expansion in which a single input can generate multiple characters.[85] Additional work is needed to determine how Wob-brock's work can be extended to cover these situations.

Software like IDA may one day assist clinicians in configuring CAT, and may also be used by clients to adjust the configuration of their technology over time. IDA is limited, however, in that the client must complete performance tests in order for IDA to collect enough data to make configuration recommendations. A more desirable approach would be for IDA to make its recommendations based on the client's performance on unconstrained real-world tasks in the normal course of computer use. Hurst and colleagues[86] have used machine-learning techniques to automatically categorize user performance on pointing tasks based on whether or not assistance with clicking on targets was likely to improve performance.

REFERENCES

1. Anson DK. Alternative computer access: a guide to selection. Philadelphia: F.A. Davis Company; 1997.
2. Chen C-L, Chen H-C, Cheng P-T, et al. Enhancement of operational efficiencies for people with high cervical spinal cord injuries using a flexible integrated point-ing device apparatus. Arch Phys Med Rehabil 2006;87:866–73.
3. Dobransky K, Hargittai E. The disability divide in Internet access and use. Inform Comm Soc 2006;9:313–34.
4. Drainoni M, Houlihan B, Williams S, et al. Patterns of Internet use by persons with spinal cord injuries and relationship to health-related quality of life. Arch Phys Med Rehabil 2004;85:1872–9.
5. Madara E. The mutual-aid self-help online revolution. Soc Policy 1997;27:20–6.
6. McKenna K, Seidman G. You, me, and we: Interpersonal processes in electronic groups. In: Amichai-Hamburger Y, editor. The social net: human behavior in cyberspace. Oxford (UK): Oxford University Press; 2005. p. 191–217.
7. McKenna K, Bargh J. Plan 9 from cyberspace: the implications of the Internet for personality and social psychology. Pers Soc Psychol Rev 2000;4:57.
8. Morahan-Martin J, Schumacher P. Loneliness and social use of the Internet. Com-put Human Behav 2003;19:656–71.
9. Stevenson B, McQuivey JL. The wide range of abilities and its impact on computer technology. Cambridge (MA): A Research Study Commissioned by Microsoft Corporation and Conducted by Forrester Research; 2003.
10. Hazell G, Colven D. ACE centre telesupport for loan equipment. Oxford: ACE Centre Advisory Trust; 2001. p. 35.
11. Raskind M. Assistive technology and adults with learning disabilities: a blueprint for exploration and advancement. Learn Disabil Q 1993;16:185–96.

12. Scherer MJ. What we know about women's technology use, avoidance, and abandonment. Women Ther 1993;14:117–29.
13. Scherer MJ, Galvin JC. In: Galvin JC, Scherer MJ, editors. Evaluating, Selecting and Using Appropriate Assistive Technology. Gaithersburg (MD): Aspen Publication; 1996. p. 1–26.
14. Phillips B, Zhao H. Predictors of assistive technology abandonment. Assist Technol 1993;5:36–45.
15. Tewey BP, Barnicle K, Perr A. The wrong stuff. Mainstream 1994;19:19–23.
16. Lysley A, Colven D, Donegan M. CATCHNET final report. Oxford (UK): ACE Centre; 1999.
17. Batavia AJ, Dillard D, Phillips B. How to avoid technology abandonment. Washington, DC: National Institute on Disability and Rehabilitation Research; 1990.
18. Riemer-Reiss M, Wacker R. Assistive technology use and abandonment among college students with disabilities. Int Electron J LeaderLearn 1999;3:23.
19. Schartz K, Schartz H, Blanck P. Employment of persons with disabilities in information technology jobs: literature review for "IT works". Behav Sci Law 2002;20:637–57.
20. Stevenson B, McQuivey JL. Examining awareness, use, and future potential. Cambridge (MA): A Research Study Commissioned by Microsoft Corporation and Conducted by Forrester Research; 2003.
21. Trewin S, Pain H. Keyboard and mouse errors due to motor disabilities. Int J Hum Comput Stud 1999;50:109–44.
22. Riemer-Reiss M. Factors associated with assistive technology discontinuance among individuals with disabilities. J Rehabil 2000;66(3):44–50.
23. Scherer M, Cushman L. Measuring subjective quality of life following spinal cord injury: a validation study of the assistive technology device predisposition assessment. Disabil Rehabil 2001;23:387–93.
24. Barker M, Cook AM. A systematic approach to evaluating physical ability for control of assistive devices. In: International conference on assistive technology for people with disabilities (RESNA). Washington, DC: RESNA Press; 1981. p. 287–9.
25. Rosen M, Goodenough-Trepagner C. The Tufts-MIT prescription guide: assessment of users to predict the suitability of augmentative communication devices. Assist Technol 1989;1:51–61.
26. Bowser G, Zabala J. SETT & Re-SETT: concepts of AT implementation. In: ConnSENSE Bulletin. 2005.
27. Cushman LA, Scherer MJ. Measuring the relationship of assistive technology use, functional status over time, and consumer-therapist perceptions of ATs. Assist Technol 1996;8:103–9.
28. Scherer MJ, Cushman LA. Predicting satisfaction with assistive technology for a sample of adults with new spinal cord injuries. Psychol Rep 2000; 87:981–7.
29. Chambers AC. Council of Administrators of Special Education and the Technology and Media Division of the Council for Exceptional Children. In: CASE/TAM Assistive Technology Policy and Practice Series: Has Technology Been Considered? A Guide for IEP Teams. Reston, VA; 1997.
30. Reed P, editor. Assessing students' needs for assistive technology. Oshkosh (WI): Wisconsin Assistive Technology Initiative; 2000.
31. Reed P, Bowser G. Education Tech Points: a framework for assistive technology planning and systems change in schools. In: Conference on technology and persons with disabilities (CSUN). Los Angeles (CA): CSUN; 1998.
32. Lee KS, Thomas DJ. Control of computer-based technology for people with physical disabilities: an assessment manual. Toronto (ON): University of Toronto Press; 1990.

33. Dumont C, Vincent C, Mazer B. Development of a standardized instrument to assess computer access performance. Am J Occup Ther 2002;56:60–8.

34. Williams WB, Stemach G, Stanger C. Lifespace access profile: assistive technology assessment and planning for individuals with severe or multiple disabilities. Irvine (CA): Lifespace Access Assistive Technology Systems; 1995.

35. Stapleton D, Garrett R, Seeger B. VOCASelect and computer access selector: software tools to assist in choosing assistive technology. In: International conference on assistive technology for people with disabilities (RESNA). Pittsburgh (PA): RESNA Press; 1997.

36. Lahm EA and Gassaway LJ. Matching assistive technology to the individual using an expert system. In: Annual meeting of the Technology and Media Division of the Council for Exceptional Children, Reston (VA). 2003.

37. Lahm EA, Gassaway LJ, Reed AG. ATES: assistive technology expert system. In: Annual meeting of the Technology and Media Division of the Council for Exceptional Children, Washington, DC. 2002.

38. LoPresti EF, Koester HH, McMillan W, et al. Compass: Software for Computer Skills Assessment. Presented at CSUN's 18 Annual Conference: Technology and Persons with Disabilities. Edinburgh (UK), March 2003.

39. Koester HH, McMillan W. Usability testing of software for assessing computer usage skills. In: International conference on assistive technology for people with disabilities (RESNA). Minneapolis, MN: RESNA Press; 1998.

40. Koester HH, McMillan W. Software for assessing computer usage skills. In: International conference on assistive technology for people with disabilities (RESNA): RESNA. 1997.

41. Ashlock G, Koester HH, LoPresti EF, et al. User-centered design of software for assessing computer usage skills. In: Simpson RC, editor. International conference on assistive technology for people with disabilities (RESNA). Atlanta (GA): RESNA; 2003.

42. Trewin S, Pain H. A model of keyboard configuration requirements. Behav Inform Tech 1999;18:27–35.

43. Lesher GW, Higginbotham DJ, Moulton BJ. Techniques for automatically updating scanning delays. In: RESNA 2000 annual conference. Orlando (FL): RESNA Press; 2000. p. 75–7.

44. LoPresti EF, Brienza D. Adaptive software for head-operated computer controls. IEEE Trans Neural Syst Rehabil Eng 2004;12:102–11.

45. McGill R, O'Beirne H, Milner M, et al. Towards the development of adaptive user interfaces for tremor disabled persons: a blackboard expert system approach. In: Annual international conference of the IEEE Engineering in Medicine and Biology Society. Atlanta, GA: IEEE Press; 1991. p. 1262–3.

46. Simpson RC, Koester HH. Adaptive one-switch row-column scanning. IEEE Trans Rehabil Eng 1999;7:464–73.

47. Tracey M, Winters J. Neuro-Fuzzy advisor for mouse setting in Microsoft Windows. In: Proceedings of the first joint BMES/EMBS conference. Atlanta (GA): IEEE; 1999. p. 664.

48. Trewin S. Automating accessibility: the dynamic keyboard. In: Assets '04: proceedings of the 6th international ACM SIGACCESS conference on computers and accessibility. Atlanta (GA): ACM; 2004. p. 71–8.

49. Trewin S. Extending keyboard adaptability: an investigation. Univers Access Inform Soc 2002;2:44–55.

50. Trewin S. Configuration agents, control and privacy. In: Conference on universal usability 2000. New York: ACM; 2000. p. 9–16.

51. Trewin S. An invisible keyguard. In: ASSETS 2002. New York: ACM; 2002. p. 143–9.

52. Trewin S. Automating accessibility: the dynamic keyguard. In: ASSETS 2004. New York: ACM; 2004. p. 71–8.
53. Trewin S, Pain H. Dynamic modeling of keyboard skills: supporting users with motor disabilities. In: 6th international conference on user modeling. New York: Springer; 1997. p. 135–46.
54. Trewin S, Pain H 1997 Dynamic modelling of keyboard skills: supporting users with motor disabilities. In: Sixth international conference on user modeling. p. 135–46
55. Koester HH, LoPresti EF, Simpson RC. Toward automatic adjustment of keyboard settings for people with physical impairments. Disabil Rehabil Assist Technol 2007; 2:261–74.
56. LoPresti EF, Koester HH, Simpson RC. Toward automatic adjustment of pointing device configuration to accommodate physical impairment. Disabil Rehabil Assist Technol 2008;3:221–35.
57. Damper RI. Text composition by the physically disabled: a rate prediction model for scanning input. Appl Ergon 1984;15:289–96.
58. Koester HH, Levine SP. Modeling the speed of text entry with a word prediction interface. IEEE Trans Neural Syst Rehabil Eng 1994;2:177–87.
59. Cronk SR, Schubert RW. Development of a real-time expert system for automatic adaptation of scanning rates. In: Annual conference on rehabilitation technology (RESNA). San Jose (CA): RESNA Press; 1987.
60. Lesher GW, Higginbotham J, Moulton BJ. Techniques for automatically updating scanning delays. In: Annual conference on rehabilitation technology (RESNA). Orlando (FL): RESNA Press; 2000.
61. Lesher GW, Moulton BJ, Higginbotham J, et al. Acquisition of scanning skills: the use of an adaptive scanning delay algorithm across four scanning displays. In: Annual conference on rehabilitation technology (RESNA). Minneapolis (MN): RESNA Press; 2002.
62. Simpson RC, Koester HH, LoPresti EF. Evaluation of an adaptive row/column scanning system. Tech Disabil 2007;18:127–38.
63. Field MJ. Telemedicine: a guide to assessing telecommunications in health care. Washington, DC: National Academy Press; 1996.
64. Burns RB, Crislip D, Daviou P, et al. Using telerehabilitation to support assistive technology. Assist Technol 1998;10:126–33.
65. Magaziner J, Zimmerman SI, Gruber-Baldini AL, et al. Proxy reporting in five areas of functional status: comparison with self-reports and observations of performance. Am J Epidemiol 1997;146:418–28.
66. Rubenstein LZ, Schairer C, Wieland GD, et al. Systematic biases in functional status assessment of elderly adults: effects of different data sources. J Gerontol 1984;39:686–91.
67. Sager MA, Dunham NC, Schwantes A, et al. Measurement of activities of daily living in hospitalized elderly: a comparison of self-report and performance-based methods. J Am Geriatr Soc 1992;40:457–62.
68. Cooper RA, Fitzgerald SG, Boninger ML, et al. Telerehabilitation: expanding access to rehabilitation expertise. Proc IEEE 2001;89:1174–91.
69. Burns R, Hauber R, Vesmarovich S. Telerehabilitation: continuing cases and new applications. In: Winters J, editor. The RESNA 2000 annual conference. Technology for the new millennium. Orlando (FL): RESNA; 2000. p. 258–60.
70. Cole E, Ziegmann M, Wu Y, et al. User of "therapist-friendly" tools in cognitive assistive technology and telerehabilitation. In: The RESNA international conference. Orlando (FL): RESNA; 2000. p. 31–3.

71. Donegan M. The TELENET project summary final report. Oxford (UK): ACE Centre; 2002.
72. Panek P, Zagler W L, Beck C, et al 2001. Providing tele-support and tele-training to severely disabled persons using ip-based networks. In: Vienna international workshop on distance education and training, Vienna, Austria.
73. Panek P, Zagler WL. Remote service of rehabilitation technology final report. Vienna, Austria: Fortec, Vienna University of Technology; 2001.
74. Panek P, Beck C, Hochgatterer A, et al. Tele-help and remote service provision using RESORT prototype system. Linz, Austria. In: Miesenberger K, editor. 8th international conference on computers helping people with special needs. AAATE. 2002. p. 635–42.
75. MacKenzie IS, Kauppinen T, Silfverberg M. Accuracy measures for evaluating computer pointing devices. In: SIGCHI conference on human factors in computing systems. Seattle (WA): ACM Press; 2001.
76. Hwang F. A study of cursor trajectories of motion-impaired users. In: Terveen L, Wixon D, editors. CHI '02 extended abstracts on human factors in computing systems. Minneapolis (MN): ACM Press; 2002. p. 842–3.
77. Hwang F. Partitioning cursor movements in "point and click" tasks. In: Cockton G, Korhonen P, editors. CHI '03 extended abstracts on human factors in computing systems. Fort Lauderdale (FL): ACM Press; 2003. p. 682–3.
78. Hwang F, Keates S, Langdon P, et al. Mouse movements of motion-impaired users: a submovement analysis. In: 6th international ACM SIGACCESS conference on computers and accessibility. Atlanta (GA): ACM Press; 2004. p. 102–9.
79. Keates S, Hwang F, Langdon P, et al. Cursor measures for motion-impaired computer users. In: Hanson VL, Jacko JA, editors. Proceedings of the fifth international ACM conference on assistive technologies. Edinburgh (UK): ACM Press; 2002. p. 135–42.
80. Keates S, Hwang F, Langdon P, et al. The user of cursor measures for motion-impaired computer users. Univ Access Inform Soc 2002;2:18–29.
81. MacKenzie IS, Soukoreff RW. A character-level error analysis technique for evaluating text entry methods. In: Bertelsen OW, editor. Proceedings of the second Nordic conference on human-computer interaction. Aarhus, Denmark: ACM Press; 2002. p. 243–6.
82. Soukoreff RW, MacKenzie IS. Measuring errors in text entry tasks: an application of the Levenshtein string distance statistic. In: Tremaine MM, editor. CHI '01 extended abstracts on human factors in computing systems. Seattle (WA): ACM Press; 2001. p. 319–20.
83. Soukoreff RW, MacKenzie IS. Metrics for text entry research: an evaluation of MSD and KSPC, and a new unified error metric. In: Cockton G, Korhonen P, editors. Proceedings of the SIGCHI conference on human factors in computing systems. Fort Lauderdale (FL): ACM Press; 2003. p. 113–20.
84. Soukoreff RW, MacKenzie IS. Recent developments in text-entry error rate measurement. In: Dykstra-Erickson E, Tscheligi M, editors. CHI '04 extended abstracts on human factors in computing systems. Vienna, Austria: ACM Press; 2004. p. 1425–8.
85. Wobbrock JO, Myers BA. Analyzing the input stream for character-level errors in unconstrained text entry evaluations. ACM Trans Comput Hum Interact 2006;13:458–89.
86. Hurst A, Hudson SE, Mankoff J, et al. Automatically detecting pointing performance. In: 13th international conference on intelligent user interfaces. Gran Canaria (Spain): ACM; 2008. p. 11–9.

Electronic Aids for Daily Living

Roger Little, MS

KEYWORDS

- X-10 • Electronic aids • Disability • Home control
- Environmental control • EADL • ECU • ECS

Electronic aids for daily living (EADLs) are devices that facilitate the operation of electrical appliances in a given environment for a person with a severe physical disability. EADLs are also referred to as environmental control units (ECUs) and, environmental control systems (ECSs). EADL has become the prevailing term over the past 10 years. According to Lange,[1] "EADL emphasizes the task performed by the individual instead of the device that it controls." She further explains that "this term helps funding sources realize the goal of the device, which is to assist in a daily living task."

EADLs have been in existence for some time. The date of origin varies greatly depending on the source. One of the earliest reported dates is the1950s[2] and the latest the 1980s.[1] The sophistication and the demands of the systems certainly have been constantly evolving as the technological age has advanced. The persons most appropriate for such devices are those with severe physical limitations such as cervical spinal cord injury, multiple sclerosis, athetoid cerebral palsy, spastic cerebral palsy, muscular dystrophy, syringomyelia, spinal muscular atrophy, and amyotrophic lateral sclerosis. Other disability groups such as those with arthritis or stroke could benefit from such devices. However, these groups have been underrepresented in EADL provision.[3]

ACTIVITIES CONTROLLED

Activities that can be supported by using an EADL include: (1) *environmental regulation* by controlling temperature (heater, air conditioner, fan, humidifier), lighting (lamps, curtains/blinds), and pressure relief (bed positions); (2) *information acquisition* by controlling audio/video equipment, page turners, and note-taking devices; (3) *safety/security* by controlling doors, door locks, monitoring the premises, and summoning emergency assistance; and (4) *communication* by controlling telephones, attendant calls, and intercoms.

Department of Rehabilitation Science and Technology, School of Health and Rehabilitation Sciences, University of Pittsburgh, Suite 5044, Forbes Tower, Atwood and Sennott Streets, Pittsburgh, PA 15260, USA
E-mail address: rlittle@pitt.edu

Phys Med Rehabil Clin N Am 21 (2010) 33–42
doi:10.1016/j.pmr.2009.07.008
1047-9651/09/$ – see front matter © 2010 Elsevier Inc. All rights reserved.

Persons who have incurred damage to the central nervous system frequently have difficulty regulating body temperature, requiring careful adjustment of the temperature to avoid medical complications and to manage comfort. Furthermore, the perceived comfort of that person may be very different from that of a caregiver or family member. Humidity control is necessary for persons with respiratory problems associated with severe disability. A person unable to independently move is unable to change positions while in bed. The ability to control bed positioning can help avoid skin break-down and pressure sores. The control of lights is important for aiding safety, maintaining sleep patterns, providing comfort, and enhancing vision.

Acquiring information through TV, radio, page turners, and so forth is important for personal enjoyment, stimulation, and quality of life. However, it is also necessary for gaining pertinent information about the weather, traffic, important happenings and for keeping apprised of community, state, national, and world events.

With regard to security, the ability to know about and control who can gain access to the home, and the ability to independently leave the dwelling may not be possible for someone with severe motor impairments. An EADL can assist in monitoring the home premises, controlling the locks, and opening doors.

The ability to communicate is essential for everyday activities such as coordinating attendant care, scheduling medical services, managing work, school, and family schedules and for requesting assistance. Communication, like information acquisition, is a key component to quality of life and avoiding isolation.

BENEFITS OF ELECTRONIC AIDS FOR DAILY LIVING

Using an EADL is not a convenience for someone with a severe disability; it is a necessity for him or her to perform many functions. The empowerment provided by such devices allows the independent performance of both urgent and repetitive tasks. Many studies have provided support for the positive psychological and functional impact of EADLs for individuals with disabilities. Ripat[4] provides a good summary table and overview of these findings. Ripat summarizes that the impact of EADLs is generally positive, and identifies independence, control, self worth, adaptability, competence, increased environmental interaction by facilitating communication, recreation, and security as important considerations for consumers. Stickel and colleagues[5] reported that consumers are generally satisfied with their EADLs, and that this satisfaction remained constant over time. Palmer and Seale[6] suggested that "users often initially see the utility in the equipment, but over time, that tool can transcend from utility into a higher level of psychological meaning for that individual." These investigators also noted that the positive feelings were generally associated with psychological and social benefits. In contrast, those who did not have EADLs expressed frustration and hopelessness, and felt restricted in terms of participating in daily activities.[5]

The areas that have been reported to be have highest functional benefit to the user of an EADL are home security, telephone, television, and attendant call.[7–9] Wolf and Roa,[9] in a qualitative study, found "the most used functions were the control of entertainment devices, TV, stereo, VCR." This finding is understandable because the study was measuring the frequency that the EADL produced each type of command, and operating electronic devices requires multiple activations.

The person using an EADL is not the only one to derive benefits from the device. The caregivers' responsibilities are also alleviated. Harmer and Bakheit[7] highlighted that a caregiver provides personal assistance and companionship as well as completion of many daily routine tasks such as placing phone calls, operating lights, and adjusting the television. Likewise, Platts and Fraser[10] noted that freeing caregivers from mundane tasks allows them to carry out other responsibilities. Making the routine tasks less burdensome will assist in obtaining the needed care that a device cannot provide. Platts and Fraser added that lessening of rote tasks will also improve the morale of the EADL user. Reducing the work load required by the family members and caregivers has also been reported to help improve the family and caregiver relationships with the EADL user.[2,11] Although the studies mentioned here all have relatively small sample sizes, the consistency of reported benefits seems to have merit.

ACCESSING ELECTRONIC AIDS TO DAILY LIVING

The user may control the EADL through several different methods, including (1) switch—single or dual, (2) touch screen, (3) voice recognition, or (4) integrated with other controls such as alternate computer access, wheelchair controls, or augmentative communication devices. Using integrated controls to operate an EADL is helpful and often necessary when a person has a limited number of switch/control sites available.

CONTROL METHODS OF ELECTRONIC AIDS FOR DAILY LIVING

EADLs can control devices through (1) direct connection, (2) infrared (IR) transmission, and (3) power line carrier (X-10). Other control protocols have been used in home automation, but these methods have not been extensively used with specialized EADLs. Each control method has benefits and limitations.

Direct connection implies that the device is wired to the EADL. Such connections may include telephone lines, intercom systems, bed control, nurse call, external speakers, IR extenders, and external relays. Directly connecting an external device is beneficial for reducing the time lag for activation, increasing the reliability of automation and controlling devices that are not suited for IR or X-10. The main disadvantage is that the EADL is tethered to the device it controls.

IR offers control of many different functions in the same way as a TV/VCR/DVD remote control. IR transmission requires "line of sight." As a result, the controlling signal cannot operate a device located in another room or even in the same room if the controller cannot "see" the device. If IR control is required and the device is located in a different room, then an IR extension cable can be used to deliver the signal to the remote area. Another alternative to controlling IR devices that are not in the line of sight is to change the IR signal into a radiofrequency (RF) signal. This change allows the control signal to pass through walls and extend in all directions. An RF receiver then captures the control signal, translates it back into an IR signal, and delivers it to the device.

The power line control method has historically been accomplished through X-10. X-10 is an industry standard for communication among devices used for home automation.[12] X-10 uses household wiring (power line) to carry short-wave RF signals to the devices to be controlled. An advantage of this type of control is that in many cases the home electrical service does not need to be modified, and no additional wires are required. Furthermore, many types of control modules are available, and the technology is relatively inexpensive. The main disadvantage of using X-10 to control devices is the less than perfect reliability. Although this type of control can dim and brighten lights, it is essentially limited to turning devices on and off.

Other control protocols are available for the home automation market, including (1) Insteon, (2) ZigBee, and (3) Z-Wave. Insteon uses both RF and power line transmission, making it more reliable than X-10. Insteon also advertises that it is compatible with X-10 devices. Both ZigBee and Z-wave use RF transmission; they are not compatible with X-10 devices. Special control units and receivers are required for each of these methods of control, and they are more expensive than X-10. There has been some preliminary work by Bessel and colleagues[13] to design a universal control module using a standard personal digital assistant and ZigBee.

EADL using these types of controls are currently not available. Nonetheless, these control methods may be appropriate for persons who are able to use the standard control interfaces.

CLASSIFICATION OF ELECTRONIC AIDS TO DAILY LIVING

Due to the diversity in the range of consumers' functional abilities, access methods, and transmission types, EADLs do not have standardized classifications. Steggles and Leslie[14] proposed a possible classification by output ability, specifically one output, two outputs, or multi outputs. Other classification systems offer a combination of functional use and output ability.[15] Information provided for EADLs often is presented by function, access method, specific devices they control, or simply by manufacturer's specifications.

ELECTRONIC AIDS FOR DAILY LIVING AND THE USER

Regardless of the classification systems that are used, of paramount importance is the usability of the system and how it meets an individual's needs. Areas to be considered include the introduction of EADLs, consumer involvement, evaluation procedures, consideration for the progression and regression of the consumer's abilities, and follow-up procedures including training, reprogramming, and accommodating the changing needs of the consumer and technology.

INTRODUCTION OF ELECTRONIC AIDS TO DAILY LIVING

Regarding the acute phase of rehabilitation, a patient's responses to using an EADL vary greatly, and the technology may even be rejected.[10,16] However, the introduction of such devices is important to provide motivation and psychological rehabilitation by providing "tangible evidence of the possibilities of overcoming physical limitations."[10] Introducing EADL technology early when someone is diagnosed with a progressive disease such as amyotrophic lateral sclerosis can also allow that person to become comfortable with the technology before his or her impairments fully develop. One report[17] recommends that the person be introduced to the EADL early in the rehabilitation process, but "the final selection of a system should wait until the person returns home and becomes familiar with patterns of care and gains some experience with their own limitations." In a study involving 8 subjects, all preferred trialing the EADL in their homes rather than in a demonstration center.[18] Maintaining consumer involvement throughout the planning and decision-making process was found to be a key to successful outcomes.[16]

Although the needs and abilities of a person will vary over time and the exact specifications of the EADL system may not be known during the early phase of rehabilitation, control of the EADL should be considered as early as possible. Other technologies such as powered seating, speech-generating devices, and computer access are often considered earlier in the rehabilitation process. Ideally, the access method of an EADL should also be considered, especially when the control sites are very limited. Control and mounting can become a tremendous challenge when considering the integration of several systems. Therefore, the usability of the EADL should be considered in the early phases of the assistive technology system. Barnes[19] commented on the necessity of EADL being considered as part of the assistive technology system and not in isolation.

ELECTRONIC AID FOR DAILY LIVING EVALUATION

The EADL evaluation should encompass the user's needs, abilities, prognosis, access options, EADL equipment options, technology integration, home/work environment, lifestyle, and the equipment that is needed to be controlled. This evaluation process can take considerable time and effort, as noted by Croser and colleagues[18] who stated that "it became apparent during the study that some of the more complex EADL required more than 2 weeks to adequately customize and trial."

When considering the functional usability of an EADL, the details of the system are important. The user of the system will likely benefit from having access to the controls while seated, in bed, in multiple rooms within the home, outside the residence, and at work. If possible, each of these scenarios should be taken into account. Furthermore, the usability of the EADL may require programming and macro-integration. Macros enable the user to carry out multiple stepped tasks by activating one command. For example, playing a DVD may require the cable, TV, and DVD to be turned on and tuned to a certain channel. Macros are useful when noise-producing devices can be muted if the phone or doorbell rings. Likewise, functions to open/close and unlock/lock a door while turning on a light may need to be controlled simultaneously. Using macros with these types of scenarios can eliminate the need for the user to access multiple menus for each function. The ability to simplify access to multiple functions can make the difference in usability, especially to a single-switch user or someone with cognitive dysfunction.

Matching personal needs with the capabilities of the EADL system is important. Not all EADLs have the same capabilities or are able to perform necessary tasks. For example, a person may need to record a phone conversation to obtain/relay information later, or they may need to use speed dials with the ability to input bank numbers/extensions and navigate through voice mail. Others may need automatic speech capabilities for emergency calls or a means to independently carry out a private conversation. The particulars of each person and system need to be matched during the evaluation.

A comprehensive evaluation that is integrated with other rehabilitation disciplines and goals from qualified evaluators will help ensure that these aforementioned areas are considered and that the equipment is properly specified. Unfortunately, this is often not the case. Novak[20] reviewed 29 ECS prescriptions. He found that 7 were not justified clinically. Of the remaining 22 justified prescriptions, 6 required complete revision and 13 systems could be substantially improved. As a result of his survey, 29 referrals for things other than ECSs were made. He also reported that of those who did need ECS, there was considerable underutilization of equipment, and that 9 of 41 room installations were not used. These findings should not be surprising because EADLs are often recommended in isolation to other rehabilitation interventions, by persons who stand to make a profit from the sale of the equipment or persons with limited knowledge and access to a wide range of EADL systems.

ELECTRONIC AIDS FOR DAILY LIVING TRAINING AND SUPPORT

Training and ongoing support are critical factors for the successful outcome of any EADL system.[20,21] However, the literature indicates that both of these key issues have been found to be inadequate. Various surveys indicate that the respondents felt that training was inadequate; 30%[17] and 70%[8]. Lack of adequate training was also reported as the third most stated reason for equipment abandonment.[22] Ongoing support is also found to be lacking. Harmer and Bakheit[7] described user and caregiver training as lasting only 1 to 3 hours, with only one training session provided.

Changes in personal abilities and technology can also have a negative impact on the performance of the user/EADL system. People with progressively deteriorating conditions will likely have decreased functional abilities after the initial setup of the system. Therefore, it is important to establish a regular follow-up procedure to meet the changing needs of the user.[7]

Wolf and Roa[9] reported that seemingly minor changes in the type or placement of the switch or display location often had major effects on the efficacy of the system. Wolf and Roa also stated that "in most cases, subjects did not complain about the problem often because they simply did not know the problem could easily be fixed."

Many times people who rely most on technology do so out of necessity, not from personal interest. Therefore, the technical knowledge and interest of each person using these systems can vary widely. Cognitive dysfunction can further complicate learning and use of the system. In addition to training the disabled person to operate the equipment, it is usually necessary to train a caregiver to operate, maintain, and adjust the system. Like the EADL user, the caregiver may not be technologically adroit or even interested in maintaining the technology.

The planning for and future accommodations of any expected deteriorating abilities and cognitive dysfunction is likewise an important concern.[11] The importance of a comprehension evaluation should also be considered in terms of future limited funding. An EADL can be expensive and difficult to fund. Therefore, replacing the equipment will likely have the same complications.[7]

ELECTRONIC AID FOR DAILY LIVING ACQUISITION CHALLENGES

Three limitations have been identified for assistive technology devices,[23] and they are especially applicable to EADLs: (1) the lack of specific knowledge/expertise, (2) limited equipment availability, and (3) limited funding sources. There is a general lack of knowledge about and specific training available for EADLs. Those engaged in the rehabilitation profession understand that rehabilitation professionals are often overburdened with other tasks, prohibiting them from spending the needed time to train with this specific equipment and learn about the technology that is available. Others have reported the same observations. McDonald and St Leger[3] note that the evaluations may include the discussion of a few options of a given system, but "the only real choice users have is whether or not they accept the system recommended by the assessor." An equally limiting factor is the lack of volume of clients that any given therapist might see for this type of intervention. With a limited volume of client cases, it is very difficult to gain needed skills and knowledge needed for competence in this area.

EADLs can be expensive for any facility to obtain/maintain, and changes in technology make it a more daunting task to keep current equipment. Most rehabilitation professionals are fortunate if they have any of the devices readily available. This limitation is further magnified by the lack of overall demand for such products and even less of a demand for one specific EADL. Manufacturers are reluctant to provide demonstration equipment to rehabilitation facilities, because these products have a low rate of turnover, the equipment may require in-depth knowledge, and the products can be expensive to manufacture.

The lack of funding for this equipment is also a major limitation, and a major reason why EADLs are not widely used.[22] Commercial insurance does not provide funding for this equipment. Because EADLs are not considered to be a medical necessity, public insurance does not supply these devices either. EADLs can be obtained via vocational rehabilitation, the Veterans Administration, certain waiver programs, workman's compensation, charities, and private pay. Most people do not have the funds to purchase an EADL from their own resources. High-end systems can cost $8,000 to $12,000 with installation and training. Perhaps third-party payers might be more likely to fund these devices if it can be demonstrated that these systems can reduce the cost of attendant care and increase the productivity of the user. These 2 elements should be the focus of future research.

EFFICACY RESEARCH
Reduction of Attendant Care

Measuring the reduction of attendant care and the increase in productivity has been quantitatively evasive. The efficacy of EADL systems has not been scientifically established.[24] Nonetheless, these 2 measures would help build the case for additional funding of this equipment.

Several studies have provided potential savings by employing EADLs. Symington and MacLean[25] extrapolated that the use of ECSs in a nursing home may have decreased the amount of nursing care needed by 1 hour per day. This study was conducted over 20 years ago in the context of an institutional setting where there was a pool of caregivers with many responsibilities, so actual costs savings in care reduction for the institution may be difficult to quantify. Other studies have also suggested some potential savings.[7,20] In one study, 2 of the disabled persons' spouses were able to continue to work as a direct result of the ECU provision. Savings have also been reported when the EADL user can be left alone for extended periods of time, especially during the night.

There are, however, expenses associated with the evaluation, purchase, training, and maintenance that also need to be considered in a fair analysis of cost savings. In addition, as pointed out by an end user (Greg Rea, personal communication, 2007), in a home setting attendant care providers are often meagerly compensated. Yet they are responsible for critical functions that must be performed at specific times on a regular basis. If the provision of an EADL is based on the requirement of reducing the amount of time that the caregiver is needed throughout the day, it could have a negative impact. For example, if overall hours are reduced for care providers, they may be required to visit the home to perform morning services and return at various times throughout the day to perform other necessary duties. The discontinuity in schedule, the increased transportation time, and the decreased billable hours would make it more difficult to provide incentives for the caregivers, and thus have a negative impact on the services available to the person with a severe disability.

Increased Productivity

There are no studies that have shown a quantitative increase in work productivity directly related to the use of an EADL. Furthermore, gaining this information will be difficult for several reasons. First, there are relatively few people who use EADLs on a regular basis for employment, and they tend to be scattered in many different locations. Second, EADL provisions vary in function and are not consistent among all areas. Third, no outcome measure exists that specifically addresses the unique benefits of an EADL. For all these reasons, gaining statistically significant, quantitative data has proven to be challenging.

Other factors contribute to the difficulties in measuring productivity benefits of EADLs. There are much higher unemployment rates among persons with disabilities compared with able-bodied persons.[26] There are also "disincentives" for persons with disabilities to work, due to the loss of their medical benefits and income support. Furthermore, the people who are most likely to need these devices will likely have major challenges with daily care needs, increased medical and transportation issues, and environmental barriers while at work. They are also likely to have a limited work tolerance, the reliance on other technologies such as wheeled mobility, speech generating devices, computer access, and the shortcomings associated with these external factors. The influence of these factors may need to be captured to gain a full appreciation of the benefits of an EADL. Standardized outcome measures specifically for EADL are being considered[27,28] and should help support the funding efforts for EADLs.[7]

SUMMARY

The independent control of many daily activities that able-bodied persons take for granted such as environmental regulation, information acquisition, personal safety, and communication is only made possible for persons with severe impairments through the use of EADLs. These specialized devices can provide tremendous psychological and functional benefits to someone with a severe disability, as well as his or her family and caregivers. These benefits can be actualized through independence and personal satisfaction for the EADL user and in the reduction of effort in repetitive tasks required of family members and caregivers. The result of these benefits can also help improve the interpersonal relationships among all involved.

Given the individual needs of each person, and the requirements and capabilities of each EADL device, it is ideal to have a comprehensive evaluation of the client, equipment, and the environment to integrate personal and assistive technology needs. The consumer should be involved throughout the entire process and be provided with as many options as appropriate. Of note, increases in independence are not always achieved by the most sophisticated electronic aid.[18] The process should not end at the delivery of equipment but should include adequate training and periodic follow-up to ensure the equipment is functioning as needed.

The antidotal, intangible benefits of EADLs can plainly be seen by anyone associated with such properly prescribed devices. However, the challenge is to expand the availability of EADLs to people who need them. Increasing the available funding for these devices may depend on the qualitative cost-saving benefits of and the increased productivity made possible with EADLs. Outcome measures that can account specifically for these benefits as well as showing the relational advantages to the user and their families may help build the case for additional funding.

To increase the appropriateness of EADL prescriptions and to provide accountability to those supplying such devices, it is recommended in the Abilities Research Centre's Report[17] that future funding decisions be based on the systematic monitoring of the end user's experiences. Novak[20] aptly wrote "environmental control systems, at their best, have a capability to substantially improve the quality of life for a number of severely disabled people and their carers, as well as achieving real cost savings in specific instances, yet, at worst to consume, without gain, considerable resources."

REFERENCES

1. Lange ML. Fundamentals in assistive technology. 4th edition. Virginia: RESNA Press; 2008.

2. Dicey R, Shealey S. Using technology to control the environment. Am J Occup Ther 1987;41:717–21.
3. McDonald P, St Leger S. Provision of environmental controls in the North West of England. J Public Health Med 1996;18(4):443–8.
4. Ripat J. Function and impact of electronic aids to daily living for experienced users. Tech Disabil 2006;18:79–87.
5. Stickel MS, Ryan S, Rigby PJ, et al. Toward a comprehensive evaluation of the impact of electronic aids to daily living: evaluation of consumer satisfaction. Disabil Rehabil 2002;24(1–3):115–25.
6. Palmer P, Seale J. Exploring the attitudes to environmental control systems of people with physical disabilities: a grounded theory approach. Tech Disabil 2007;19:17–27.
7. Harmer J, Bakheit AMO. Benefits of environmental control systems as perceived by disabled users and their carers. Br J Occup Ther 1999;62:394–8.
8. McDonald DW, Boyle MA, Schumann TL. Environmental control unit utilization by high level spinal cord injury patients. Arch Phys Med Rehabil 1989;70:621–3.
9. Wolf WM, Roa RL. Usage patterns of environmental control units by severely disabled individuals in their homes. IEEE Trans Rehabil Eng 1995;3(2):222–7.
10. Platts R, Fraser M. Assistive technology in the rehabilitation of patients with high spinal cord lesions. Paraplegia 1993;313:280–7.
11. Wellings DJ, Unsworth J. Fortnightly review: environmental control systems for people with a disability: an update. BMJ 1997;315:409–12.
12. Wikipedia. Available at: http://en.wikipedia.org/wiki/X10_(industry_standard). Accessed May 2, 2009.
13. Bessel T, Randell M, Knowles G, et al. Connecting people with the environment—a new accessible wireless remote control. Available at: http://www.e-bility.com/arataconf06/paper/environmental_control/ec_hobbs_paper.doc. Accessed April 8, 2009.
14. Steggles E, James Leslie. Electronic aids to daily living: an equipment classification. RESNA proceedings. 2000. p. 180–2.
15. Available at: http://www.atilange.com. Accessed April 8, 2009.
16. Phillips B, Zhao H. Predictors of assistive technology abandonment. Assist Technol 1993;5:36–45.
17. Ability Research Centre environmental control systems for people with spinal injuries; a report on research undertaken by the Ability Research Centre, September 1999. Available at: http://www.abilitycorp.com.au/ftp/research/environmental_controls_systems_report.pdf. Accessed April 8, 2009.
18. Croser R, Garrett R, Seeger B, et al. Effectiveness of electronic aids to daily living: increased independence and decreased frustration. Aust Occup Ther J 2001;48: 35–44.
19. Barnes MP. Switching devices and independence of disabled people. BMJ 1994; 309:1181–2.
20. Novak SA. Environmental control systems—an audit of existing provision in three inner London districts. Clin Rehabil 1998;12:88. doi:10.1191/026921598671164157. Available at: http://cre.sagepub.com/cgi/content/abstract/12/1/88. Accessed April 8, 2009.
21. Maguire SM, McCann JP. An audit of the provision of environmental control systems in Northern Ireland, 1992-1997. Clin Rehabil 2001;15:320–3.
22. Holme SA, Kanny EM, Gurthrie MR, et al. The use of environmental control units by occupational therapist in spinal cord injury and disease services. Am J Occup Ther 1997;51:42–8.

23. Platts RGS, Andrews K. How technology can help rehabilitation? BMJ 1994;309: 1182–3.
24. Craig A, Tran Y, McIsaac P, et al. The efficacy and benefits of environmental control systems for the severely disabled. Med Sci Monit 2004;11:32–9.
25. Symington D, MacLean J. Environmental control systems in chronic care nursing homes. Arch Phys Med Rehabil 1986;67:322–5.
26. Available at: http://www.bls.gov/cps/cpsdisability.htm. Accessed May 15, 2009.
27. Rigby P, Campbell K, Cooper B, et al. Measuring the cost utility of electronic aids to daily living. RESNA Proceedings. 2002. p. 143–5.
28. Tam C, Rigby P, Ryan SE, et al. Development of the measure of control using electronic aids to daily living. Tech Disabil 2003;15:181–90.

Advances in Augmentative and Alternative Communication as Quality-of-Life Technology

Katya Hill, PhD, CCC-SLP[a,b],*

KEYWORDS

- Augmentative and alternative communication • Quality of life
- Evidence-based practice • Performance measurement
- Language representation methods

Augmentative and alternative communication (AAC) is a field of endeavor addressing the expressive communication needs of people with significant speech disability. AAC interventions range from unaided methods using no technology (gestures, signs) up to high technology voice output communication systems. Over a lifetime, an individual may be recommended several AAC systems with the goal, as identified by the American Speech-Language-Hearing Association,[1] to optimize communication for the highest quality of life (QOL) possible. Use of AAC technology has been shown to enhance QOL for children as young as 32 months,[2] adults with amyotrophic lateral sclerosis (ALS),[3,4] children with autism spectrum disorder,[5] adolescents and adults with developmental disabilities,[6] family networks,[7] and adults with aphasia or other acquired neurologic conditions.[8,9] The evidence base indicates that the life experience of people who use AAC is determined by their ability to achieve the highest performance communication possible. People who use AAC say that the two most important values in their use of AAC are saying exactly what they want to say and saying it as fast as they want.[10]

Applying the principles of evidence-based practice (EBP) is expected to achieve the most effective communication. AAC stakeholders participating on AAC evaluation teams have become aware of the limitations of expert opinion as the basis for

[a] Communication Science and Disorders, School of Health and Rehabilitation Sciences, 6017 Forbes Tower, University of Pittsburgh, Pittsburgh, PA 15260, USA
[b] AAC Institute, 1000 Killarney, Pittsburgh, PA 15234, USA
* Communication Science and Disorders, School of Health and Rehabilitation Sciences, 6017 Forbes Tower, University of Pittsburgh, Pittsburgh, PA 15260.
E-mail address: khill@pitt.edu

Phys Med Rehabil Clin N Am 21 (2010) 43–58
doi:10.1016/j.pmr.2009.07.007
1047-9651/09/$ – see front matter © 2010 Elsevier Inc. All rights reserved.

pmr.theclinics.com

decisions on the selection of AAC technology. Yet, many individuals receive an unsystematic or idiosyncratic approach to AAC system selection.[11] The model for matching the person with technology (MPT) systematically integrates personal, clinical, and external evidence into the AAC assessment process.[12] By placing the client's benefits first, practitioners pose specific questions of direct practical importance, gather objectively and efficiently the current best evidence, and take appropriate action guided by the evidence.[13] EBP integrates personal data about an individual's values, preferences, and expectations, with clinical data about the individuals abilities, skills, and performance, and an appraisal of the research evidence that matters.[14] Consequently, AAC intervention is data-driven and consumer-centered. This poses a challenge to AAC rehabilitation, because practitioners must make clinical decisions that involve the identification, selection, and implementation of various AAC technology solutions based on evidence when minimal external evidence may be available.[15]

FRAMEWORKS FOR IMPROVING QUALITY OF LIFE

The World Health Organization's International Classification of Functioning, Disability, and Health (ICF)[16] provides a framework for representing the relationship among body or health status, activities, participation, and environmental and personal factors. AAC intervention can be placed within the ICF framework to show the interaction among the components influencing function.[17] Identifying and defining the set of AAC system characteristics are critical to meeting the needs of individuals who rely on AAC and achieving long-term outcomes expected of the ICF framework.[18–20] AAC system characteristics include a long list of technology features and components that are updated and released frequently that could influence activities and participation performance positively or negatively.

The MPT and the AAC language-based assessment models provide for a systematic and principled approach for selecting and evaluating AAC system characteristics in the face of continued progress in technology research and development. Each model reflects principles common to the ICF framework and EBP. The MPT is a set of person-centered measures that examine self-reported perspectives of individuals regarding strengths/capabilities, needs/goals, preferences and psychosocial characteristics, and expected technology benefits.[21] In addition, a companion form is available so that provider perspectives can be assessed to ensure collaboration in the matching process. The AAC language-based assessment model conceptualizes a methodical approach to evaluate and select AAC interventions and technology.[22,23] In a retrospective study involving an archival clinical data review, Hill and Scherer[24] reported on the complex nature of the AAC assessment, including the MPT process, and the complex nature of selecting and integrating the full range of AAC system technology interventions. In addition, use of personal and clinical evidence provided data to support decisions when patient-oriented research evidence was lacking. Finally, the results showed that identified outcomes were achieved when AAC components were grouped based on patient priorities and influences on communication performance.[25] The remainder of this article will address advances to primary, secondary, and tertiary components of state-of-the art AAC systems classified as QOL technology with the acknowledgment that not all innovations can be covered in the space provided.

ADVANCES TO PRIMARY COMPONENTS

The software designs of the AAC systems have made significant advances in performance because of improvements to how language is represented and generated using technology. The primary components of AAC technology are related to how the system can perform the functions of a natural language (**Fig. 1**). Having the features of language available is critical to achieving the goal of AAC and providing the most effective communication possible. Language performance is influenced by the availability of the three AAC language representation methods (LRMs), the selection and organization of vocabulary, and the method of constructing messages/utterances.[26]

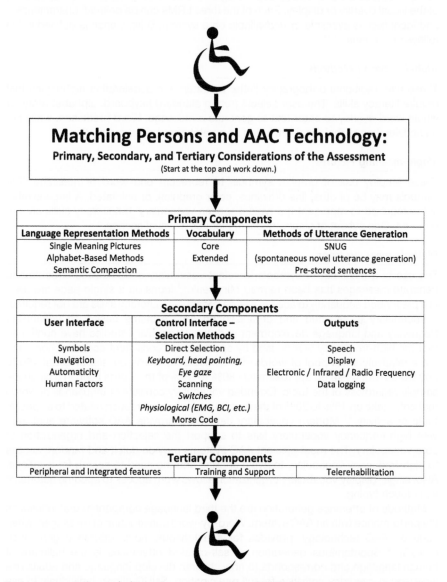

Fig. 1. Augmentative and alternative communication (AAC) primary, secondary, and tertiary components considered by AAC team members (such as speech language pathologists, occupational and physical therapists, rehabilitation engineers and counselors, educators and administrators, and consumers and families) during the Matching Persons and Technology (MPT) process.

These language-based components of the technology generally influence communication performance more than any other components.

In evaluating the full range and large variety of AAC systems available, all AAC systems support only up to three language representation methods (LRMs): (1) alphabet-based methods, (2) single-meaning picture symbols, and (3) multiple-meaning symbols. The three AAC LRMs may be available singularly or as a combination of methods simultaneously depending on the software program and appearance of the visual overlay or display. Each of the three LRMs can be defined, characterized, and identified as available or unavailable on a system. Briefly, each is defined in the following sections.[23,27]

Alphabet-based Methods

These use traditional orthography (letter-by-letter) and acceleration techniques that require literacy skills. The user selects from a standard keyboard, alphabet array, or whole word overlay to enter text to generate a message. Word prediction, while not an acceleration technique, is included as an alphabet-based method.

Single-meaning Pictures

These employ use of graphic symbols to represent one word or message. The symbols may be photos, line drawings, color graphics, or animated. A large symbol set is required to represent the typical spoken vocabulary, but literacy skills are not required. One subset of single-meaning pictures is visual scenes.

Multiple-meaning Icons

The use of a small set of symbols to select vocabulary and linguistic structures to generate messages has been termed Minspeak.[28] Icons on a single page are used in a prescribed sequence to access a large vocabulary. Literacy skills are not required.

Vocabulary is selected and organized on AAC systems based on vocabulary frequency and language development and use. Vocabulary studies have confirmed that the high-frequency words used by speakers are consistent across cohorts and are a relatively small pool of words.[29–32] These core words consist of about 450 to 500 words, but make up approximately 80% to 85% of the words used in a language sample regardless of the topic. Extended vocabulary consists of thousands of words that only make up 15% to 20% of the words used in a conversation related to a specific topic or activity.[33] Modern vocabulary databases provide AAC software engineers with high-frequency vocabulary lists to support the selection and organization of core vocabulary. The most efficient AAC systems provide quick and random access to high-frequency vocabulary to avoid spelling and the need to search for locations. Also, single-display vocabulary organization allows word access to become automatic as in touch typing.

Methods of utterance generation are the third language component that influences the performance with an AAC system. Word-by-word construction of messages, when used on AAC technology, provides for spontaneous, novel utterance generation (SNUG).[34] Spontaneous generation of self-created utterances is the hallmark of human language and corresponds to how children develop language and adults use language in everyday activities for full participation. SNUG allows individuals to say exactly what they want and intend to say. The design considerations regarding availability of the AAC LRMs and organization of core vocabulary influence SNUG. The use of prestored messages provides an alternative to spontaneous self-generated text and communication, but has several important performance issues.

Advances in computer speed and memory have provided the means to incorporate sophisticated algorithms for predicting language units longer than single words.[27] Pre-programmed phrase and utterance-based programs may aid literate individuals who use AAC to engage in social conversations and structured situations.[35,36] As the term implies, the quick-hit or quick-fire features, depending on the product, support pragmatic language functions. These one-hit prestored messages allow individuals convenient and prompt selection of prestored social comments, interjections, polite remarks, and conversational fillers to provide for turn-taking and topic maintenance during conversations. **Fig. 2** shows an AAC system that has, among its other communication modes, programming to support social language use by prestored utterances and scripts appropriate for specific topics and situations or general conversational turn taking.

In summary, today's AAC language software is multifaceted with complex programming that provides for the characteristics of a natural language. The MPT process starts with prioritization of the primary language considerations by ensuring the individuals are informed fully of all available options and performance information. Rehabilitation clinicians, however, must be careful when appraising the evidence base. For example, several studies have shown that word prediction is not any faster than spelling.[37,38] Yet, word prediction is referenced routinely as a rate enhancement strategy in some product literature and textbooks. Because word prediction reduces the number of key strokes for text entry, the feature still may be recommended for patients who fatigue with AAC technology use. **Fig. 3** shows the communication rates (words per minute) by LRM during a one-on-one conversation for 20 (N = 20) individuals using an AAC language application program supporting all three LRMs.[34] The results show an average of a 282% (range 166% to 717%) communication rate advantage for multiple-meaning icons (semantic compaction) over spelling with no significant difference in communication rates between spelling and word prediction. These results demonstrate the importance of measuring these language components on an individual basis.

Finally, several language applications are based on similar LRM configurations, but do not have performance data available for consumers to make comparisons. These language applications may be installed on different user interfaces with different selection interfaces (as the secondary components described in the next section), further influencing performance and outcomes. For example, although the participants in the study represented in **Fig. 3** were using different versions of the same language

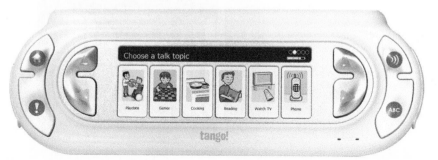

Fig. 2. Augmentative and alternative communication (AAC) system fashioned after a gaming device, among the communication modes, offers preprogrammed scripted messages (Tango! courtesy Blink Twice; with permission.)

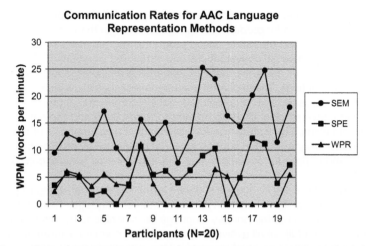

Fig. 3. Comparison of communication rates by language representation methods based on conversational language samples by twenty (N = 2) adults using augmentative and alternative communication (AAC) systems. *Abbreviations:* SEM, semantic compaction; SPE, spelling; WPR, word prediction.

application program, the versions all supported access to the three LRMs with 128 locations. Current versions of this language application provide the choice of 144, 84, 60, or 45 locations. Other language application programs with other LRM availability offer different numbers of locations or visual scenes, but similar performance data have not been reported. Thus, software innovations have made gains beyond the pace that quantitative performance and outcomes data have been reported.

ADVANCES TO SECONDARY COMPONENTS

Frequently, advances to AAC hardware components and access technology create dramatic first impressions and even may make the evening news. Yet, the technology in and of itself still takes second place to language components (**Figs. 4** and **5**).

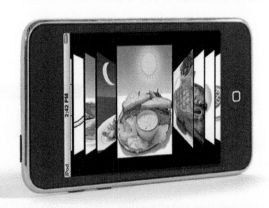

Fig. 4. Augmentative and alternative communication (AAC) language software loaded on iPod touch screen (Smalltalk *courtesy of* Lingraphica; with permission.)

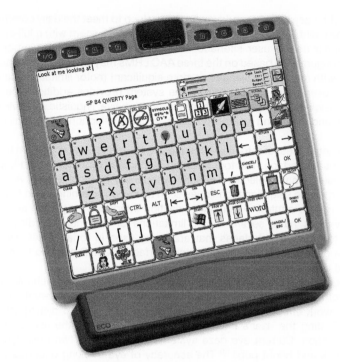

Fig. 5. Augmentative and alternative communication (AAC) system with touch screen user interface and various selection interfaces available (ECO-14 with ECOpoint courtesy of Prentke Romich Company; with permission.)

Looking at the hardware of AAC systems of even a decade ago, however, would convince anyone that QOL for people who rely on AAC has been impacted positively by the progress. Looking back 20 years is even more impressive as a testament to AAC technology developments. For this article, the following secondary features are highlighted: (1) user interface (symbols, navigation, automaticity, and human factors), (2) selection techniques (eye gaze and brain computer interface), and (3) outputs (speech and logged data).

By way of background, the user interface refers to the interaction between the user and the AAC system. Generally, this is the point at which the user is sending information to the AAC system that will result in communication being generated. The user interface, however, occasionally includes the sending of information back to the user. When a visual display is involved, the common implementation is use of a touch screen. This allows user input and feedback to the user. For users with visual impairment, auditory and/or tactile methods are employed. Consequently, the user interface includes various features and functions that may be present or absent, and when present these can vary widely in application across products.

Recently, AAC language software applications have been installed on cell phones or PDAs (personal digital assistants) for highly mobile clients. **Fig. 4** represents an AAC system based on the iPod touch or iPhone (Lingraphica®, Princeton, NJ) for use with patients with aphasia who have good fine motor dexterity. Individuals benefiting from phrase sets to use in situations such as doctors' appointments, playing bridge, shopping, or ordering at restaurants may prefer this type of technology. Considered a mobile accessory, an AAC system with a cell phone as the user interface is very portable, light, easy to carry, and may be determined to meet the daily communication needs of the client. **Fig. 5**, however, represents an AAC system with a full-sized touch screen monitor as the user interface. Various language application programs with different configurations based on the three AAC LRMs may be installed on this system. Individuals with mobility challenges or more significant motor limitations can operate this type of user interface. In addition, the system provides additional flexibility for meeting possible changing needs (eg, physical, cognitive, linguistic, or environmental) of a client and changing uses, computer access, telephoning, or environmental controls.

Selection interfaces refer to the technique used to make selections from those available in the user interface. The touch screen technology represented in **Figs. 4** and **5** allows the user to make selections directly by touching the display. Most AAC systems provide for multiple selection techniques such as switch scanning, head tracking, and joystick or mouse control. Alternative selection interfaces frequently are warranted when individuals have severe motor limitations or degenerative disorders. Two advances to selection interfaces that are being used in today's AAC systems are remote eye gaze and the brain–computer interface (BCI). These two techniques will be covered in more detail.

The process of making a selection using remote eye gaze technology is quite different from how eyes are used as a perceptual organ for observation.[39] Consequently, to work effectively, remote eye gaze must be able to distinguish between a gaze indicating the user's interest and a gaze indicating the user's intention to make a selection. Current eye gaze systems are based on two main types of eye tracking: dark and bright pupil.[40] The accuracy of eye tracking depends very much on successful calibration for each user. Potential variables influencing the user's ability to achieve calibration may include the background lighting, use of eyeglasses, a pupil that is blocked by a droopy eyelid, or inability to maintain head position. **Fig. 5** shows an AAC system with an eye gaze camera module attached beneath the touch screen. Such technology is improving the QOL for individuals with significant motor limitations such as ALS in that it has the potential to outperform other alternative access methods or provide the opportunity to continue use of an AAC system when other methods are no longer functional.

A BCI creates a no-muscular output channel for the brain. Instead of being executed through peripheral nerves and muscles, the user's selections are conveyed by brain signals (such as electroencephalogram [EEG]), not dependent on neuromuscular activity.[41] Use of brain signals and not neuromuscular activity is the significant benefit offered by BCI technology. For people who are totally paralyzed (ie, locked in), the BCI makes it possible to communicate with the outside world. **Fig. 6** represents the basic process for using a BCI as the selection interface of an AAC system, although the user interface must be configured to support target acquisition. Current BCI systems require good technical and supportive care, because the person depends on someone to set up technology, and training is needed to ensure that the caregiver or partner can manage the system independently. BCI, however, is not a technology of the future. Although limited in availability, the Wadworths Center in Albany, New York reports success by a small number of people already using BCI systems for spoken and written communication and computer access.[42] Performance evidence, however, is not widely available.

Recent innovations in output relate to speech synthesis, voice banking, and data logging. Synthesized voice technology rather than recorded human speech is needed to provide for a text-to-speech function. People relying on AAC and family members have advocated for improving the voice quality of speech output in terms of

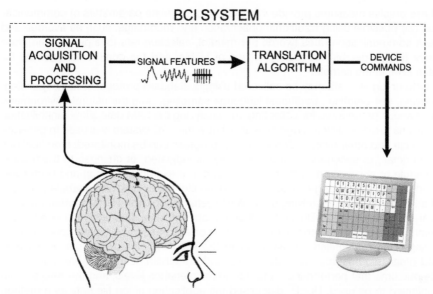

Fig. 6. Basic diagram of the brain–computer interface (BCI) process. Signals reflecting brain activity are acquired from the scalp, from the cortical surface, or from within the brain and are analyzed to measure signal features (ie, electroencephalogram [EEG] rhythms) that reflect the user's intent. These features are translated into commands that operate an AAC system.

naturalness (intonation, stress, and expression of emotion). Individuals with degenerative conditions want to be able to record or bank their natural voice for use when their natural speech is no longer intelligible. Advances in speech output have found their applications in reading skill enhancement, telephone and integrated voice response systems, multimedia CD-ROMs, kiosk information systems, talking World Wide Web pages, emergency notification systems, proofreading programs, vehicular guidance systems, and real-time language translators.[43] These synthesized voices, along with voice banking, are available on AAC systems. People may select from various male, female, children's or banked voices for a more natural sounding speech output.

PERFORMANCE MEASUREMENT

EBP is the application of external, clinical, and personal evidence to make data-driven decisions about AAC interventions. Current high technology AAC systems provide for built-in monitoring as a secondary output component to consider in the MPT process. Efforts to automate logging of data have been integral to specific communication or writing systems and vary in the degree of comprehensiveness of the log file data.[37,44–47] The term language activity monitoring (LAM) was coined to focus on recording how language is generated using AAC systems, and provides for efficient and cost-effective tracking.[48] The LAM format was developed for clinical application with a time stamp, a mnemonic to indicate the LRM, and a single field for the recorded activity. For a language event, the protocol is: Hour:Minute:Second (HH:MM:SS) "LRM code" "any continuous text that is transmitted by the AAC device."[49]

When uploaded into a computer, the start and end times for various communication activities during the time the LAM feature was active can be viewed and analyzed.

These precise measures provide information to calculate parameters of communication not possible using traditional observation and recordings, such as average and peak communication rates (words per minute), selection rate (bits per second), rate index (words per bit), frequency of use of LRMs, and the communication rate for each LRM in the sample.

LAM or log file data may be collected using a standard protocol of tasks (pointing, copying, self-creating), traditional language sampling, or in the natural environment. The various procedures for collecting and analyzing the LAM data allow rehabilitation clinicians to make clinical judgments about how the AAC system was used to generate language and other events. Consequently, progress can be monitored; modifications to a primary or secondary component may be indicated, or changes to the training schedule or approach may be recommended. For example, Tullman and Hurtubise[2] used LAM to collect language samples and monitor the expressive vocabulary usages of a 32-month-old child relying on an AAC system. Cook and Hill[50] reported on a 70-year-old man with ALS. During late-stage treatment, LAM data showed decreases in communication rate (words per minute) and selection accuracy. When performance changes were identified, adjustments to the scanning speed, number of rescans, and other features such as auto repeat and on-screen scanning were made, with the outcome that performance returned to maintenance levels, and the AAC system continued to be used. Hurd[51] discussed the application of log file data as a method to report progress on curriculum goals and objectives identified in the individualized education program (IEP). In summary, this innovation moved data logging from the research laboratory into clinical practice, and has provided rehabilitation clinicians with valuable performance data to guide decisions about intervention and compare AAC systems to identify which system will produce the best outcomes for a client.

ADVANCES TO TERTIARY COMPONENTS

The consideration and availability of tertiary features may seem an afterthought to many and go unidentified until expected performance and outcomes are not achieved. A review of the literature found that the main factors leading to AAC abandonment were related to lack of support and training, poor maintenance and adjustments to the AAC system, and generally a poor match between the person and the technology.[52,53] **Fig. 1** identifies tertiary features integral to the MPT process and notes that they are similar to those identified as contributing to disuse when not ameliorated. Peripheral features include such consideration as switches, mounts, positioning, transporting, and portability. For example, poor switch and site selection for a user can result in slow speed, fatigue, and increased inaccuracies in accessing an AAC system, causing overall frustration and a feeling of lack of success. Training and on-going support, including periodic maintenance and adjustments to the equipment, are required for most long-term users of AAC.

Advances in telerehabilitation technology provide opportunities to improve training and support for AAC users, thus not only reducing a major cause of disuse, but also potentially increasing achieved communication effectiveness and improved QOL. Telerehabilitation is the provision of rehabilitation services at a distance using electronic communication and information technologies. Several studies report that the provision of telerehabilitation services resulted in comparable performances or gains relative to traditional treatments.[54–56] The propitious availability of LAM resources gives rehabilitation clinicians practical tools to monitor AAC performance remotely. In addition, patients who rely on AAC frequently experience transportation challenges or live at distances away from centers of AAC excellence. Telerehabilitation provides real-time videoconferencing that allows patients to receive specialist consultations or specialist input.[57] Provision of AAC telerehabilitation treatment is not limited by the technology, but restricted by service delivery models and policies slow on the uptake of integrating today's Internet-based applications and technologies into daily clinical practice.

External evidence documenting the rapid innovations of integrating AAC systems with computer-based applications and functions has not kept pace with customer demands. Many AAC systems previously labeled as dedicated devices now run Microsoft Windows or mobile applications and have InfraRed (IR) or Bluetooth capabilities to support wireless computer access and environmental controls. With computer access, individuals are using AAC systems to access the Internet, send and receive emails, and use mobile telephones. As previously stated, **Fig. 4** shows an AAC application that runs on a cell phone with all the phone functions available, and **Fig. 5** is an AAC system that provides for computer, Internet, and phone functions. The user can switch conveniently between using the system for spoken communication and other forms of written communication (eg, word processing or E-mail and telecommunication).

DISCUSSION

Today's AAC systems include such major technology innovations, that traditional approaches to selecting components and intervention services no longer apply. Or do they? Although recent technology innovation has been significant, the language components continue to drive AAC decisions. Early AAC electronic solutions were primitive compared with current computer-based technologies. Outcomes to improve functional communication for expressing basic daily living and medical needs were considered an achievement then. Yet service delivery models and funding policies are responsible for this needs-based, medical necessity framework being perpetuated. QOL is multidimensional in nature, and is composed of the same factors for people with disabilities that are important to people without disabilities.[7] Practices should not limit the possible outcomes for people with disabilities without taking into consideration the ICF framework, QOL domains, and advances to AAC assistive technology.

The ICF model acknowledges the fundamental premise of AAC practice to facilitate interactive communication, and thus, participation.[20] The first factor contributing to AAC success is more naturalistic interactions of using the AAC system, while the second factor involves the numerous daily instances of using the AAC system for communication, education, and employment successfully and substantively.[53] Three factors stand out as important for AAC rehabilitation clinicians to consider: (1) the performance being achieved by the AAC system, (2) use of the AAC system for multiple communication tasks, and (3) ecological approaches to services.

Service delivery reimbursement often limits contact with patients in traditional settings, and funding policies for AAC technologies sometimes limit the selection of AAC systems. Generally, one device per patient is funded every 5 or more years. This is problematic, especially for patients with progressive degenerative disorders. If improvement to QOL is the ultimate desired outcome of AAC services and interventions,[58] then this formula for service is not likely to result in the highest QOL possible for a patient with ALS, for example. If the MPT process ignores the current funding policies, a patient with ALS might rely on several AAC systems through the course of the disease process. Before the onset of speech disturbances, the patient may record his or her natural speech using a voice-banking feature. As a first AAC device, the patient might select a highly portable AAC system or one with a standard keyboard as natural speech is declining, but before motor skills have deteriorated. This mobile or easy-to-carry device could transition to a more complex, flexible AAC system as needs change. The patient can transition from direct keyboard selection to alternative selection interfaces with the onset of significant motor limitation. Eventually, the patient may be recommended a remote eye gaze add-on module or a BCI interface. With each of these changes to the selection interface, the primary language components have been managed to allow as seamless as possible a transition to the user interface. In addition, besides spoken communication, the AAC technology is integrated to support computer access, E-mail, telephone, calendar, and daily reminder functions. Clinical services are delivered through telerehabilitation or videoconferencing, with LAM data being sent to the clinician to monitor any changes in performance. Management or instructions for modifying, customizing, troubleshooting, or upgrading the AAC system can be handled remotely.

The Pittsburgh Employment Conference (PEC) for Augmented Communicators, organized by Support Helps Others Use Technology (SHOUT), has been the world's largest gathering of individuals who rely on AAC for over 19 years (**Fig. 7**). Jennifer Lowe,[59] executive director of SHOUT and an augmented communicator, states that the most important aspect of the conference is that it has created a forum for people who rely on AAC to express their opinions: "common for many, but liberating for us!" Complementing PEC is the AAC Evidence-Based Practice Symposium organized by a parent as a conference for consumers, family members, and practitioners to appraise together the evidence regarding AAC interventions, performance, and outcomes.[60] Although these international conferences mirror the values achieved by many adults who rely on AAC QOL technology, many individuals relying on outdated technology can outperform individuals using the most technologically up-to-date AAC systems. Observations on achieving enhanced fluency by competent communicators

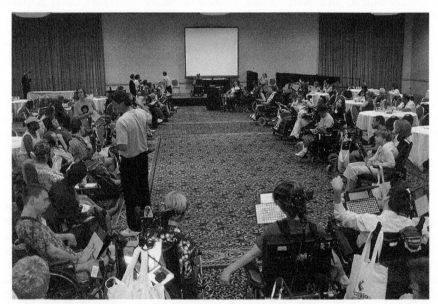

Fig. 7. The Pittsburgh Employment Conference (PEC) for Augmented Communicators reflects the quality of life achieved by many individuals with various disabilities who rely on AAC (PEC Town Hall Meeting *courtesy of* SHOUT).

have been attributed to the language or linguistic program and teaching supports as central to this phenomenon.[61] Consequently, consumers and families alike express the opinion that more individuals who use AAC should be achieving optimized communication for QOL.

SUMMARY

A component of the field of AAC involves the research and development of technology innovations that lead to effective communication and an improved QOL.[15] The major technology innovations to AAC systems are prioritized as primary, secondary, and tertiary components or functions. This article, however, was more informative than empiric regarding the effectiveness of innovations to AAC treatment. Although the evidence base supports the premise that AAC systems enhance QOL, outcomes in important life domains are generally discouraging for some populations who rely on AAC.[62] The gap between achieving optimized communication and continued advances in AAC QOL technology will not be closed by impressions of what is an effective innovation, but by using quantitative data or evidence to guide clinical decision making about AAC interventions.

ACKNOWLEDGMENTS

The author would like to thank Laura Murphy, graduate student, and Tom Kovacs, doctorate student, both research assistants at the AAC Performance and Testing (PAT) Teaching Lab, Department of Communication Science and Disorders, University of Pittsburgh, for their assistance in the review of AAC products, research and development tasks, and evidentiary base that supported this article. A special expression of gratitude goes out to the augmented communicators and families who shared their life experiences with AAC systems and rehabilitation services as the manuscript was developed.

REFERENCES

1. American Speech-Language-Hearing Association. Preferred practice patterns for the profession of speech–language pathology. Available at: www.asha.org/policy.
2. Tullman J, Hurtubise C. Language activity monitoring on a young child using a VOCA. In: Proceedings of the 9th Biennial Conference of the International Society for Augmentative and Alternative Communication. Washington, DC: ISAAC; 2000. p. 310–3.
3. Hill K, Jans D. AAC outcomes in persons with ALS/MND. In: Proceedings of the 11th Biennial ISAAC Conference. Toronto, Canada: ISAAC; 2004. CD-ROM.
4. Brownlee A, Palovcak M. The role of augmentative communication devices in the medical management of ALS. Neuro Rehabilitation 2007;22(6):445–50.
5. Halloran J, Emerson M. LAMP: language acquisition through motor planning. Wooster (OH): Prentke Romich Company; 2006.
6. McNaughton D, Bryen DN. AAC technologies to enhance participation and access to meaningful societal roles for adolescents and adults with developmental disabilities who require AAC. Augment Altern Commun 2007;23(3): 217–29.
7. Saito Y, Turnbull A. Augmentative and alternative communication practice in the pursuit of family quality of life: a review of the literature. Research & Practice for Persons with Severe Disabilities 2007;32(1):50–65.

8. Beukelman DR, Fager S, Ball L, et al. AAC for adults with acquired neurological conditions: a review. Augment Altern Commun 2007;23(3):230–42.

9. Johnson RK, Hough MS, King KA, et al. Functional communication in individuals with chronic severe aphasia using augmentative communication. Augment Altern Commun 2008;24(4):269–80.

10. Hill K, Romich B. AAC evidence-based practice: four steps to optimized communication. Pittsburgh (PA): AAC Institute Press; 2007.

11. Glennen S. AAC assessment myths and realities. Paper presented at: the ASHA SID 12 Leadership Conference on Augmentative. Sea Island (GA), January, 2000.

12. Hill K, Scherer M. Matching persons and technology: data-driven AAC assessments. In: Proceedings of the 23rd Annual International Conference on Technology and Persons with Disabilities. Los Angeles (CA): CSUN; 2008. Available at: www.csun.edu/cod/conf/2008/proceedings.

13. Gibbs LB. Evidence-based practice for the helping professions: a practical guide with integrated multimedia. Pacific Grove (CA): Thompson Brooks/Cole; 2003.

14. Dollaghan CA. The handbook for evidence-based practice in communication disorders. In: Paul H, editor. Baltimore, MD: Brookes Publishing Company; 2007.

15. Hill K. Augmentative and alternative communication (AAC) research and development: the challenge of evidence-based practice. International Journal of Computer Processing of Oriental Languages 2006;19(4):249–62.

16. World Health Organization (WHO). The international classification of functioning, disability, and health (ICF). Available at: http://www.who.int/icidh/index.html. Accessed June 3, 2009.

17. Huer M, Hill K, Loncke F. AAC: an international community, an international field, an international market. Presented at the RESNA Annual Conference. Atlanta (GA), June 22–26, 2006.

18. Cook AM, Hussey SM. Assistive technologies: principles and practices. 2nd edition. St Louis (MO): Mosby Incorporated; 2002.

19. Huer MD, Hill K. AAC and the rights and dignity of persons with disabilities. Presented at the RESNA Annual Conference. Phoenix (AZ), June 15–19, 2007.

20. Raghavendra P, Bornman J, Granlund M, et al. The World Health Organization's international classification of functioning, disability, and health: implications for clinical and research practice in the field of augmentative and alternative communication. Augment Altern Commun 2007;23(4):349–61.

21. Scherer MJ, Craddock G. Matching person and technology assessment process. Technol Disabil 2002;14:125–31.

22. Hill K. Achieving success in AAC assessment and intervention. Wooster (OH): AAC Institute Press; 2002. p. 1–5.

23. Hill K, Baker B, Romich B, et al. Augmentative and alternative communication (AAC) technology. In: Cooper R, Ohnabe H, Hobson D, editors. Introduction to rehabilitation engineering. London: Institute of Physics Publishing; 2006.

24. Hill K, Scherer M. Applying evidence-based practice and the matching persons & technology model to augmentative and alternative communication (AAC). Disability and Rehabilitation, in revision.

25. Cooper RA, Brewer BR, Cooper R, et al. Seating, assistive technology, and equipment. In: Stein J, Harvey RL, Macko RF, editors. Stroke recovery and rehabilitation. New York: Demos Medical Publishing; 2009. p. 543–68.

26. Romich B, Vanderheiden G, Hill K, et al. Augmentative communication. In: Bronzino JD, editor. The biomedical engineering handbook. 3rd edition. Boca Raton (FL): CRC Press; 2005.

27. Beukelman DR, Mirenda P. Augmentative and alternative communication: supporting children and adults with complex communication needs. 3rd edition. Baltimore (MD): Paul H. Brookes Publishing Company; 2005.
28. Baker B. Using images to generate speech. Byte 1986;11:160–8.
29. Mein R, O'Connor N. A study of the oral vocabularies of severely subnormal patients. J Intellect Disabil Res 1960;4(2):130–43.
30. Beukelman DR, McGinnis J, Morrow D, et al. Vocabulary selection in augmentative and alternative communication. Augment Altern Commun 1991;7:171–85.
31. Balandin S, Iacono T. A few well-chosen words. Augment Altern Commun 1998; 14(3):147–61.
32. Banajee M, Dicarlo C, Stricklin SB, et al. Core vocabulary determination for toddlers. Augment Altern Commun 2003;19(2):67–73.
33. Baker B, Hill K, Devylder R. Core vocabulary is the same across environments. In: Proceedings for Technology and Persons with Disabilities Conference. Northridge (CA): CSUN; 2000.
34. Hill K. The development of a model for automated performance measurement and the establishment of performance indices for augmented communicators under two sampling conditions. Dissertation Abstracts International 2001; 62(05):2293.
35. Todman J, Alm N. Modeling conversational pragmatics in communication aids. Journal of Pragmatics 2003;35:523–38.
36. Higginbotham DJ, Lesher, Moulton, et al. The frametalker project: building an utterance-based communication device. In: Proceedings of the 2005 CSUN Conference. Los Angeles: CSUN; 2005.
37. Koester HH, Levine SP. Modeling the speed of text entry with a word prediction interface. IEEE Trans Neural Syst Rehabil Eng 1994;2(3):177–87.
38. Venkatagiri HS. Effect of window size on rate of communication in a lexical prediction AAC system. Augment Altern Commun 1994;10:105–12.
39. Majaranta P, Räihä K. Text entry by gaze: utilizing eye tracking. In: Mackenzie IS, Tanaka-Ishii K, editors. Text entry systems: mobility, accessibility, universality. New York: Morgan Kaufmann Publishers; 2007. p. 175–87.
40. Lin A, Weaver J, Aedo L. Eye tracking technology: overview of current systems. Presented at the annual CSUN conference. Los Angeles (CA), March 16–21, 2009.
41. Wolpaw J, Birbaumer D, McFarland G, et al. Brain–computer interfaces for communication and control. Clin Neurophysiol 2002;113:767–91.
42. Kübler A, Nijboer F, Mellinger J, et al. Patients with ALS can use sensorimotor rhythms to operate a brain–computer interface. Neurology 2005;64:1775–7.
43. Bauer SM, Drenchek JA, Panchura CA, et al. Available at: http://t2rerc.buffalo. edu/pubs/forums/aac/forum/output/white_paper.htm. Accessed June 3, 2009.
44. Higginbotham DJ. The interplay of communication device output mode and interaction style between nonspeaking persons and their speaking partners. J Speech Hear Disord 1989;54:320–33.
45. Miller LJ, Damasco PW, Elkins RA. Automatic data collection and analysis in an augmentative communication system. In: Proceedings of the thirteenth annual RESNA conference. Arlington, VA: RESNA; 1990. p. 99–100.
46. Ahlsen E, Stromqvist S. ScriptLog: A tool for logging the writing process and its possible diagnostic use. In: Loncke J, Clibbens H, Arvidson LL, editors. Augmentative and Alternative Communication: New Directions in Research and Practice. Proceedings of the 1998 ISAAC Research Symposium. London: Whurr Publisher; 1999. p. 144–9.

47. Copestake A, Flickinger D. Evaluation of NLP technology for AAC using logged data. In: Proceedings of the 1998 research symposium. Dublin (Ireland): London Whurr Publishers; 1999.
48. Hill K. AAC evidence-based practice and language activity monitoring. Topics in Language Disorders: Language and Augmented Communication 2004;24: 18–30.
49. Hill KJ, Romich BA. A language activity monitor for supporting AAC evidence-based clinical practice. Assistive Technology 2001;13:12–22.
50. Cook S, Hill K. AAC performance data for an individual with amyotrophic lateral sclerosis. In: Proceedings of the RESNA Annual Conference. Arlington (VA): RESNA Press; 2003.
51. Hurd R. AAC and the IEP. Perspectives on augmentative and alternative communication. 2009;18:65–70.
52. Kraskowsky LH, Finlayson M. Factors affecting older adults' use of adaptive equipment: review of the literature. Am J Occup Ther 2001;55(3):303–10.
53. Johnson JM, Inglebret E, Jones C, et al. Perspectives of speech language pathologists regarding success versus abandonment of AAC. Augment Altern Commun 2009;22(2):85–99.
54. Brennan D, Georgeadis A, Baron C, et al. Telerehabilitation tools for the provisions of remote speech–language treatment. Topics in Stroke Rehabilitation 2004;8(4):71–8.
55. Georgeadis AC, Brennan DM, Barker LM, et al. Telerehabilitation and its effect on story retelling by adults with neurogenic communication disorders. Aphasiology 2004;18:639–52.
56. Hill A, Theodoros DG, Russell TG, et al. An Internet-based telerehabilitation system for the assessment of motor speech disorders: a pilot study. Am J Speech Lang Pathol 2006;15:45–56.
57. Savard L, Borstad A, Tkachuck J, et al. Telerehabilitation consultations for clients with neurologic diagnoses: cases from rural Minnesota and American Samoa. NeuroRehabilitation 2003;18(2):93–102.
58. Schlosser R. Outcome measurement in AAC. In: Light J, Beukelman D, Reichle J, editors. Communicative competence for individuals who use AAC. Baltimore (MD): Paul H. Brookes; 2003. p. 479–513.
59. Lowe J. Why attend PEC? Around the water cooler. Pittsburgh, PA: AAC Institute; 2009.
60. Hurd R. Coming changes in the field of AAC: Pittsburgh employment conference symposium on evidence-based practice. In: AAC Institute parents corner 2005. Available at: http://www.aacinstitute.org/Resources/ParentsCorner/2005March. html. Accessed June 10, 2009.
61. Klein C, Baker B, Stump B. The social impact of rate enhancement in augmentative communication. Presented at the annual RESNA conference. New Orleans (LA), June 24–26, 2009.
62. Hamm B, Mirenda P. Postschool quality of life for individuals with developmental disabilities who use AAC. Augment Altern Comm 2006;22(2):134–47.

Recent Trends in the Development and Evaluation of Assistive Robotic Manipulation Devices

Sonya Allin, PhD[a],*, Emily Eckel, MS[b],
Heather Markham, MS[c], Bambi R. Brewer, PhD[c]

KEYWORDS

- Assistive robotics • Robotic arms
- Upper extremity prostheses
- Assistive device outcomes

The last 15 years have seen the development of several robotic arms to support activity and occupation of individuals with limb loss or motor disabilities. New, lightweight robotic arms, like the SensorHand SPEED and i-LIMB, can provide good function and cosmesis for individuals with upper limb amputation or deficiency. Heavier robotic arms, even industrial arms, may also support object manipulation by people with motor disabilities. Robotic arms that may be too heavy to be worn on the body may be mounted to desktops,[1,2] wheelchairs,[3] or overhead workstations.[4,5] In these configurations, robotic arms can support manipulation required for office work,[4–6] to eat,[7,8] or to operate devices like a TV remote control. Many arms specifically designed for use by people with disabilities are, in fact, now commercially available, including the ARM and Raptor manipulators.[3,9] Commercially available industrial robotic arms are also seeing use in the context of assistive applications, including the Puma robotic arm.[10,11]

Utility of robotic arms can be judged along many dimensions. A robotic arm may be useful in that it demonstrably enhances the operator's ability to interact with the physical environment or participate in occupation, for example. Alternatively, it may reduce

[a] Department of Occupational Science and Occupational Therapy, Intelligent Assistive Technology and Systems Laboratory (IATSL), University of Toronto, 160 - 500 University Avenue, Toronto, Ontario M5G 1V7, Canada
[b] Occupational Therapy Program, Chatham University, Woodland Road, Pittsburgh, PA 15232, USA
[c] Department of Rehabilitation Science and Technology, University of Pittsburgh, 5044 Forbes Tower, Pittsburgh, PA 15260, USA
* Corresponding author.
E-mail address: s.allin@utoronto.ca (S. Allin).

Phys Med Rehabil Clin N Am 21 (2010) 59–77
doi:10.1016/j.pmr.2009.09.001
1047-9651/09/$ – see front matter © 2010 Elsevier Inc. All rights reserved.
pmr.theclinics.com

cost associated with providing assistive care or visits to a hospital or clinic. Finally, a robotic arm may enhance feelings of personal well-being or confidence in activities that require the device as well as those that do not. These dimensions of device "utility" have recently been codified into the CATOR taxonomy of assistive device outcomes,[12] which organizes outcomes according to device effectiveness, social significance, and impact on subjective well-being. Device effectiveness reflects measures of impact on user functioning and activity participation as well as impact on the accessibility of a users' environment. Social significance includes measures of impact on society more generally; these may reflect the labor of caregivers, use of the health care system, or housing cost. Finally, subjective well-being measures focus on individuals' satisfaction with a device, and with their lives, more generally, after device adoption.

The purpose of this review is to explore recent trends in the development and evaluation of assistive robotic arms, both prosthetic and externally mounted. Evaluations of the devices have been organized along the axes of the CATOR taxonomy. Questions that have informed the review include:

- Are robotic arms being comprehensively evaluated along axes of the CATOR taxonomy?
- Are definitions of effectiveness in accordance with the priorities of users?
- What gaps in robotic arm evaluation exist, and how might these gaps be best addressed?
- What further advances can be expected in the *next* 15 years?

To perform the review, a literature search was performed in the following research databases: IEEE Explore, PubMed, Cinahl, PsycInfoNet, Ovid, and Embase. Keywords used to guide the searches included combinations of "assistive," "disability," "user trial," "robotic arm," "robotic manipulator," "upper extremity," and "prosthesis." Several articles were iteratively added to the review based on references contained in previously selected articles. Articles were selected based on the following criteria:

- Published in the last 15 years (ie, 1994 or later)
- Include evaluation of specific assistive robotic arms, either prosthetic or externally mounted
- Include evaluation based on the experience of potential adult users

Five hundred and seven articles were retrieved as a result of the search. Articles that related to orthotic devices were excluded, as were articles with a therapy focus, review articles, and articles in which users were exclusively children. The remaining 51 articles included evaluations of commercial devices based on user trials and surveys, evaluations of devices still in the research and development phase, and evaluations of novel interfaces to existing commercial devices.

EXTERNALLY MOUNTED MANIPULATORS
Overview

Robotic manipulators that are not attached directly to an individual's arm can loosely be organized into 3 categories: those that connect to a wheelchair[3,13]; desktop-mounted arms embedded in activity-specific workstations[5,14]; or arms that move about the room on their own mobile base.[15,16] The same devices, moreover, can be organized according to the range of their functionality. Some devices are designed for a single purpose, like self-feeding,[7] whereas others are capable of performing a variety of tasks within a particular activity context, like the office.[17] Finally, general purpose robotic arms exist, and hold the potential to perform a wide range of functional manipulations in many contexts, including factory environments[18] and homes.[19]

Many externally mounted manipulation aids are now commercially available; their cost is governed, at least in part, by their functionality. Commercially available tools include the ARM (Assistive Robotic Manipulator, Exact Dynamics; formerly the MANUS) (**Fig. 1**) and Raptor robotic arms, the MASTER/EPI-RAID system (sold as the AFMaster, Afma Robots, France[20]), the DeVAR system (sold by The Tolfa Corporation, Palo Alto, CA[21]) and various desktop-mounted feeders (examples include HANDY, Rehab Robotics, UK[2]; Neater Eater, Neater Solutions Ltd, UK[22]; My Spoon, SECOM Co. Ltd, Tokyo[23]; and Winsford Feeder, Winsford Products Inc, Pennington, NJ[8]) (**Fig. 2**). As is perhaps to be expected, the more functionality provided by a particular system, the higher its cost. Feeders start at roughly $2500. The HANDY costs $6300 yet supports a range of functional activities in addition to eating, like shaving, painting, and applying make-up. The Raptor and ARM arms, which are intended for general-purpose manipulation, retail at $12,000 and $35,000, respectively. Finally, workstation robots that include a general-purpose robotic arm tend to be most costly. In 2004, the AFMaster retailed for $50,000. Costs of several devices, drawn from Hillman,[24] are indicated in **Table 1**.

Widespread access to commercially available robotic manipulators is governed partly by recommendations of health care service providers and partly by reimbursement policies. For costly devices, reimbursement potential exists only for limited groups of devices and users. The ARM robotic arm, for example, has received reimbursement support from the government of the Netherlands; between 2001 and 2004 this was provided through an exploratory government grant and since 2004 it has been provided formally by the country's health care system. There are now more than 150

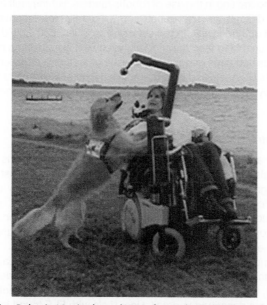

Fig. 1. The Assistive Robotic Manipulator (ARM, formerly MANUS), a wheelchair-mounted robotic arm. (*Courtesy of* Exact Dynamics, *from* Assistive Robotic Manipulator (ARM) aka Manus mobile rehabilitation robot. 2004. Available at: http://www.exactdynamics.nl/english/index.html. Accessed June 15, 2009.)

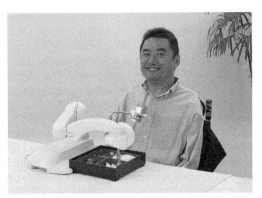

Fig. 2. MySpoon, an example of a feeder robot. (*Courtesy of* SECOM Co. Ltd, Tokyo, *from* SECOM: Meal-assistance robot MySpoon. 2009. Available at: http://www.secom.co.jp/english/myspoon/index.html. Accessed June 22, 2009.)

ARM arms owned by individual users.[24] Comparable reimbursement support from United States insurance providers, however, does not exist at present. Evidence that might support reimbursement in the United States for similarly priced systems has been mixed; in 1994, for example, evaluators from the United States Veterans Affairs found the DeVAR desktop workstation insufficiently robust and overly task limited to be considered medically prescribable.[11]

In the United States, use of robotic manipulation aids has additionally been limited by a lack of standardized prescription protocols among service providers. A 1996 study of 12 United States care facilities,[11] for example, found occupational therapists received little or no training in the use of robotic feeders, yet they felt the devices to be too expensive, difficult to use, unattractive, unreliable, inconvenient, or time consuming to set up and install. In the surveyed facilities, 920 individuals were found to be completely unable to feed themselves, yet only 3 were using a powered feeding device. These aids had been acquired as a result of factors like device availability and the motivation of individuals and their therapists. None of the centers had a standardized procedure by which clients' needs or appropriateness for robotic feeders was evaluated.

Manipulator Control

Unlike prosthetic arms, control of externally mounted robotic arms is rarely driven by myoelectric signals (see Kyberd and Chappell[25] for an exception). Instead, users must supply control signals to the robots using a variety of possible input devices, which may include voice input, head-mounted switches, track balls, joysticks, mice, keyboards, or touchscreen devices. The robotic device El-E additionally allows users to input control commands using a laser pointer, which may be mounted to the ear or controlled with the hand.[15]

The choice of input device depends on users' comfort and physical capacity. In the study by Tijsma and colleagues,[26] prototypical development of a wide range of potential input devices, like large lapboard mounted push buttons and individually molded hand-held grips, are described in detail. User trials with El-E found input device preference among users with amyotrophic lateral sclerosis (ALS) to be partially explained by levels of functional arm impairment recorded on the Revised ALS Functional Rating Scale (ALSFRS-R). Those with higher "handwriting" scores on the ALSFRS-R were

Table 1
Device profiles and cost

Robotic arm name	ARM (MANUS)	HANDY	IRVIS	ProVAR	Winsford feeder
Arm profile	6 DOF manipulator 1 DOF grip	5 DOF manipulator 1 DOF "scoop"	5 DOF manipulator No grip	6 DOF manipulator 1 DOF grip	2 DOF manipulator 1 DOF "scoop"
Category	Wheelchair mount	Desktop mount (feeder)	Desktop mount (vocational)	Desktop mount (vocational)	Desktop mount (feeder)
References	6,9,13,14,18,19,26,28,29,32	7,8,31	30	4,5	8
Cost	$35,000	$6300		ProVAR is not sold commercially; DeVAR, which was extended by ProVAR, sold for $50000–100000	$2500

Robotic arm name	BEESON FEEDER	MOVAID	EL-E	MASTER/EPI-RAID	HELPING HAND/RAPTOR
Arm profile	2 DOF manipulator 1 DOF "scoop"	8 DOF manipulator 1 DOF grip	5 DOF manipulator 1 DOF grip	6 DOF manipulator 1 DOF grip	5 DOF manipulator 1 DOF grip
Category	Desktop mount (feeder)	Autonomous mobile	Autonomous mobile	Desktop mounted (vocational)	Wheelchair mounted
References	8	16	15	17,36	3
Cost	No longer sold			$50000	$12000

Costs in US dollars are derived from Hillman.[24]

more likely to prefer controlling a laser pointer input with the hand; those with lower scores were more likely to prefer a pointer mounted to the ear.[15]

Inputs to robotic manipulators may also be constrained by cognitive factors. The standard interface to the ARM, for example, requires an individual to activate a switch to select which degree of freedom (DOF) he or she would like to manipulate; after selection, this DOF may be manipulated independently of the others. The ARM may alternatively be controlled in Cartesian coordinates, using a similar "switching" form of control. Using either switching method, performing a complex task like grasping and lifting a glass of water requires many DOF switches and an ability to plan the order of these switches, which typically results in lengthy task times. In the study by Mokhtari and colleagues,[19] for example, a user's effort to grasp a remote control was found to take more than 9 minutes with the ARM. Task performance may be further complicated by the fact that, like most prosthetic arms, externally mounted robotic arms typically do not provide force-feedback to the user. Tijsma and colleagues[26] designed several training tasks in an effort to demonstrate to users the vertical forces they were applying to objects with the robot. The ability to translate what was learned during these training tasks to novel tasks, however, depended on the cognitive abilities of the user.

To reduce physical and cognitive demands associated with device control, many systems employ varying degrees of abstraction in their command structure. El-E, for example, takes commands in the form of a gesture to an object on the floor, and this gesture can be made using a laser pointer or touch screen device. Robot navigation to the object and grasp are then entirely automated. Even for devices that must currently be manually controlled, some degree of abstraction may be preferred by users. Eftring and colleagues[14] found that roughly 50% of task time with the ARM, on average, related not to moving the robot's end effector but to the execution of grasping. Users indicated they would prefer the device with an automated grasp, were it to exist.

ProVAR, MASTER/EPI-RAID, and Movaid all feature task-level degrees of abstraction in the control of a robotic arm. Using MASTER/EPI-RAID, for example, a user may grasp a book from the bookshelf by selecting prerecorded locations of books from a pull-down menu; alternatively, he or she may select a book by title.[27] Movaid similarly allows users to control a moving robot to execute tasks, like operating a microwave, with abstract and task-level commands.[16] ProVAR not only allows users to invoke prerecorded activities, but to visually draft new task "plans" by manipulating a virtual arm via click and drag operations or keyboard inputs of joint angles.[4,5] Actions on the virtual arm can be refined until they meet a user's needs, then stored and played on the physical arm at any point in the future. Visualizing 3-dimensional kinematics of the virtual arm on a 2-dimensional screen has, however, proven to be difficult for some users.[4,5]

Trends in Manipulator Evaluation

Users and environments explored

Studies that have evaluated external assistive manipulators have generally taken place in clinical environments, yet many evaluations now focus on use in homes.[6–8,17,19,28,29] Comparatively few evaluations have taken place in vocational environments. Exceptions can be found,[18,30] although results from these studies relate to the experience of a relatively small number of users (less than 5). Both MASTER/EPI-RAID and ProVAR, however, have been fairly extensively evaluated in clinics[4,5,17,27] and hold potential to be evaluated in working offices. DeVAR, the device that later evolved into ProVAR, was in fact deployed at the Pacific Gas and Electric Company during its evaluation.[24]

Users typically include severely disabled individuals with spinal cord injuries, spina bifida, ALS, cerebral palsy, and traumatic brain injuries, as well as others. For the most part, user studies with externally mounted arms have been performed on small populations, typically less than 15 in number. Notable exceptions relate user studies with MASTER/EPI-RAID,[17] the ARM,[9] Movaid,[16] and HANDY[1] robots.

Use of the ARM robot was evaluated in the context of user trials by the Netherlands. Gelderblom and colleagues[9] describe 2 sets of year-long experiments. One compared 13 users of the ARM to a disability-matched control group of 21 nonusers, and the other introduced the ARM to 10 novel users with disabilities. Comparisons in the latter study were made within subjects, before and after device acquisition. Results focused on the degree to which individuals could perform activities independently and whether the device replaced or minimized required care. Users without the ARM were found to receive an average of 3.7 hours of caregiver assistance daily, whereas those with the device required 2.8. In addition, provision of an ARM to novel users reduced dependence on a caregiver by 0.7 to 1.8 hours per day. Reduced dependence on a caregiver was estimated to translate into a saving, per client, of between 7000 and 18,000 euros annually.

In a similarly large study,[17] use of the MASTER/EPI-RAID was evaluated by 91 users with tetraplegia in France. MASTER/EPI-RAID was installed at various locations for a year, including clinics and individual homes. In these locations, users were asked to evaluate the device's support of their leisure, vocational, and domestic activities. Results indicated several leisure activities, like turning pages of a magazine and setting up a television, to be both effectively implemented by the device and of high priority to users. Among domestic tasks, using the refrigerator and serving guests were similarly viewed as both extremely important and well implemented.

Evaluations on this scale and of this time duration have resulted from various European funding initiatives including SPARTACUS in France, TIDE in the European Union, and funding from the Netherlands government. No comparably large or long-term evaluations of nonprosthetic assistive robotic devices were found to have taken place in North America in the last 15 years. The largest North American evaluations have focused on the ProVAR workstation[5] and off-the-shelf feeding devices[8]; in each of these studies, 12 users provided data regarding device effectiveness and usability. Durations of both studies were less than 1 week.

Popular evaluation metrics

Many evaluations of externally mounted assistive arms focus on device effectiveness. Task success rates and times to complete a task, for example, are measures of device effectiveness, either quantitatively or qualitatively.[3,8,14,15,19,26,30,31] To evaluate functional impact on users, standardized occupational therapy assessments were used to evaluate the ASEL fixed workstation arm.[22]

Evaluations of the social significance of robotic manipulators, by comparison, are relatively infrequently performed. Training time and the level of caregiver prompting required to effectively use a device are measured in several studies[4,5,7–9,17,31,32]; results from these studies, however, are mixed. Gelderblom and colleagues[9] found that required activities of daily living (ADL) assistance dropped when the ARM was introduced to a home by as much as 1.8 hours in a day. By contrast, queried caregivers felt the HANDY was time consuming to set up and clean, and did not reduce time assisting with meals.[7] In the study by Hermann and colleagues,[8] however, 92% of clients and their assistants indicated use of a feeding device was an improvement over the way meals had previously taken place. Device setup and cleanup time in this study were found to be, on average, less than 4 minutes, whereas meals lasted 30 to 40 minutes. Of all surveyed studies, only Gelderblom and colleagues[9] evaluated the monetary costs associated with device use in terms of reduced caregiver assistance. Cost savings for individual care resulting from device use were estimated to be able to pay for the device within 3 years.

Many of the studies included some measure of subjective well-being attributable to device use, although the precise measures used vary substantially. Several studies[7–9,29] include, in their evaluations, some measure as to users' satisfaction with devices, more often than not a Likert scale. Standardized device evaluation measures, like the Quebec User Evaluation of Satisfaction with Assistive Technology (QUEST 2.0),[33] were used in the evaluation of the ARM.[9]

Opportunities for Future Research

Several robotic manipulators are on the market and are reasonably affordable (several feeders cost less than $5000) and at least one general-purpose robotic arm retails for less than $15,000. Along with increasingly moderate price tags, there is evidence to suggest that devices like robotic feeders and general-purpose arms reduce the amount of care required by an individual and increase his or her independence. Nevertheless, robotic manipulation devices have yet to see widespread use in North America.

Comprehensive evaluation and effective dissemination of information to health care practitioners may promote increased use. Cost savings associated with the ARM device, for example, have been demonstrated in the European Union,[9] but have yet to be translated into a North American context. Device evaluations that span longer time periods can also provide information needed to gauge costs associated with device maintenance and repair.

Consumer perception of factors that effect long-term use of robotic arms have been identified and prioritized; these may prove to be valid predictors of device acceptance and reduce the rate of device abandonment. For robotic arms, the 5 most important factors are device effectiveness, operability, dependability, affordability, and flexibility.[34]

PROSTHETIC DEVICES
Overview

In current clinical practice, there are 2 main methods of controlling upper extremity prostheses. Body-powered prostheses are controlled via a harness worn by the user. Movements of the user, typically glenohumeral flexion and biscapular abduction, pull on a cable connected to the harness; this cable opens the terminal device and also flexes the elbow in the case of a transhumeral amputation. Most often, an individual with a transhumeral amputation uses a second cable to lock the elbow into position so that the terminal device can be operated.

Externally powered prostheses, on the other hand, use motors to operate the terminal device. The input to the motors is usually controlled via myoelectric signals. A typical fitting uses only 2 myoelectric sites, typically an agonist/antagonist pair of muscles. These 2 sites can control up to 2 DOF, for example, the opening and closing of the prosthetic hand and pronation/supination of the wrist. However, 2 DOF cannot be controlled simultaneously. Typically, the user must position the wrist, then switch modes to use the hand.

Two examples of the current state of the art in commercially available prostheses are the SensorHand SPEED and the i-LIMB. In addition to the single open/close DOF of the hand, the SensorHand SPEED from Otto Bock incorporates a sensor to detect slip; when an object begins to slip in the hand's grasp, the grip force is automatically increased to stop the object from falling. The i-LIMB, which is commercially available through Hanger, has 5 independently powered digits, but this device still uses only 2 myoelectric sites that open and close the hand with a single DOF (**Table 2**).

Thus, in current clinical practice users can actively control only 2 DOF in an upper extremity prosthesis, a far cry from the 21 DOF of the human hand and wrist.[35] Further, these 2 DOF must be controlled sequentially rather than simultaneously, which makes using an upper extremity prosthesis time consuming and unintuitive. In the last 15 years, most of the research in upper extremity prosthetics has focused on addressing these control problems, although a few articles have also been published on the development of new components.[25,36]

Targeted Muscle Reinnervation

A major area of recent research has focused on targeted muscle reinnervation. In 2002, researchers at the Rehabilitation Institute of Chicago performed the first targeted reinnervation to improve myoelectric control.[37] This technique involves the transfer of nerves from the residual limb to muscle groups in the upper arm, chest, or back.[38] Functional results have been reported for 6 individuals, 3 with shoulder disarticulation and 3 with transhumeral amputation.[39] Before the surgery, each individual was fitted with an externally powered device that was controlled using conventional myoelectric sites and external sensors. After the surgery, each individual used a prosthesis with 3 powered DOF; these DOF were controlled by a combination of conventional myoelectric sites, myoelectric sites resulting from the reinnervation

Table 2				
State of the art in commercially available prostheses				
Hand	**Manufacturer**	**Control Method**	**DOF**	**Special Features**
Commercially available				
Sensor hand SPEED	Otto Bock[65]	Electromyography	1	Slip detection prevents dropped objects
i-LIMB	Touch Bionics Inc.[66]	Electromyography	1	Five individually powered digits
Motion control ETD/Hand	Motion control Inc.[67]	Electromyography	1	Optional flexion wrist
In development				
Proto 2	Applied Physics Laboratory, John Hopkins University[68]	Electromyography (targeted muscle reinnervation)	25	Provides sensory feedback
DEKA arm	DEKA R&D Corp.[58]	Electromyography (targeted muscle reinnervation), foot pad in shoe	18	Currently beginning clinical trials
MANUS-HAND	Pons et al[69]	Electromyography	3	Design based on user input

procedure, and external sensors. Subjects showed improvements ranging from 95% to 271% on a modified version of the Box and Blocks Test, and reported that the re-innervation procedure made control of the prosthesis easier and faster because the terminal device and the elbow could be operated simultaneously.

Pattern Recognition

Targeted muscle reinnervation results in a greater number of myoelectric sites available for prosthesis control. If each site is used to control a single DOF, 3 or 4 DOF can potentially be controlled. However, machine-learning techniques can be used to identify patterns of activity across multiple electrodes that correspond to a particular movement. These techniques, known as pattern recognition, have the potential to enable prosthetic control of upwards of 10 DOF. This topic has been widely studied in individuals without amputation; only the results for individuals with upper extremity amputation are reported here.

To use pattern recognition, electromyography (EMG) data must be used to calculate features. The features considered can range from straightforward quantities such as the mean absolute value of the signal and the number of zero crossings[40] to more complicated values such as the coefficients used to decompose the EMG signal using wavelets.[41]

Zhou and colleagues[42] report pattern recognition results for 4 individuals after the targeted reinnervation procedure. Each individual was asked to imagine 16 different movements (8 DOF) of the arm, wrist, and hand and to try to accomplish these movements using the amputated limb. During this process, the activity of the reinnervated muscles was measured with a very large number of surface electrodes (79–128, depending on the individual; **Fig. 3**). Pattern recognition (specifically, linear discriminant analysis) was able to correctly classify 95% to 96% of movements based on the EMG data recorded. Because the large number of electrodes used was not currently practical for clinical practice, Huang and colleagues[43] investigated ways to reduce the number of electrodes needed while maintaining classification accuracy. These investigators found that 10 to 12 surface electrodes chosen from a high-density electrode array by an automated optimization procedure could be used to correctly

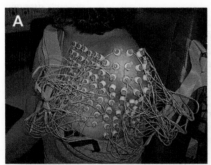
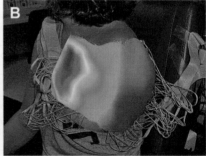

Fig. 3. (*A*) Placement of electrodes for surface electromyography. (*B*) Map of surface electromyogram amplitude during hand closure. Pattern recognition is the association of different patterns of activation with particular movements of the hand and arm. (*Reprinted from* Kuiken TA, Miller LA, Lipschutz RD, et al. Targeted reinnervation for enhanced prosthetic arm function in a woman with a proximal amputation: a case study. Lancet 2007;369(9559):371–80; copyright 2007, Elsevier; with permission.)

classify 93.0% of movements for 8 DOF. When the same number of electrodes was placed according to a clinical protocol, 88.7% of movements were correctly classified.

Kuiken and colleagues[38] report similar results for 5 individuals with targeted muscle reinnervation. Each individual wore 12 electrodes placed by clinicians over the reinnervated areas. The subject imagined and tried to perform 10 movements while EMG data was recorded. The classifier trained from this data had a mean classification accuracy of 88%. In addition, the classifier was then used to enable the individual to control a virtual prosthesis. The subject was asked to perform the 10 movements with the virtual prosthesis, and the investigators measured the time required to correctly select and complete movements, as well as the completion rate. The mean time required to select the appropriate movement was 0.22 seconds for the elbow and wrist and 0.38 seconds for the hand, whereas the corresponding mean times to complete the appropriate movement were 1.29 seconds and 1.54 seconds, respectively. A total of 96.3% for movements of the elbow and wrist and 86.9% for movements of the hand were completed within 5 seconds.

Pattern recognition has also been investigated as a method for increasing the number of prosthetic DOF that can be controlled by an individual who has not had targeted muscle reinnervation. Sebelius and colleagues[44] describe an experiment with 6 individuals with transradial amputation or limb deficiency. Eight electrodes were placed on the residual limb, and EMG recordings were made while subjects performed 10 movements with the contralateral hand and attempted to perform the same movements with the residual limb. An artificial neural network was trained to identify various movements based on the EMG signal. The network was able to successfully classify 6 movements for the best user, and the system successfully classified approximately 3 movements for any of the individuals. Ajiboye and Weir[45] demonstrate that fuzzy logic may provide comparable or better classification performance relative to strategies used in current commercial devices. In addition, Momen and colleagues[46] show that a classifier for EMG signals can be trained based on any patterns of activation chosen by the individual.

Alternative Control Techniques

Although electromyography remains the most popular control method for externally powered prostheses, researchers have considered a variety of other options. A sensor incorporating a magnet has been used to measure the change in muscle dimension that occurs with contraction.[47] This sensor was used with 6 subjects with transradial amputation, and subjects were able to control a single DOF. Mechanomyography, the measurement of the sound produced by contracting muscles, has also been used to control a single DOF.[48] Abboudi and colleagues[49] used pneumatic sensors to measure the pressure exerted by the residual limb on the socket. Experiments with 3 subjects with transradial amputation showed that 3 pneumatic sensors were sufficient to control 3 DOF corresponding to the movement of the thumb, index finger, and small finger of an experimental prosthesis. An additional sensor was used to change the grasping mode of the hand. Similar results were reported for 2 subjects by Curcie and colleagues.[50]

Sensory Feedback

Users of body-powered prostheses receive some force-feedback from the harness as they operate the prosthesis, whereas current users of externally powered prostheses must operate the device using only visual feedback. Pylatiuk and colleagues[51] designed and studied the use of force-feedback closed-loop controls for users with myoelectric hands to more naturally grasp objects. The system consisted of a force sensor, an electronic board, and a vibration motor. The pilot study with 5 myoelectric arm users investigated both direct feedback onto nearby skin and indirect feedback into the prosthetic hand. Results showed a reduction in mean forces required to grasp an object by 54% and 37%, respectively. The users were most receptive of the technology when the vibration was applied indirectly to the prosthetic hand, and users reported that the sensory information provided a sense of confidence in their movements. Lundborg and colleagues[52] used piezoresistive sensors to create artificial sensibility in 4 persons with median/ulnar nerve injury and 1 person with a myoelectric arm. Spatial resolution in nonsensate digits and regulation of the power pinch grip were studied, with significant improvements in both categories by all subjects. Weir and colleagues[53] identified the possibility of using multiple, small muscle cineplasties to control prosthetic components while simultaneously providing force-feedback. Dhillon and Horch[54] investigated the use of implanted electrodes into the fascicles of severed nerves to determine if sensory feedback could be transmitted. Finally, sensory reinnervation of the target muscle by the transferred nerve can occur with targeted muscle reinnervation[38,55]; stimulation of this area could provide tactile feedback to these individuals. Although a variety of options for force and tactile feedback have been investigated, to this point there has been little work examining how tactile feedback could improve the functional performance of individuals using an upper extremity prosthesis.

Opportunities for Future Research

For prosthetic arms, features heavily prioritized by consumers include comfort, durability, function, appearance, and cost.[56] Functional priorities for prosthetics include gripping, steadying, and manipulating objects, as well as conveying body language.[56] To accurately express body language and manipulate complex objects, devices with DOF that mimic the human hand are required.

Current research results show that the number of prosthetic DOF that can be controlled by a user can be increased using pattern recognition based on the EMG signals from 8 to 12 electrodes. This technique is particularly effective after the use of targeted muscle reinnervation to separate the nerves of the residual limb. Clinical use of these advances, however, requires prostheses with 3 or more powered DOF. Miller and colleagues[57] constructed a 3-DOF prosthesis from commercially available components, although one component was custom modified; the investigators also report preliminary use of a 6-DOF prosthesis that includes prototype components. Recently, the Department of Veterans Affairs announced clinical trials of the DEKA arm,[58] which features 10 powered DOF and 6 grasp modes (**Fig. 4**). If the tests of this device are successful, it may represent a way to apply the current research in targeted muscle reinnervation and pattern recognition in such a way as to dramatically improve the quality of life of individuals with upper extremity amputation.

SUMMARY
Are Robotic Arms Being Comprehensively Evaluated Along All Three Axes of the CATOR Taxonomy?

The CATOR taxonomy of assistive device outcomes[59] organizes outcomes according to device effectiveness, social significance, and impact on subjective well-being. Device effectiveness seeks to measure the impact on user functioning, activity participation, and accessibility of a user's environment. Social significance includes measures of impact on society, including changes in labor required of caregivers, use of the health care system, or housing cost. Finally, subjective well-being measures focus on individuals' satisfaction with a device, and with their lives more generally, after device adoption.

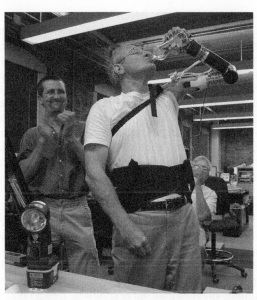

Fig. 4. Frederick Downs Jr. of VA tries the DEKA prosthetic arm for the first time at the company's New Hampshire headquarters. (*Courtesy of* the Office of Research and Development, Department of Veterans Affairs; *from* VA conducting "optimization study" of advanced prosthetic arm. VA Research Currents, Research News from the US Dept of Veterans Affairs 2009;1, 3, 6, 7. http://www.research.va.gov/resources/pubs/docs/va_research_currents_may_09. pdf. Accessed 11 June 2009.)

Several standardized outcome assessments measure assistive device outcomes, yet these have not been frequently employed by recent studies. The Psychosocial Impact of Assistive Devices Scale (PIADS), for example, is a 26-item self-report questionnaire that assesses changes in functional independence, well-being, and quality of life that result from assistive technology use. It has been demonstrated to be a good predictor of device use or abandonment.[12] QUEST 2 is a related, 12-item measure that assesses user satisfaction with the device and its related service. This scale is intended to be used as both a clinical and a research tool,[33] and has been used to assess the impact of the ARM during user testing in the Netherlands.[9] The QUEST is based on the "Matching Person and Technology" model, which posits that goodness of fit between consumer and technology "requires attention to aspects of the environments in which the technology will be used, the needs and preferences of the user, and the functions and features of the technology."[60] For evaluation of prosthetics, the Prosthesis Evaluation Questionnaire exists as a standardized instrument; this consists of 82 questions that measure user perception of device effectiveness and impact on quality of life.[61]

At present, device effectiveness is typically assessed with study-specific measures that may include task success, the time to complete tasks, or the number of switch inputs required to operate a device. The effect of a device on user functioning is sometimes measured with standardized occupational therapy assessments like the Jebson Hand Test, the Box and Block Test, or the Minnesota Rate of Manipulation Test. As an example, these measures were used to evaluate the functional effectiveness of the ASEL fixed workstation arm to perform manipulative tasks.[55] Increased use of standardized measures that are familiar to occupational therapists may ultimately enhance communication between engineers and clinicians, and improve the market acceptance of devices.

Assessments of social significance, which include measures of the saved assistance or economic cost, are not routinely performed. However, methodology to holistically measure cost effectiveness of assistive technology has been developed.[62] This methodology measures the long-term costs associated with an assistive device user's current situation (occupational priorities, adaptive equipment, and environment). Computed costs are then compared with the long-term costs of enabling a user's participation in occupational priorities with optimal assistive devices and environments. As a result, an understanding of the societal cost of providing versus not providing assistive technology can be built and potentially used to structure policy. Cost analyses are, in fact, of vital importance to insurance providers and can be used to argue for device reimbursement. The lack of these kinds of analyses in research may partially explain why whereas robotic manipulation devices are increasingly available and affordable, they have yet to see widespread use in North America.

Are Definitions of Effectiveness in Accordance with the Priorities of Users?

Design criteria emphasized by users for externally mounted arms differ from those for prosthetic arms. Users of prosthetics are individuals with amputation, who may or may not have additional injuries or disabilities. Users of externally mounted arms typically include severely disabled individuals with spinal cord injuries, spina bifida, ALS, cerebral palsy, and traumatic brain injuries, among others. Design priorities vary accordingly. For externally mounted arms, tasks prioritized by users relate to ADL and instrumental ADL, with eating and drinking, personal hygiene, object retrieval from shelves and the floor, food preparation, housework, and recreational activities weighted heavily.[63] Top arm priorities for these users include effectiveness, operability, dependability, and affordability.[34] Despite the difficulty with the current control of devices like the ARM, however, many users indicate they believe the device increases their independence.[9] The device, then, may be difficult to control yet is tolerable to users based on other properties and benefits.

For prosthetic arms, features prioritized include comfort on the body, durability, function, appearance, and cost.[56] Functional priorities for prosthetics include gripping, steadying, and manipulating objects, as well as conveying body language.[56] The more DOF that need to be replaced by a prosthetic arm, however, the less likely it is a potential user will accept a prosthetic over the long term.[56] This finding indicates that easy control of many DOF is a heavily weighted determinant of device acceptability among individuals with amputation, in whom it may be less heavily weighted by users of externally mounted devices.

In 1996, consumer functional priorities for research and development of prosthetics included the ability to move digits separately, ability to perform movements with less visual attention, ability to perform two coordinated movements at one time, more DOF at the wrist, more forceful grip, and the ability to perform vigorous tasks.[64] Despite 9 years of prosthetic research, in 2007 consumer areas of dissatisfaction echo the same priorities. Dexterity, sensory feedback, coordination of multiple joints, wrist movement and control, ability to keep objects from slipping, and grasp of awkward shapes are still research priorities for prosthetics consumers.[56] Additional consumer priorities are reducing the weight of the prosthetic, the durability of the glove, the device cost, heat, reduction of unplanned movements, cosmesis, and reliability.[56] Although not a priority, some consumers have expressed interest in additional functionality such as MP3 players, watches, cell phones, flashlights, and so forth.[56]

Consumer priorities obviously inform device acceptance, yet they are not always intuitively represented in popular outcome measures for user studies. The relationship between task time and consumer opinion of effectiveness, for example, likely exists but is not necessarily intuitive. A relationship between user priorities and tasks commonly selected for evaluation, like building a tower of blocks[29] or lifting a cup,[14] is also not necessarily given. Finally, the length of time devices are commonly evaluated is typically less than 6 months, which may not be sufficient to accurately gauge other features important to users, like dependability or reliability.

What Gaps in Robotic Arm Evaluation Exist, and How Might These Gaps be Best Addressed?

A few recommendations based on the literature review include:

Use of standardized outcome measures

The use of existing standardized instruments in all 3 domains of the CATOR taxonomy can improve communication among stakeholders. Appropriate standardized instruments are available, including the PIADS, QUEST 2.0, and occupational therapy hand manipulation tests such as the Jebson Hand Test, the Box and Block Test, and the Minnesota Rate of Manipulation Test.

Emphasis on measures of social significance, particularly cost

Cost-based assessments are required to ensure that potential funding sources for devices can make well-informed decisions about risks and benefits associated with device use. This same information allows stakeholders to more strongly advocate for funding.

Emphasis on measures of quality of life

The impact of device adoption on the quality of life of the user is also not currently consistently measured. It is, however, ultimately the user of the robotic arm who makes the decision as to whether the device will be used or abandoned.

What Further Advances can be Expected in the Next 15 Years?

A significant amount of recent research and development has been dedicated to producing more comfortable, efficient control of robotic arms to enable improvements in task performance. Trends in this development, however, differ based on whether the arms are prosthetic or externally mounted. For prosthetic arms, research has focused on leveraging signals produced by muscle contraction for the control of increasing numbers of DOF of the limb. Much of this research has specifically focused on development of increasingly sophisticated pattern recognition techniques to translate EMG signals to the control of increased DOF. For externally mounted arms, research has focused on providing increasingly intelligible user interfaces so that users may comfortably and intuitively use available degrees of freedom with a keyboard, mouse, touchpad, or alternative input device.

Whereas much research has been dedicated to interface and control details, much less research has focused on the development of novel manipulators. Gaps, then, exist not only in the evaluation of current devices but in the form of the devices themselves. Of prosthetic devices profiled, for example, those that are commercially available tend to have 1 DOF whereas those under development have between 18 and 25 DOF. There is obviously room for devices with intermediate DOF; the precise relationship between DOF and usability or user satisfaction, however, remains to be explored.

For externally mounted arms, payloads must be increased; the Raptor, for example, currently has a 1-kg payload, which is not sufficient to lift a gallon of milk. The ARM is similarly limited, with a 1.5-kg payload. To save costs, the Raptor has sacrificed a certain degree of intuitive control; the Raptor can currently only be controlled by manipulating each joint individually, one at a time, not by specifying the Cartesian coordinates of the end effector. It is not yet clear whether users are willing to accept decreased functionality in exchange for lower cost.

The authors have reviewed recent research (post 1994) in the development and evaluation of assistive arms, both prosthetic and externally mounted. Analysis of the articles highlights a need for increased standardization of evaluation methods; several potential standard outcome measures, like the PIADS or QUEST, have the potential to fill some evaluation gaps. In addition, these studies demonstrate a need for an increased emphasis on the social significance (ie, social cost) of devices in particular, so as to enable health care practitioners to more adequately advocate for device reimbursement. It is hoped that increased standardization and increasingly comprehensive evaluation will enable better communication between engineers and clinicians and increased funding for large-scale and long-term user tests, as well as more adequate reimbursement of devices that have already been proven and which are currently on the market.

REFERENCES

1. Topping M. The development of Handy 1, a robotic aid to independence for the severely disabled. Paper presented at the Mechatronic Aids for the Disabled, IEE Colloquium. Dundee, Scotland; May 17, 1995.
2. Topping M. An overview of the development of Handy 1, a rehabilitation robot to assist the severely disabled. J Intell Robotic Syst 2002;34(3):253–63.
3. Sheredos SJ, Taylor B, Cobb CB, et al. Preliminary evaluation of the helping hand electro-mechanical arm. Tech Disabil 1996;5(2):229–32.
4. Wagner JJ, Wickizer M, Van Der Loos HFM, et al. User testing and design iteration of the ProVAR user interface. Robot and human interaction, 1999. RO-MAN '99. 8th IEEE International Workshop on. vol. Pisa, Italy1999:18–22.
5. Wagner JJ, Van der Loos HFM. Training strategies for the user interface of vocational assistive robots. Paper presented at the Engineering in Medicine and Biology Society, 2004. IEMBS '04. 26th Annual International Conference of the IEEE 2004. September 1–5, 2004.
6. Mahoney RM, Dallaway JL. Robotic vocational accommodations in manufacturing jobs. Tech Disabil 1996;5:167–76.
7. Smith J, Topping MJ. Study to determine the main factors leading to the overall success of the Handy 1 robotic system. Paper presented at the ICORR'97 International Conference on Rehabilitation Robotics. Bath Institute of Medical Engineering, Bath University, Bath, UK; April 14–15, 1997.
8. Hermann RP, Phalangas AC, Mahoney RM, et al. Powered feeding devices: an evaluation of three models. Arch Phys Med Rehabil 1999;80(10):1237–42.
9. Gelderblom GJ, de Witte L, van Soest K, et al. Cost effectiveness of the Manus robot manipulator. Paper presented at the ICORR 2001 International Conference on Rehabilitation Robotics. Institut National des Télécommunications, Evry, France; July 9–12, 1996.
10. Engelhardt KG, Awad R, Perkash I, et al. Interactive evaluation of a robotic aid: a new approach to assessment. Paper presented at the 2nd Annual International Robot Conference. Long Beach, CA; March 13–15, 1984.
11. Van der Loos HFM. VA/Stanford rehabilitation robotics research and development program: lessons learned in the application of robotics technology to the field of rehabilitation. IEEE Trans Rehabil Eng 1995;3(1):46–55.

12. Jutai J, Day H. Psychosocial Impact of Assistive Devices Scale (PIADS). Tech Disabil 2002;14(3):107–11.
13. Romer GRBE, Stuyt HJA, Peters A. Cost-savings and economic benefits due to the assistive robotic manipulator (ARM). Paper presented at: Rehabilitation Robotics, 2005. ICORR 2005. 9th International Conference. Chicago, Illinois; June 28–July 1, 2005.
14. Eftring H, Boschian K. Technical Results from Manus User Trials. Paper presented at: 1999 ICORR International Conference on Rehabilitation Robotics 1999; Stanford University, Palo Alto, CA; July 1–2, 1999.
15. Choi YS, Anderson CD, Glass JD, et al. Laser pointers and a touch screen: intuitive interfaces for autonomous mobile manipulation for the motor impaired. Paper presented at the 10th International ACM SIGACCESS conference on Computers and accessibility. Halifax, Nova Scotia, Canada Oct 15–17, 2008.
16. Dario P, Guglielmelli E, Laschi C, et al. A personal robot in everyday life of disabled and elderly people. Tech Disabil 1999;10(2):77–93.
17. Busnel M, Cammoun R, Coulon-Lauture F, et al. The robotized workstation "MASTER" for users with tetraplegia: description and evaluation. J Rehabil Res Dev 1999;36(3):217–29.
18. Kang JW, Kim BS, Chung MJ. Development of assistive mobile robots helping the disabled work in a factory environment. Paper presented at: Mechtronic and Embedded Systems and Applications, 2008. MESA 2008. IEEE/ASME International Conference on 2008; July 15–17, 2008.
19. Mokhtari M, Didi N, Roby-Brami A. A multi-disciplinary approach in evaluating and facilitating the use of the Manus robot. Paper presented at the Robotics and Automation, 1999. Proceedings: 1999 IEEE International Conference. Detroit, Michigan; May 10–15, 1999.
20. AFMASTER. 2009. Photo of MASTER desktop robot. Available at: http://www.laas. fr/iarp-france/devices/afmaster.html. Accessed June 15, 2009.
21. Schraft RD, Schmeirer G. Service robots. First edition. AK Peters, editor. Buxton, UK; 2000.
22. Neater Solutions, Ltd. Available at: http://www.neater.co.uk/. Accessed June 12, 2009.
23. SECOM. Meal-assistance robot MySpoon. 2009. Available at: http://www.secom. co.jp/english/myspoon/index.html. Accessed June 22, 2009.
24. Hillman M. Rehabilitation robotics from past to present: a historical perspective. In: Bien ZZ, Stefanov D, editors. Advances in rehabilitation robotics: human-friendly technologies on movement assistance and restoration for people with disabilities, vol. 306. Berlin/Heidelberg: Springer; 2004. p. 25–44.
25. Kyberd PJ, Chappell PH. The Southampton Hand: an intelligent myoelectric prosthesis. J Rehabil Res Dev 1994;31(4):326–34.
26. Tijsma HA, Liefhebber F, Herder JL. Evaluation of new user interface features for the MANUS robot arm. Paper presented at: Rehabilitation Robotics, 2005. ICORR 2005. 9th International Conference. Chicago, Illinois; June 28–July 1, 2005.
27. Eftring H. Robot control methods using the RAID workstation. Paper presented at the 4th International Conference on Computers for Handicapped Persons. Vienna, Austria; September 14–16, 1994.
28. Lopez N, di Sciascio F, Soria C, et al. Robust EMG sensing system based on data fusion for myoelectric control of a robotic arm. Biomed Eng Online 2009; 8(1):5.
29. Buhler C. Integration of a robot arm with a wheelchair. Paper presented at: Intelligent Robots and Systems '94. 'Advanced Robotic Systems and the Real World',

IROS '94. Proceedings of the IEEE/RSJ/GI International Conference. Munich, Germany; September 12–16, 1994.

30. Driessen B, Liefhebber F, Kate TT, et al. Collaborative control of the MANUS manipulator. Paper presented at: Rehabilitation Robotics, 2005. ICORR 2005. 9th International Conference. Chicago, Illinois; June 28–July 1, 2005.

31. Tsui K, Yanco H, Kontak D, et al. Development and evaluation of a flexible interface for a wheelchair mounted robotic arm. Paper presented at the 3rd ACM/IEEE International Conference on Human Robot Interaction. Amsterdam, The Netherlands, 2008; May 12-15, 2008.

32. Kwee H, Quaedackers J, van de Bool E, et al. Adapting the control of the MANUS manipulator for persons with cerebral palsy: an exploratory study. Tech Disabil 2002;14(1):31–42.

33. Demers L, Weiss-Lambrou R, Ska B. The Quebec User Evaluation of Satisfaction with Assistive Technology (QUEST 2.0): an overview and recent progress. Tech Disabil 2002;14:101–5.

34. Batavia AI, Hammer GS. Toward the development of consumer-based criteria for the evaluation of assistive devices. J Rehabil Res Dev 1990;27(4):425–36.

35. Jones LA, Lederman SJ. Evolutionary development and anatomy of the hand. New York, NY: Human Hand Function Oxford University Press US; 2006. p. 10–23.

36. Cupo ME, Sheredos SJ. Clinical evaluation of a new, above-elbow, body-powered prosthetic arm: a final report. J Rehabil Res Dev 1998;35(4):431–46.

37. Kuiken TA, Dumanian GA, Lipschutz RD, et al. The use of targeted muscle reinnervation for improved myoelectric prosthesis control in a bilateral shoulder disarticulation amputee. Prosthet Orthot Int 2004;28(3):245–53.

38. Kuiken TA, Li G, Lock BA, et al. Targeted muscle reinnervation for real-time myoelectric control of multifunction artificial arms. JAMA 2009;301(6):619–28.

39. Miller LA, Stubblefield KA, Lipschutz RD, et al. Improved myoelectric prosthesis control using targeted reinnervation surgery: a case series. IEEE Trans Neural Syst Rehabil Eng 2008;16(1):46–50.

40. Hudgins B, Parker P, Scott RN. A new strategy for multifunction myoelectric control. IEEE Trans Biomed Eng 1993;40(1):82–94.

41. Boostani R, Moradi MH. Evaluation of the forearm EMG signal features for the control of a prosthetic hand. Physiol Meas 2003;24:309–19.

42. Zhou P, Lowery MM, Englehart KB, et al. Decoding a new neural machine interface for control of artificial limbs. J Neurophysiol 2007;98(5):2974–82.

43. Huang H, Zhou P, Li G, et al. An analysis of EMG electrode configuration for targeted muscle reinnervation based neural machine interface. IEEE Trans Neural Syst Rehabil Eng 2008;16(1):37–45.

44. Sebelius FCP, Rosén BN, Lundborg GN. Refined myoelectric control in below-elbow amputees using artificial neural networks and a data glove. J Hand Surg Am 2005;30(4):780–9.

45. Ajiboye AB, Weir RF. A heuristic fuzzy logic approach to EMG pattern recognition for multifunctional prosthesis control. IEEE Trans Neural Syst Rehabil Eng 2005; 13(3):280–91.

46. Momen K, Krishnan S, Chau T. Real-time classification of forearm electromyographic signals corresponding to user-selected intentional movements for multifunction prosthesis control. IEEE Trans Neural Syst Rehabil Eng 2007;15(4):535–42.

47. Kenney LPJ, Lisitsa I, Bowker P, et al. Dimensional change in muscle as a control signal for powered upper limb prostheses: a pilot study. Med Eng Phys 1999;21(8):589–97.

48. Silva J, Heim W, Chau T. A self-contained, mechanomyography-driven externally powered prosthesis. Arch Phys Med Rehabil 2005;86(10):2066–70.

49. Abboudi RL, Glass CA, Newby NA, et al. A biomimetic controller for a multifinger prosthesis. IEEE Trans Rehabil Eng 1999;7(2):121–9.
50. Curcie DJ, Flint JA, Craelius W. Biomimetic finger control by filtering of distributed forelimb pressures. IEEE Trans Neural Syst Rehabil Eng 2001;9(1):69–75.
51. Pylatiuk C, Kargov A, Schulz S. Design and evaluation of a low-cost force feedback system for myoelectric prosthetic hands. J Prosthet Orthot 2006;18(2):57–61.
52. Lundborg G, Rosén B, Lindström K, et al. Artificial sensibility based on the use of piezoresistive sensors. Preliminary observations. J Hand Surg Br 1998;23(5):620–6.
53. Weir RF, Heckathorne CW, Childress DS. Cineplasty as a control input for externally powered prosthetic components. J Rehabil Res Dev 2001;38(4):357–63.
54. Dhillon GS, Horch KW. Direct neural sensory feedback and control of a prosthetic arm. IEEE Trans Neural Syst Rehabil Eng 2005;13(4):468–72.
55. Schuyler JL, Mahoney RM. Assessing human-robotic performance for vocational placement. IEEE Trans Rehabil Eng 2000;8(3):394–404.
56. Biddiss E, Beaton D, Chau T. Consumer design priorities for upper limb prosthetics. Disabil Rehabil Assist Technol 2007;2(6):346–57.
57. Miller LA, Lipschutz RD, Stubblefield KA, et al. Control of a six degree of freedom prosthetic arm after targeted muscle reinnervation surgery. Arch Phys Med Rehabil 2008;89(11):2057–65.
58. VA conducting 'optimization study' of advanced prosthetic arm. VA Research Currents, Reserach News from the US Dept of Veterans Affairs; 2009. 1, 3, 6, 7 Available at: http://www.research.va.gov/resources/pubs/docs/va_research_currents_may_09.pdf. Accessed June 11, 2009.
59. Jutai JW, Fuhrer MJ, Demers L, et al. Toward a taxonomy of assistive technology device outcomes. Am J Phys Med Rehabil 2005;84(4):294–302.
60. Scherer MJ, Craddock G. Matching Person & Technology (MPT) assessment process. Tech Disabil 2002;14(3):125–31.
61. Prosthesis Evaluation Questionnaire (PEQ). 1998. Available at: http://www.prs-research.org/htmPages/PEQ.html. Accessed June 15, 2009.
62. Schraner I, Jonge D, Layton N, et al. Using the ICF in economic analysis of assistive technology systems: methodological implications of a user standpoint. Disabil Rehabil 2008;30(12–13):916–26.
63. Stanger CA, Anglin C, Harwin WS, et al. Devices for assisting manipulation: a summary of user task priorities. IEEE Trans Rehabil Eng 1994;2(4):256–65.
64. Atkins D, Heard D, Donovan W. Epidemiologic overview of individuals with upper-limb loss and their reported research priorities. J Prosthet Orthot 1996;8(1):2–11.
65. Otto Bock—SensorHand Speed 2009; technical description. Available at: http://www.ottobockus.com/cps/rde/xchg/ob_us_en/hs.xsl/5735.html?openteaser=1. Accessed June 22, 2009.
66. Touch Bionics: The i-LIMB Hand. The worlds first fully articulating and commercially available bionic hand. 2009. Available at: http://www.touchbionics.com/professionals.php?section=5. Accessed June 22, 2009
67. The Motion Control ETD Electric Terminal Device. 2009. Technical specifications. Available at: http://www.utaharm.com/etd.php. Accessed June 22, 2009.
68. Adee SA. "Manhattan Project" for the next generation of bionic arms. IEEE Spectrum. 2009;2008. Available at: http://www.spectrum.ieee.org/biomedical/bionics/a-manhattan-project-for-the-next-generation-of-bionic-arms/0. Accessed June 22, 2009.
69. Pons JL, Rocon E, Ceres R, et al. The MANUS-HAND dextrous robotics upper limb prosthesis: mechanical and manipulation aspects. Autonomous Robots 2004;16(2):143–63.

Joystick Control for Powered Mobility: Current State of Technology and Future Directions

Brad E. Dicianno, MD[a,b,c,d,*], Rory A. Cooper, PhD[b,d,e,f], John Coltellaro, MS, ATP[c]

KEYWORDS

• Control interface • Joystick • Power mobility
• Switch control • Wheelchair

By 2010, approximately 4 million Americans will be users of wheeled mobility devices in community settings, with approximately 17% using electric power wheelchairs (EPW) or scooters.[1,2] The number of device users continues to grow,[3] as does the number of people who cannot use the technology currently available. A survey study by Fehr et al[4] demonstrated that approximately one quarter of a million individuals cannot use EPWs because of various impairments in motor function, sensation, or cognition. The authors concluded that approximately half of the individuals who

Work presented in this article is partially supported by The National Institutes of Health, Rehabilitation Medicine Scientist Training Program (Grant #K12 HD001097-09, Grant # K12-HD1097-11, and Grant #1R21HD050717-01A1-1), the National Science Foundation (Grant# EEC-0540865), and The Department of Veterans Affairs (Grant #B3142C and Grant #B3287R).

[a] Department of Physical Medicine and Rehabilitation, University of Pittsburgh Medical Center (UPMC), Kaufmann Medical Bldg, Suite 202, 3471 5th Avenue, Pittsburgh, PA 15213, USA

[b] Department of Rehabilitation Science and Technology, University of Pittsburgh, PA, USA

[c] UPMC Center for Assistive Technology, 3010 Forbes Tower, 4020 Forbes Tower, Pittsburgh, PA 15260, USA

[d] Department of Veterans Affairs, Human Engineering Research Laboratories (HERL), Pittsburgh, VA Pittsburgh Healthcare System. 7180 Highland Drive, 151R-1, Pittsburgh, PA 15206, USA

[e] Department of Bioengineering, 306 CNBIO, 300 Technology Drive, University of Pittsburgh, PA 15219, USA

[f] Department of Physical Medicine and Rehabilitation, University of Pittsburgh, PA, USA

* Corresponding author. University of Pittsburgh Medical Center, Department of Physical Medicine and Rehabilitation, Kaufmann Medical Bldg, Suite 202, 3471 5th Avenue, Pittsburgh, PA 15213.

E-mail address: dicianno@pitt.edu (B.E. Dicianno).

Phys Med Rehabil Clin N Am 21 (2010) 79–86
doi:10.1016/j.pmr.2009.07.013   pmr.theclinics.com
1047-9651/09/$ – see front matter. Published by Elsevier Inc.

cannot currently operate an EPW by conventional methods could benefit if new technology were developed that could accommodate their needs and abilities.

Most classic research on control interfaces in general has focused on unimpaired individuals such as surgeons, pilots, and computer operators.[5–7] These studies demonstrated the ability of control interfaces to distinguish between intentional and unintentional movements. Although some conventional control interfaces on the market today can compensate for some unintentional movements, such as small amplitude tremor, during tasks such as EPW driving, we do not yet have the technology that can accommodate many severe movement disorders, such as larger amplitude tremor or involuntary movements like severe athetosis. Riley and Rosen[8] showed that customization of a joystick to an individual user can significantly improve an individual's performance with that control interface. In the last 5 years, more research has focused on combinations of hardware, and specialized software applications could theoretically be used to create a customized device for each individual user. Although newer joysticks allow customization of various features, completely customizable joysticks for EPWs are not yet a reality in clinical practice. Later in this article we discuss novel research aimed to make this customization possible. First, we examine the current state of control interface technology.

PROPORTIONAL CONTROL

The standard EPW joystick commonly prescribed in the clinic is a type of proportional control, so named because the device's output (the wheelchair's velocity) increases as the stick is progressively moved away from center. These devices also can be referred to as movement-sensing joysticks (MSJ) because the stick physically moves as a user exerts force on it. Other proportional input devices, such as trackballs, some head arrays, and touchpads, are also available. Similar controls used by unimpaired individuals are automobile accelerator pedals and video game joysticks. Efficient use of proportional controls generally requires a certain amount of intact proprioception, joint mobility, and dexterity.

Individuals who do not have the ability to operate proportional controls must use a combination of switches with or without scanning control. Although discussion of switch and scanning control is outside the scope of this article, the reader should be aware that many options are available besides the technology mentioned in this article, and switches can be added to some of the newer joysticks.

PROFILES AND FEATURES OVERVIEW

Most joysticks have a variety of profiles that can each contain a plethora of different parameter settings.[9] What follows is a detailed description of the most common parameters and features used to date. Some devices contain off-the-shelf profiles such as those for a new user, which can be used as a starting template. A clinician may want to have available a wide array of profiles set up to appropriately evaluate clients for power mobility. Each consumer may want more than one profile to accommodate for variations in his or her condition (eg, to accommodate for fatigue or during times of disease flares). The number of parameter combinations is almost limitless, so it is important to have a few standard templates established as a starting point for further customization. Decisions about the types of devices and settings to select for an individual depend on a person's current level of function and the individual's prognosis. Underuse of these features is probably one of the biggest obstacles to harnessing the potential of modern joystick technology.

CONTROLLERS

The joystick is composed of the interface between the user and the device (ie, the stick) and a controller that acts as the intermediary between the human input on the stick and the output of the EPW. Controllers contain the electronics and software, modify the signals from the interface, and convert them to output that is passed along to the device being controlled. The controller can be integral (ie, the main controller is integrated into the chair and used by the client) or remotely placed, such as one used by an attendant. A nonexpandable controller regulates the speed and direction of the power wheelchair drive mechanism and can be used to control up to 2 power seating actuators that allow the user to change the orientation of the seat. Typically, nonexpandable controllers can accept only a proportional joystick as an input device. An expandable controller can accommodate many other proportional input devices besides a standard joystick, such as a touchpad or proportional head array, and non-proportional input devices, such as a sip and puff or head array switches. This type of controller also operates 3 or more power seating actuators, sometimes requiring an additional component to do so. An expandable controller may be used to operate such devices as a separate display for a different control interface, an alternative and augmentative communication device, a computer, or an attendant control.

MOUNTING AND COMPATIBILITY ISSUES

Appropriate mounting of the input devices is critical to functional operation for any user and requires a thorough clinical assessment to determine the best access point for the device. Some joysticks have a built-in handrest for stability, and the shape of the stick often can be changed to accommodate the body part that is being used to operate it. Not all control interfaces can be used with all EPW bases. Intellectual property issues and incompatibility issues between components and brands limits a clinician's ability to create a truly fully customizable device, which is another hurdle to advancements in this field. Software also must be updated frequently, which may require a secure digital (SD) card, a flash upgrade, or download via computer. Some systems, when taken "off the shelf" have factory settings, and a programmer or SD card may be needed to modify the device for a particular user. On the other hand, some systems are "plug and play," which means that some of the modules can be recognized and programmed automatically.

PROGRAMMING

Many different joystick parameters can be programmed or customized. Usually a separate programming device is used to program these features, but some parameters can be programmed through the display on the input device itself. In other cases, programming files can be transferred by mini-USB or memory stick. Some devices may allow memory back-up of a program for later use. This feature may be particularly important for clinicians who spend a great deal of time creating a custom program and want to use it for similar clients or tweak it later for the same clients. Occasionally, a new programming device may be needed if the control interface technology changes substantially. If an input device is not programmed appropriately, the device may be difficult to control, which could result in the client appearing to fail an initial assessment for power mobility, an unsafe driving condition, or fatigue during use.

Some programming devices also allow programming of parameters during use of the EPW so they can be tested in real time. Diagnostics may be available that can help the programmer troubleshoot errors. Parameters such as the wheelchair speed or angle of seat tilt sometimes can be monitored in real time.

Several different parameters can be programmed. Changing torque can provide more power at lower speeds. Sensitivity and acceleration also can be set, which controls how quickly the EPW responds to the user input. Some manufacturers refer to changing the sensitivity as "tremor damping"; however, this use of the term does not refer to filtering a specific frequency of movement. The dead zone (also sometimes called the deadband or neutral zone) is the distance through which the joystick can be moved but for which no EPW output is generated. Some models offer an alternate mode in which the EPW's other features, such as a communication device, can be used but the chair is disabled from driving mode. Another difference among interfaces is the tracking technology, which is used to reduce the compensatory movements a user must make, such as for caster alignment after making a turn.

DISPLAY AND ACCESS METHODS

The joystick display may be in color or black and white, and some are backlit. Generally, several different languages are supported and font or style can be changed. The display screen on some models is difficult to view for individuals with low vision. Some models display pictures or symbols, which can be helpful for clients who cannot read or have low vision. Audible displays are not yet conventionally available. Some models also have clocks, odometers, or auxiliary modes for storage and display of image files such as photos or object images, which clients may desire not only for "leisure" but also to assist with communication.

ADDITIONAL FEATURES

Various buttons, dials, and toggle switches may allow the user to switch modes, shortcut to a different function, control power or speed, access different profiles or power seat functions, or allow the joystick to operate as either a proportional control or a switch. Additional switch jacks may be available to allow additional switches to be added. Newer models may contain an infrared output signal that can control end devices such as televisions or telephones, X-10 control, which allows for control of some appliances, or Bluetooth to control an on-screen keyboard or full, "un-tethered" mouse control.

THE FUTURE OF JOYSTICK TECHNOLOGY

Isometric controllers for power mobility devices are not yet commercially available but are emerging as an alternative input device with much promise, especially for users with spasticity or complex movement disorders.[10] Isometric joysticks (IJs), as opposed to proportional joysticks, are noncompliant devices that sense force exerted on them; they do not change position perceptively when a subject applies force. An automobile brake pedal is an example of an isometric control. Once the brake engages, the pedal barely moves, but pressing harder with the foot proportionally increases the braking action. IJs can detect intent of motion by sensing force without the need for large displacements of the stick. That is, IJs require only the production of a simple, graded muscle force rather than the movement of multiple joints in the forearm and hand. Zhai et al[11] showed that although isometric controls are initially less intuitive to use, once mastered, they may be less fatiguing and produce smoother movement trajectories.

A few previous studies have compared IJs to MSJs and have shown that IJs have better accuracy in tasks such as computer target acquisition.[12–15] These studies also reported that because IJs lack damping features, they were very poor at attenuating unintentional movements, however. Thus, IJs were initially thought to be too sensitive in the face of movement disorders and even in normal physiologic tremor. For individuals already familiar with MSJs, it was thought that proportional control may still be the best option. Because of the desirable features of IJs that allow them to be operable by individuals with limitations in range of motion and motor control, however, our work has focused on improving these types of controls.

We have developed the Human Engineering Research Laboratories (HERL) IJ[16–21] (Fig. 1), which uses a programmable embedded microcontroller that provides some flexibility in how the user's input is interpreted. The HERL IJ has been tested in computer access tracking tasks and in real-world driving by subjects with and without upper limb impairments. In prior work, subjects who used the IJ had quicker trial times and fewer movement errors during forward and circular driving than when they used the MSJ.[17,18] To allow better customization of the IJ, Spaeth and colleagues[22] developed a force-sensing algorithm that allows an IJ to act as a simple isometric device and a variable-gain algorithm that allows an IJ to simulate many of the features of an MSJ.

For the purposes of our initial work[10] we wished to compare a customized IJ to standard of care (ie, a conventional joystick that consumers receive in the clinic). This study showed that if an IJ is customized appropriately, it has a short learning curve and its performance is on par with that of an MSJ. One drawback to isometric control is a user's tendency to overexert force on the device, much more than what is needed to control it. Our subsequent research showed that this is likely a factor that can be mediated with much less training than was once thought, however.[23]

Additional parameters are also emerging as ways to further customize joysticks.[10] When individuals exert force in forward, reverse, or side directions, their movement axes are sometimes biased away from 90-degree angles. We developed tuning software that can bias the axis angles to align directional movement of the chair with the intentional directions of the user. As mentioned previously, dead zones are also being used; however, current devices on the market allow limited customizability of dead zones, which are usually circular in shape. We have developed tuning software that allows for more complex dead zone shapes. We also have found that customizing gain is important for persons with impaired strength or motor control and that the

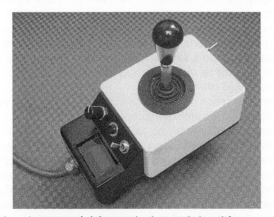

Fig. 1. Human engineering research laboratories isometric joystick.

mechanical template inside the joystick case that limits stick excursion may not be adequate to control force production in some situations, such as outdoor driving.[23] It may be necessary to customize the template or the maximum force on the joystick that should be recognized in each direction. These parameters can be programmed virtually for IJs although the sticks have no observable excursion. We have investigated various correction algorithms that can significantly decrease the error and variability in movement produced during joystick use.[24]

Some standard proportional joysticks contain low-pass filters, and some have built in damping features because of the nature of the rubber boot around the joystick post.[25] These filters allow damping of high frequencies such as those from environmental vibrations; however, low-pass filters are often inadequate for filtering some human unintentional movement, such as tremor. If the filter is set in the range of human tremor, inevitably some intentional human movements are also cancelled. One solution involves use of adaptive notch filters, which can dampen frequencies within a small range. This method has been useful for surgeons performing microsurgery[6] but has not always been sufficient when tested in individuals with disability and tremor.[25] Future research should focus on creating a "smart filter" that could continuously monitor the vibration frequencies from various sources and adjust accordingly. Previous research on dynamic coupling principles might also be applied to help overcome the effects of frequencies that are transmitted to the hand when EPWs are driven over rough terrain.[26]

We have collected large amounts of data from individuals with such diagnoses as athetoid and spastic cerebral palsy, multiple sclerosis, and various forms of tremor and from control subjects, and future work is aimed at comparing tuning parameters to identify overarching themes that are common to each diagnostic group. Identification of such parameters would allow for development of a series of default tuning parameters that could be available as software packages for particular diagnostic groups and could be further customized according to individual user needs.

One useful addition to joysticks may be haptic feedback in the form of vibration or audio signals that indicate when users have produced adequate force to about half of the template maximum or when they are exceeding the threshold needed to control it. This technology may allow gain to be adjusted and counteract some of the effects that are caused by limited proprioception. It may be worthwhile to consider using a joystick with variable compliance, such that the stiffness of the joystick varies along a spectrum from an MSJ to an IJ. As our control interfaces advance, so must the controllers. As more complex algorithms are developed, the need for more advanced controllers that can handle the mathematics will increase. Most current EPW controllers also ignore the wheelchair dynamics, making them unable to ensure the same performance with variations in loads or terrain. Cooper and colleagues[27] are developing an advanced controller based on a kinematic and dynamic model of a wheelchair (NIH R03 HD048465-01) that will be able to be augmented with advanced algorithms and accommodate a variety of interfaces.

Another worthwhile direction of future research is developing a device for recording the signals generated from control interfaces—not only joysticks but also other input devices such as switches. Currently, no technology allows clinicians to observe and analyze the signals generated by the user. Access to such data would allow clinicians to custom tune the interface, identify algorithms that could be applied (eg, tremor filter), identify targets for training (eg, excessive use of force on a joystick that results in arm fatigue), and identify efficacy of treatment on functional use of an interface (eg, medications or interventional injections for spasticity). We aim to design and develop a technology (I-Log) that can record and analyze input signals.

It is likely that in the future, people will be able to use a single device not only for their computers and wheelchair driving but also for environmental control of many target devices, such as garage doors, keyless entry, home lighting, heating and air conditioning thermostats, and a universal remote for home entertainment products, portable augmentative communication aids, and alternative methods of operating a mobile phone. The development of integrated controls would offer third party payers the option of funding single multifunctional controls rather than separate and would benefit the many users who lack funding for the different devices they may need in their everyday lives.

The overall goal of improving control interface technology is to allow individuals who might otherwise not be able to drive an EPW to have independent mobility and to give marginal drivers better control over their EPWs and other end devices. Developing better control interfaces that can be used despite motor impairments and movement disorders may improve computer access, mobility, community interaction, and ultimately quality of life for millions of individuals.[4]

REFERENCES

1. McNeil J. Household economic studies, current population reports P70-73, Americans with disabilities: Washington, DC: U.S. Census Bureau; 1997.
2. Available at: http://www.ap.buffalo.edu/idea/Anthro/spacerequirementsforwheeledmobility.htm. Accessed July 5, 2009.
3. Kaye H, Kang T, LaPlante M. Mobility device use in the United States. US department of education. National Institute on Disability and Rehabilitation Research Disability Statistics Report 2000;14:1–60.
4. Fehr L, Langbein W, Skaar S. Adequacy of power wheelchair control interfaces for persons with severe disabilities: a clinical survey. J Rehabil Res Dev 2000;37(3): 353–60.
5. Lifshitz S. Adaptive suppression of biodynamic interference in helmet-mounted displays and head teleoperation. J Guid Contr 1991;14:1173–80.
6. Riviere C, Rader R, Thakor N. Adaptive canceling of physiological tremor for improved precision in microsurgery. IEEE Trans Biomed Eng 1998;45(7):839–46.
7. Bootsma RJ, Marteniuk RG, MacKenzie CL, et al. The speed-accuracy trade-off in manual prehension: effects of movement amplitude, object size and object width on kinematic characteristics. Exp Brain Res 1994;98(3):535–41.
8. Riley P, Rosen M. Evaluating manual control devices for those with tremor disability. J Rehabil Res Dev 1987;24(2):99–110.
9. Lange M. New power wheelchair electronics: from overview to controlling external AT using drive control. International Seating Symposium Lecture. Orlando (FL), 2009.
10. Dicianno BE, Spaeth DM, Cooper RA, et al. Advancements in power wheelchair joystick technology: effects of isometric joysticks and signal conditioning on driving performance. Am J Phys Med Rehabil 2006;85(8):631–9.
11. Zhai S. Human performance in six degree of freedom input control [thesis]. Toronto: graduate department of industrial engineering, University of Toronto; 1995.
12. Rao RS, Seliktar R, Rahman T, et al. Evaluation of an isometric joystick as an interface device for children with CP. Arlington (VA): RESNA Press; 1997. p. 327–9.
13. Rao RS, Seliktar R, Rahman T. Evaluation of an isometric and a position joystick in a target acquisition task for individuals with cerebral palsy. IEEE Trans Rehabil Eng 2000;8(1):118–25.

14. Stewart H, Noble G, Seeger B. Isometric joystick: a study of control by adolescents and young adults with cerebral palsy. Aust Occup Ther J 1991;39(1):33–9.
15. Pellegrini N, Guillon B, Prigent H, et al. Optimization of power wheelchair control for patients with severe Duchenne muscular dystrophy. Neuromuscul Disord 2004;14(5):297–300.
16. Cooper R. Intelligent control of power wheelchairs. IEEE Eng Med Biol Mag 1995; 14(4):423–31.
17. Cooper R, Widman L, Jones D, et al. Force sensing control for electric powered wheelchairs. IEEE Trans Control Syst Tech 2000;8(1):112–7.
18. Cooper R, Jones D, Fitzgerald S, et al. Analysis of position and isometric joysticks for powered wheelchair driving. IEEE Trans Biomed Eng 2000;47(7):902–10.
19. Cooper R, Spaeth D, Jones D, et al. Comparison of virtual and real electric powered wheelchair driving using a position sensing joystick and an isometric joystick. Med Eng Phys 2002;24(10):703–8.
20. Jones D, Cooper R, Albright S, et al. Force sensors for control of power wheelchairs. J Rehabil Res Dev 1997;35(Suppl):262.
21. Jones DK, Albright S, Cooper RA, et al. Computerized tracking using force and position sensing joysticks. Arlington (VA): RESNA Press; 1998. p. 176–8.
22. Spaeth D. Evaluation of an isometric joystick with control enhancing algorithms for improved driving of electric powered wheelchairs [doctoral dissertation]. Pittsburgh (PA): department of rehabilitation science and technology, University of Pittsburgh; 2002.
23. Dicianno BE, Spaeth DM, Cooper RA, et al. Force control strategies while driving electric powered wheelchairs with isometric and movement-sensing joysticks. IEEE Trans Neural Syst Rehabil Eng 2007;15(1):144–50.
24. Mahajan HP, Waaser R, Dicianno BE, et al. Isometric joystick performance and error correction during computer access tasks. Presented at the proceedings of the 2009 RESNA conference. New Orleans (LA).
25. Dicianno BE, Sibenaller S, Kimmich C, et al. Joystick use for virtual power wheelchair driving in individuals with tremor: pilot study. J Rehabil Res Dev 2009;46(2): 269–75.
26. Kotovsky J, Rosen MJ. A wearable tremor-suppression orthosis. J Rehabil Res Dev 1998;35(4):373–87.
27. Wang H, Salatin B, Grindle GG, et al. Real-time slip detection and traction control of electrical powered wheelchairs. Presented at the 2009 RESNA conference. New Orleans (LA).

Advances in Lower-limb Prosthetic Technology

Justin Z. Laferrier, MSPT, OCS, SCS, ATP, CSCS[a,b,*], Robert Gailey, PhD, PT[c,d]

KEYWORDS

- Prosthesis • Ossesointegration • Microprocessor
- Silicone • Negative Pressure • Elastomer

Throughout history, most advances in technology and health care occur during wartime for tactical reasons and for the care of the wounded. The Civil War was the bloodiest war in the history of the United States and resulted in more than 30,000 Union soldiers and 40,000 Confederate soldiers losing their limbs in the 4 years between 1861 and 1865. In World War I (WWI), 4403 American soldiers suffered amputations. During World War II (WWII), there were 14,912 US service members with amputations and more than 1 million worldwide. Between 1961 and 1975, the Vietnam War resulted in 5283 amputations, with 1038 service members with multiple amputations.[1] Although survival rates are increasing due to advances in early battlefield medical care and improvements in combat vehicles and personal armor, this corresponds to an increased number of veterans who are living with a variety of severely disabling conditions including amputations.[2–5]

The younger age, higher functional status, and desire to return to these veterans to their premorbid level of function has led to an explosion of technological and rehabilitative advancements. During the last 30 years there have been far-reaching developments in battlefield care, amputation surgery, rehabilitation, and prosthetic technology, allowing individuals with limb loss to return to functional levels once believed improbable. The development of technology has increased the diversity of prosthetic components and fabrication techniques used in assisting people with limb loss to achieve maximum functional performance. The most recent advancements in surgery, socket design, and prosthetic components are now providing

[a] Department of Research and Development, Human Engineering Research Laboratories, VA Rehabilitation Research and Development Service and VA Pittsburgh Healthcare System, 7108 Highland Dr., BLDG 4, Pittsburgh, PA 15260-1260, USA
[b] Department of Rehabilitation Science and Technology, Forbes Tower 5044, University of Pittsburgh, Pittsburgh, PA 15260, USA
[c] Department of Research and Development, Functional Outcomes Research and Evaluation Center, VA Miami Health Care System, 1201 N.W. 16th Street, Miami, FL 33125, USA
[d] Department of Physical Therapy, University of Miami Miller School of Medicine, 5915 Ponce De Leon Blvd., Coral Gables, FL 33146-2435, USA
* Corresponding author. Human Engineering Research Laboratories, 7108 Highland Dr., BLDG 4, Pittsburgh, PA 15260-1260.
E-mail address: jzl15@pitt.edu (J.Z. Laferrier).

Phys Med Rehabil Clin N Am 21 (2010) 87–110
doi:10.1016/j.pmr.2009.08.003
1047-9651/09/$ – see front matter. Published by Elsevier Inc.

amputees with more options, such as better stability, improved comfort, increased responsiveness, and generally better performance, potentially with a reduction in stresses on the body.

The advances in prosthetic technology have been possible through the concerted efforts of multiple disciplines in response to the demands of our active-service members and veterans. The continued collaboration and expertise of a variety of disciplines, including orthopedic surgery, rehabilitation medicine, physical therapy, occupational therapy, biomedical engineering, prosthetics, and orthotics have narrowed the gap between what is imagined and what is real.

HISTORY

Prostheses were developed out of necessity to replace the function of lost limbs, and to return individuals to a productive state within the social structure. There is evidence for the use of prostheses from as early as the fifteenth century BC. One of the earliest examples of prosthetic usage was found in the eighteenth dynasty of ancient Egypt in the reign of Amenhotep II. A mummy on display in the Cairo Museum had his right great toe amputated and replaced with a prosthesis manufactured from leather and wood.[6]

During the Dark Ages, armorers developed prostheses for warriors who had been injured during combat. These early prosthetics were developed to allow soldiers to return to battle and hide deformity.[7] They were constructed with the most advanced materials available at the time; namely wood, leather, and metal. Unfortunately, these devices were clumsy and heavy, with little functional value. The first prosthetics that demonstrated a sound understanding of basic biomechanical functions were developed by French army barber-surgeon Ambroise Pare. Dr Pare designed upper- and lower-limb prostheses. His "Le Petit Lorrain", a mechanical hand operated by catches and springs, was worn in battle by a French Army captain, with limited success.[7]

Advances in medical science, such as the invention of the tourniquet, anesthesia, analeptics, blood clotting styptics, and disease-fighting drugs during the 1600s to the early 1800s improved amputation surgery and, subsequently, the function of prostheses. These advancements allowed surgeons to make residual limbs more functional, enabling prosthetists to make more usable prostheses.[7–9] In 1858, Dr Douglas Bly patented his "anatomic leg," which used a series of cords to control the ankle motions. A few years later J.E. Hanger, after losing his leg at the beginning of the Civil War in 1861, introduced an artificial foot that used rubber bumpers to control ankle motion. Dr Bly and Hanger competed fiercely for contracts with Walter Reed Medical Army Hospital to provide services to returning soldiers who lost limbs during the war. By 1863, the care of returning veterans led to numerous prosthetic patents, such as Dubois D. Parmelee's suction socket for arms and legs, which used pressure to suspend the sockets of lower and upper limb amputees. His work with suction sockets was abandoned some years later, but the fabrication of better, more functional, artificial limbs had begun. WWII produced the second largest number of amputees from war in the United States. Because of the vigorous protest by the returning veterans about the prosthetic devices they were receiving, in 1945 the National Academy of Sciences National Research Council, at the request of Norman Kirk, Surgeon General of the Army, established the Committee on Prosthetic Devices, later known as the Prosthetic Research Board.[1] During the following decade, numerous prosthetic devices were developed worldwide and became the standard of care for more than 50 years.

SURGERY
Amputation Surgery

Amputation surgery was once revered as a surgery for only the highly skilled surgeon; before the Civil War, only 500 of the 11,000 northern physicians and 27 of the 3000 southern physicians had performed surgery. The mortality rate from a primary amputation was 28%; if a second amputation was performed, it rose to 58%, and if an infection such as pyemia occurred, the mortality rate was more than 90%.[1] During WWI, the concept of debridement with antiseptic technique and delayed primary closure began to replace prophylactic amputation of war extremity injuries.[9]

Currently, newer body armor, protecting the head and thorax, and the immediate use of powerful antibiotics have led to a remarkable survival rate, with the wounded/dead ratio before body armor being 3:1, compared with the current figure from Iraq of 10:1. As a result of body armor, most trauma is to the exposed limbs, but, because of the outstanding medical triage of care, and better control of secondary complication due to infection, there are more injured in need of care.[1,4,9]

In January 2006, the American Association of Orthopedic Surgeons (AAOS) and the Orthopedic Trauma Association (OTA) cosponsored a symposium titled "Extremity war injuries: state of the art and future directions." Military and civilian orthopedic surgeons convened to define the current knowledge of the management of extremity war injuries. As of June 2009, more than 950 American service members have sustained injuries resulting in major limb loss.[10] Resuscitation of an injured soldier begins in the field with the use of special tourniquets, if necessary, to prevent exsanguination. Antibiotics are given early in the evacuation chain. Thorough irrigation and debridement are performed, usually within 2 hours of wounding. Redebridement is performed every 48 to 72 hours as the patient travels to higher echelons of care. All viable tissue is preserved. Fractures are immobilized with plaster or external fixation, and all wounds are left open before transport. Amputations are determined by the level of soft-tissue injury, not the level of fracture. Flaps of opportunity, split-thickness skin grafting, and free tissue transfers are frequently used for coverage.[11]

Osseointegration

Osseointegration was originally defined as a direct structural and functional connection between ordered living bone and the surface of a load-carrying implant.[12] During the 1950s, it had been shown by P.-I. Brånemark that chambers made of titanium could become permanently incorporated into bone, and that the 2 could not be separated without fracture.[13] Osseointegration has been used in several different situations, including dental implants, facial prostheses, and hearing aids. Osseointegration has recently been proposed to create an improved interface between a residual limb after amputation and a prosthetic limb. The main obstacles to prosthetic use are the problems encountered at the stump-socket interface. Poor socket fit can lead to instability, tissue damage, and pain, leading to the rejection of the prosthesis. Osseointegration integrates titanium implants into the medullary cavity of the bone; however, the implants extend from the bone, emerging through the skin to create an anchor for the prosthetic limb. This method bypasses skin contact with the prosthesis, reducing pain and tissue damage.

Another feature reported by the proponents of osseointegration is the improved ability to identify tactile stimuli transmitted through the prosthesis. This "osseoperception" has been studied in dentistry and orthopedics. A recent study conducted by Jacobs and colleagues[14] reported that bone-anchored prostheses yielded better perception than socket prostheses. This finding could prove invaluable to the amputee by improving kinesthetic awareness and increasing the overall responsiveness of limbs.

The technique has raised concerns, however, because it destroys the barrier function provided by skin, which prevents contamination of the internal environment by the external environment. When pathways develop around the implant through the soft tissues, infection and metal corrosion can result, which in turn can lead to additional loss of bone in residual limbs. One research focus at the Center for Restorative and Regenerative Medicine (CRRM; a collaborative research initiative that includes the Providence VA Medical Center, Brown University, Massachusetts Institute of Technology (MIT), and other VA hospitals including the Salt Lake VA in Utah) is to develop an environmental seal, integrating skin and dermis with the metal implant by promoting adhesion to, or growth into, porous prosthetic surfaces.

Limb Lengthening

A difficult socket fitting and biomechanical problem for traumatic amputees is short residual limbs. A person with a short residual limb after transfemoral amputation may have difficulty with prosthetic fitting because of the complexities of obtaining adequate suspension or pain from greater forces to the smaller surface of bony areas. Likewise, the higher amputation requires a heavier prosthesis, with reduced anatomic force production because of loss of femur and muscle tissue, which conversely decreases mobility and functional ability.

One alternative is to lengthen a short residual limb by surgically lengthening bone. This is accomplished by creating an osteotomy and separating the bone ends by gradual distraction, a process called distraction osteogenesis.[15–17] The history of surgical limb lengthening dates back to the turn of the twentieth century when Codivilla published the first article on the subject in 1905.[15] Limb lengthening has been performed using several techniques, each with its own complications and failures. A breakthrough came with a technique introduced by the Russian orthopedic surgeon Gavril Ilizarov in 1951. Ilizarov developed a procedure based on the biology of the bone and on the ability of the surrounding soft tissues to regenerate under tension; the technique involved an external fixator, the Ilizarov apparatus, structured as a modular ring.[16] Ilizarov's method of distraction osteogenesis still had several complications, but it was the safest and most effective method of the time.[17]

One complication of distraction osteogenesis is delayed bone healing, which leads to functional deficits such as contractures and muscle atrophy. Researchers at the CRRM have investigated techniques of accelerating or augmenting bone healing, including the use of biomimetic scaffolds, growth factors, demineralized bone matrix, gene therapy, and interaction with physical stimuli, such as mechanical, ultrasound, and electrical energy. These tissue engineering strategies hold the promise of accelerating the rate of elongation, maximizing the length of regenerated bone, and diminishing osteoporosis and refracture.[18]

SUSPENSION SLEEVES AND LINERS

Some of the most significant developments in recent years have occurred with the interface systems between the residual limb and the socket. The 2 most common interface systems are suspension sleeves and liners. The primary function of the suspension sleeve is to hold the socket in place or suspend the socket, whereas the liner is designed to provide padding or cushioning for the residuum. The properties of suspension sleeves and liners may be combined to create suspension liners, an interface system that provides suspension and padding. In the early days of prosthetic development, protection of the residual limb was achieved by lining the socket with animal fur.[19] Today, many variations of suspension sleeves and liners are available in a prefabricated form or they can be custom manufactured. There are numerous material variations available, such as closed-cell foam, urethanes, silicone elastomers, silicone gels, and many combinations of materials.

Silicone liners, and suspension systems and liners, have seen a steady increase in use since their introduction 1970s.[20,21] Several advantages have been reported with the use silicone liners, including improved socket interface, greater comfort, decreased pain, and greater skin protection.[22,23] Dasgupta[22] found an increase in distance walked with a prosthesis with a decrease in assistive device use and increased comfort in liner users. Datta and colleagues[23] reported that some transtibial amputees using silicone suspension experienced improved prosthetic control with a decrease in skin abrasion and irritation, and a reduction in phantom limb pain.

Elastomeric liners have been reported to have high coefficients of friction when in contact with skin, reducing localized skin tension and shear, and therefore decreasing slippage. Moreover, there is an increase in the total surface area contact of the residuum with the socket, leading to increased pressure distribution, compared with a conventional closed-cell foam material. It is reasoned that, with the high coefficient of friction (COF) with the skin, and low compressive stiffness, elastomeric liners experience minimal displacement relative to residual-limb skin during walking. This effect helps to maintain total contact, and is believed to reduce localized skin tension and shear, making the liner more comfortable to the amputee.[22]

Sanders and colleagues[24] compared the compressive stiffness, COF, shear stiffness, and tensile stiffness of 15 commonly prescribed elastomeric liner products with a skin-like material. In general, silicone gels had a lower compressive, shear, and tensile stiffness than did silicone elastomers. The difference between silicone elastomers and silicone gels is found in their cross-linking and fluid-retention properties. Silicone elastomers are extensively cross-linked and contain little free polydimethylsiloxane (PDMS) fluid, which allows them to retain their fluid under stress. Silicone gels have lightly cross-linked polysiloxane networks, swollen with PDMS fluid that causes them to bleed on loading.[25]

Materials with a high COF will allow the liner to "stick" to the skin better, therefore reducing localized shear stress in the form of slippage between the socket and residual limb, which improves fit during prolonged ambulation. This improvement is important for all amputees, but especially for those with weak or adherent tissue. Compressive stiffness should be considered based on the soft-tissue properties of the residual limb. An individual with a boney residual limb would benefit from a liner with a low compressive stiffness that would allow the residual limb to "sink" further into the liner and provide more cushioning. However, an individual with excessive soft tissue would gain a better sense of control from a liner with a high compressive stiffness.

Shear stiffness is another important material property to be considered with prosthetic liners. Low shear stiffness will allow the residual limb to sink further into the prosthetic socket whereas high shear stiffness will not. For the individual with the boney residual limb, a liner with low shear stiffness would allow a safe amount of movement between the residual limb and the socket during weight bearing. Tensile stiffness must also be considered. High tensile stiffness will improve suspension and fit by decreasing pistoning or slippage. As illustrated in the earlier examples, there are many factors to consider when selecting liners and sleeves for the individual with a lower-limb amputation. Through advances in material science, most amputees can be comfortably and functionally accommodated through comprehensive clinical evaluation by an experienced clinician.

SOCKET

The prosthetic socket is generally considered the most important component of a prosthesis. As a human-prosthesis interface, the socket should be designed properly to achieve satisfactory load transmission, stability, and efficient control for mobility.[26] The functionality of a socket extends beyond simply accommodating the load or forces of the anatomy of the residuum in a comfortable manner. For example, when an able-bodied person takes a step, signals from the central nervous system (CNS) stimulate the muscles to produce a biomechanically efficient gait pattern, and the body operates on a feed-forward system to adapt to obstacles and varied terrain. There is little conscious effort. When a person with limb loss takes a step, the musculature of the residual limb develops a compensatory contraction strategy to first create a closed kinetic chain environment within the socket for anatomic stability, and then a series of contractions to maintain prosthetic control during functional movements. The configuration of the socket's structural design has been reported to influence the length/tension ratio of muscle, the movement of the femur, and movement of the residual limb, all of which would affect gait and other gross functional movements.[26]

Another important consideration in socket design is the understanding that the skin and underlying soft tissue of the residual limb are not designed to sustain the range of pressure variations and repetitive forces encountered during prosthetic usage. As the understanding of residual limb anatomy and soft-tissue biomechanics have evolved, socket design has progressed to provide the most effective transfer of forces from the prosthesis through the residual limb to support prolonged activity without damaging soft tissue, skin, or producing discomfort.

Because each residual limb is unique and prone to change over time, some consider prosthetic socket design to be as much an art as it is a science. However, many within the profession believe that there is a need for the fabrication of well-fitting sockets that can be replicated and quantified.

With the development of computer-aided design and computer-aided manufacturing (CAD/CAM) technology, computational modeling has become a tool to generate a quantitative mathematical model of the residual limb during the time of imaging. Modifications can be made to the image, similar to the modifications made on a plaster positive mold. The computer models that are made and stored electronically by the clinician can be used as a reference for changes to the residual limb over time. Currently, more robust CAD/CAM systems are being developed that use computerized tomography (CT) scans or magnetic resonance imaging (MRI) in addition to the mechanical or laser input modeling used today. Furthermore, with additional computer-generated computations, values with respect to load transfer between the socket and the residual limb for the purpose of optimal socket design and objective evaluation of the fit may be incorporated as diagnostic tools.[26] Although the use of CAD/CAM technology has increased the repeatability of socket design, inconsistencies in the software and carving hardware continue to complicate the issue.[27]

The fluctuation in residual limb volume is typically greatest during the first year post-amputation as the limb heals from surgery and the muscle first atrophies, and then often hypertrophies, as prosthetic use and restoration of function increases. After the first year, residual limb volume stability varies among amputees. Some people have little change in volume, whereas others will fluctuate during the course of the day. Designing a socket shape and method of suspension for the potential short- and long-term changes in residual limb volume has long been a challenge for prosthetists.[27–29] During ambulation, the continual changes in forces through the prosthetic limb during stance and swing subjects the residual limb to a repetitive cycle of positive and negative pressures.[21,30–31] Positive pressures during the stance phase are believed to be the result of compression to the soft tissues, occluding the small lymph and blood vessels moving fluid out of the residual limb's periphery. Conversely, negative pressures are present within the socket during swing phase when the socket walls are drawn away from the residuum, allowing the same fluids to fill the small vessels of the limb's periphery. Most amputees experience some degree of volume change during activity, with some active amputees experiencing significant volume change (usually a reduction) that drastically alters socket fit and stability. To better manage, or even reduce, the consequential changes in limb volume, Carl Caspers developed the concept of using a vacuum to maintain a more constant environment within the socket. By using a small pump to create a vacuum, a more constant environment of negative pressure is produced by drawing the skin and soft tissues to the walls of the socket. Reducing the positive forces that occlude the vessels and allowing the vessels to move fluids through the soft tissues at a continual rate, a theoretical state of homeostasis is created within the residuum while in the socket. Conceptually, by maintaining a constant limb volume control throughout the day, there is a no longer a need for stump socks, and, because of the improved fit and socket suspension, the amputee would have better comfort. Board and colleagues[32] found that positive pressures during stance were significantly lower, and negative pressures during swing phase were significantly greater, with the vacuum-assisted socket. The vacuum-assisted socket has shifted the balance of this fluid movement from a net loss to a net gain. A reduction in positive pressure has been found to reduce skin irritation and tissue breakdown.[33,34] The increased negative pressure has been hypothesized to improve circulation within the residual limb, which increases nutrition to the tissues, facilitating improved health of the tissues or more rapid healing if a wound were present.[35]

The Harmony (Otto Bock), which was the first commercially available vacuum socket system, has a small pump attached to the prosthesis to maintain a 508-mm Hg (20 inches of mercury) environment of vacuum. Currently there are several other custom fabricated and commercially available negative-pressure or vacuum-assistive socket systems for clinicians to choose from. Because few scientific data are available regarding long-term use or the relationship of negative-pressure sockets in dysvascular residual limbs and other potentially at risk populations, patients fitted with these socket systems should be monitored carefully for adverse events.

Research is currently being conducted on sensors embedded in socket liners that will automatically adapt to fluctuations in body volume. Self-adjusting sockets could make the device more comfortable and prevent sores, bruises, and other complications. The leg socket will adjust to the changing diameter of the wearer's residual limb during the course of a day.

PROSTHETIC KNEES
The Microprocessor Knee

The development of microprocessor technology in prosthetics dates back to the late 1940s when Professor John Lyman at University of California Los Angeles introduced the first microprocessor prosthesis with integrated circuits for upper limb prosthetics. Upper limb amputees have commonly used myoelectric prosthetics, but not until the

1990s was microprocessor technology successfully transferred to lower-limb amputees. Microprocessor controls used in prosthetic knees use sensors to continuously monitor knee position, time, velocity, and forces and moments during ambulation. The microprocessor then calculates comparisons between steps, and routinely adjusts the resistance to control the mechanical knee. Microprocessor knee (MPK) units all work on the same principals and are different only in the medium used for cadence control and microprocessor speeds. The resistance for swing or stance is maintained by different cadence control mediums, depending on the manufacturer. The 3 cadence control media commonly used in MPKs are pneumatics, hydraulic fluid, and magnetorheological fluid. The sensors located within the knee unit or pylon determine the load or force placed through the prosthetic limb during stance. The microprocessor then adjusts the flow of fluid for the required knee stability, especially when walking down ramps or uneven terrain. As the amputee rolls over the prosthetic foot, the microprocessor senses that the limb is moving into swing and adjusts the fluid resistance to accommodate the speed of ambulation. Most MPKs use "step averaging" or adjust the knee resistance based on the last few steps, so, as the amputee walks slower or faster, the prosthetic knee flexion will be equal to that of the anatomic knee (**Table 1**).

Evidence suggests that there are minimal kinematic and kinetic differences,[36] and no reduction in the metabolic cost of ambulating between mechanical knees and MPK.[37–40] The major advantages seem to be increased stability when descending ramps, a decrease in stumbles and falls, with an increase in confidence during activities.[41]

The Power Knee II

The Power Knee is the only commercially available prosthetic knee that uses a motor to actively control knee position (**Fig. 1**). An array of onboard sensors relay a continuous stream of information to the microprocessor, which in turn sends output to the harmonic drive motor, powering the knee to the desired position. Technological advancements have allowed the second generation of the Power Knee to meet the requirements of many amputees for size, weight, and battery life.

The effects of powered knee joints on the gait of transfemoral, hip disarticulation, and hemipelvectomy amputees has not yet been documented; however, it has been observed that the knee motion in stance and swing phase can reduce the requirements for the use of hip power and other compensatory movements to control knee position. This reduction in turn may assist in the prevention of short- term injuries through falls and long-term repetitive stress on the intact joints and muscles. In addition, the use of knee power has been observed to enable ambulation in individuals who would be unsafe or unable to do so with a passive prosthesis.

The powered knee extension has also been seen to assist in a variety of movements typical in daily activities. Dynamic assistance during walking assists with limb advancement and prevention of knee buckling, and powered knee extension in stance can assistance the user when rising from a chair, walking up gradients or stairs, and if they stumble or slip.

FOOT AND ANKLE SYSTEMS

In the summer of 1945, Howard Eberhart, a military engineer, was setting up a research project on the landing gear of B-29s when his left leg was crushed beneath one of the testing trucks. The Naval Surgeon, Dr Verne Inman, who performed his amputation suggested that, as part of Eberhart's occupational therapy, he join another engineer,

Table 1
Commonly used MPK knee units

Product Name	Manufacturer	Cadence Control Medium	Processor Speed	Features	Reference
C-Leg	Otto Bock	Hydraulics	50 Hz	Offers several functional modes. The first 2 modes can be set for various activities. A new "standing" mode lets you lock the leg between 7 and 70°. Switch between modes with a wireless handheld control	http://www.ottobockus.com
Rheo	Ossur	Magnetorheological	1000 Hz	MR fluid moves between blades that, when charged, bind the MR fluid for resistance. The advantage is that with slow movements in confined quarters, there is no minimum resistance as with fluids that move through ports and cylinders	http://www.ossur.com
Adaptive	Blatchfords	Hybrid (hydraulic/pneumatic)	62.5 Hz	Two stepper motor valves operated by the microprocessor. The hydraulic part of the system controls stance, flexion, and terminal impact. The pneumatic part of the system controls swing phase and extension assistance	http://www.amputeeresource.org
Agility	Freedom	Hydraulics	1000 Hz	Actuator response time (ART), supported by advanced microprocessor programming, allows the knee to make nearly instantaneous adjustments to knee position and velocity. Increased water resistance	http://www.freedom-innovations.com

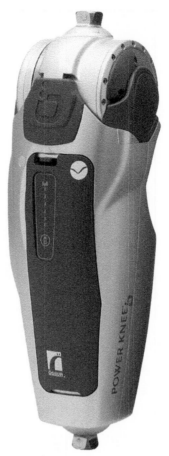

Fig. 1. The Power Knee. (*Courtesy of* Ossur Americas, www.ossur.com, Foothill Ranch, CA; with permission.)

Eugene Murphy, to help design a new prosthetic foot.[41,42] Together with a team of notable researchers, they made many contributions to the science of prosthetics, one of the most notable being the development the solid ankle cushioned heel (SACH) foot. The SACH foot would soon become the standard prosthetic foot for returning service members who had lost a lower limb, and today it continues to be the most commonly used foot worldwide.

It was not until the 1980s that any significant research examining prosthetic foot and ankle components was published. A review of the literature comparing prosthetic feet suggests that J-shaped energy storing and return (ESAR) feet are more beneficial than conventional prosthetic feet such as the SACH foot and many single-axis feet.[44–47] ESAR feet with a J-shaped pylon design seem to promote a faster walking speed. This may be because the Flex-Foot has repeatedly demonstrated the greatest peak dorsiflexion moment of any prosthetic foot.[43,47,48] The increased dorsiflexion occurs because of the larger moment arm created by the pylon and foot plate being constructed as a single section, permitting the body's weight to progress over the stationary foot and allowing the pylon to mimic the tibia's forward progression. Because of the greater dorsiflexion, there is greater movement of the center of pressure farther forward.[48,49] The ability of the center of pressure to move farther forward is also a product of the foot plate extending to the toe of the prosthetic foot. Because the body's weight passively produces the force that dorsiflexes the J-shaped foot, the amputee does not have to provide any additional muscular effort during single-limb support. As a result of the increased dorsiflexion and the extended foot plate, the rate of progression of the center of pressure moves faster from the rear foot to the forefoot at slow and fast walking speeds.[43,49]

The increase in walking speed with the Flex-Foot was found to be related to the significantly longer duration of swing with the sound limb. The greater swing time suggests that there is greater stability when standing on the Flex-Foot, because the ability to balance longer over the prosthetic foot during late stance permits the sound limb to take a slower and longer step.[50] Torburn and colleagues[43] found that the SACH and single-axis feet had a more rapid progression during terminal double-limb support or pre-swing than the Flex-Foot. Therefore, it seems that, when using prosthetic feet with shorter keels that do not extend to the toe, the amputee is "falling" off the end of the foot. Lehmann and colleagues[48] confirmed the falling onto the sound limb with the SACH foot, reporting a difference of aft shear impulse on the prosthetic side and the fore shear impulse on the sound foot, with the smallest shear values for the Flex-Foot and the greatest shear values for the SACH foot. The SACH feet also had a greater vertical force-loading peak, a greater plantar flexion moment, and an increased knee flexion moment on the sound limb, which may explain the greater transfer of loading to the sound limb during initial contact, due to the ineffective push-off on the prosthetic side. The inability to push off after foot flat in prosthetic feet with short keels or limited dynamic capabilities, the "drop-off" phenomenon becomes even more evident when amputees try to walk fast or run with conventional-keel prosthetic feet.[51] Consequently, some amputees may limit their walking speed in an effort to reduce the drop-off effect and lessen the forces placed on the sound limb.

Many of the new generation of prosthetic feet have taken into consideration prior research and anecdotal reports from the users. For example, most new prosthetic feet have several key elements in their design, such as a version of the J-shaped ankle or pylon, heel-to-toe foot plates, carbon graphite materials for greater energy return, split toe, or some mechanism for ankle mobility. In addition, many manufacturers have taken into consideration Hansen's[52] work on roll-over shape of the prosthetic foot, and the relation to the anatomic limb, when designing a foot. The SACH foot and the early generation of ESAR have been replaced at military hospitals by the new generation of prosthetic feet that provide maximal energy return, shock absorption, and quick response time. Most prosthetic feet worn by service members with lower-limb loss have the J-shape design with a heel-to-toe foot plate, and are made of carbon fiber.

The expectation is no longer just the ability to walk, but to have a prosthesis that allows the amputee to move quicker, and even run, the moment they need or want too. Moreover, people with lower-limb loss at an early age are at great risk for degenerative joint disease at the sound limb knee or hip, and back pain.[53,54] Although no cause and effect evidence currently exists for the increase incidence of secondary conditions related to the sound limb and spine, prosthetic feet that tend to reduce the vertical and shear forces to the sound limb, promote equal stance time, and promote overall symmetry between lower limbs may have longitudinal benefits that have not yet been realized.

The use of microprocessor, or bionic, technology in prosthetic feet has produced only 1 foot that is currently commercially available. There are several other feet currently in development with government funding, but only a small percentage of prosthetic devices mature from the stage of prototype development to become commercially viable products that are economically manufactured and clinically accepted. For this reason, it would not be prudent to describe in any detail those devices that are not currently available to the general public.

The Proprio Foot (Ossur) (**Fig. 2**) was introduced in 2006 as the first of the bionic, or microprocessor, prosthetic feet. The Proprio uses accelerometers to sample ankle motion at 1000 Hz, identifying specific events during the gait cycle, such as heel strike and toe off, to enable a timely response to variations in terrain and activity. The constant stream of signals to a microprocessor controls the linear actuator, which in turn produces ankle movements designed to allow a lightweight stepper motor to replicate the anatomic ankle. Benefits of the microprocessor-controlled ankle movements include the ability to identify slopes and stairs after a few steps, permitting active plantarflexion or dorsiflexion, enabling the prosthetic foot to be flat on the surface for better single limb balance over the prosthetic limb. During sitting, the user can hold the prosthetic foot off the ground briefly to activate active plantarflexion, which permits the foot to rest flat on the surface. When rising from a chair, a tap of the heel on the ground activates dorsiflexion so that the foot remains flat on the floor as the amputee rises out of the chair. The advantage of having both feet firmly on the surface is greater symmetry between the lower limbs regarding foot pressures and timing when rising from a chair.[55] For diabetic amputees at risk for foot ulcers, any reduction in abnormal plantar pressures would be beneficial. The Proprio seems to be more appropriate for community ambulators and people with limb loss who desire improved balance and a more natural appearance when walking and sitting.

Prosthetic Ankle/Foot Systems in Development

Promising technology in development includes The Power Foot and SPARKy. The Power Foot is a powered ankle-foot prosthesis designed by MIT research group

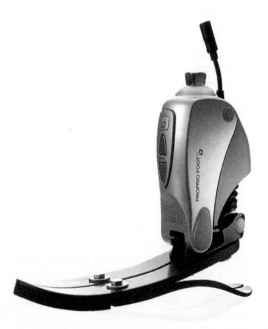

Fig. 2. The Proprio Foot. (*Courtesy of* Ossur Americas, www.ossur.com, Foothill Ranch, CA; with permission.)

Biomechatronics. It comprises a unidirectional spring, configured in parallel with a force-controllable actuator with series elasticity. The prosthesis is controlled to mimic the normal human ankle walking behavior[56] (**Fig. 3**). The Spring Ankle with Regenerative Kinetics (SPARKy) was designed by the Arizona State University Human Machine Integration Laboratory with team members from Arise Prosthetics, Robotics Group, Inc., and St. Louis University Human Performance Laboratory. SPARKy 3 is a 2 degrees of freedom (DOF) device incorporating active control of inversion and eversion, plantarflexion, and dorsiflexion. The design combines the power of regenerative kinetics, twin brushless direct current (DC) motors, and long-lasting rollerscrews (**Fig. 4**).[57]

SPORT PROSTHETIC COMPONENTS

There are few sport specific prosthetic feet, as most sports do not require a specialized prosthesis. A well-fitting everyday prosthesis that either offers the dynamic response or the required mobility will allow participation in most sports with few limitations. The source and degree of mobility available in prosthetic feet have changed greatly through the years. The motion no longer comes from only the ankle, the "split toe" found in some foot plates permits frontal motions, yet do not absorb as much elastic energy as the rubber bumpers typically used in ankle joints. The advantage is motion with limited loss of dynamic properties. The use of an elastomer pad is another design that has become popular, in which the hard rubber is sandwiched between a primary and a secondary foot plate. The frontal, and some transverse plane, ankle motion can be mimicked while maintaining foot dynamics.

The degree of motion required should be determined for the sport or recreational activities in which the amputee will participate. A golfer who plays on hilly courses may want a fairly large degree of motion in all planes to negotiate hills when walking, adopting a stance on uneven terrain, or to permit some rotation during the swing. A bowler may require a significant degree of sagittal plane movement, with dorsiflexion and plantarflexion, but a reduced frontal or transverse plane motion. Boaters, however, want to keep their prosthetic feet flat on the deck of the boat, but would prefer some motion at the ankle to absorb the rocking motion of the boat for better balance.

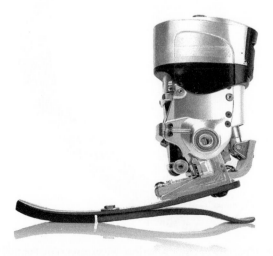

Fig. 3. The Power Foot. (*Courtesy of* Hugh Herr, PhD, Boston, MA.)

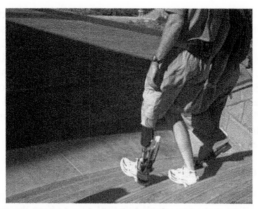

Fig. 4. SPARKy. (*Courtesy of* Thomas Sugar, PhD, Mesa, AZ.)

Although there has been much controversy in recent years, the current running prostheses do not match the human foot in terms of energy efficiency, and, due to having to reduce loading on their residual limb, amputees cannot compensate enough at the hip to match the total energy generated in a human limb.[58] In short, there is no advantage for an amputee using a sprinting or running prosthesis and, under most circumstances, they are still at a significant disadvantage.

The Cheetah (Ossur) (**Fig. 5**) was originally designed primarily for unilateral and bilateral transtibial amputations (TTAs), but recently it has also become the prosthetic foot of choice for transfemoral amputees. The Cheetah is plantar flexed and does not have a heel to keep sprinters on their toes. The distal posterior pylon is severely bowed, lengthening the foot plate to increase the moment arm for maximal deflection so

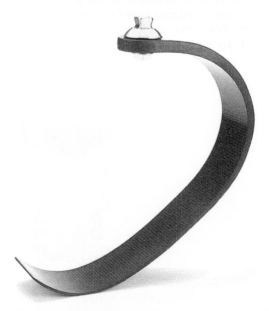

Fig. 5. The Cheetah. (*Courtesy of* Ossur Americas, www.ossur.com, Foothill Ranch, CA; with permission.)

that, as the material energy is returned, it will propel the athlete's limb into the acceleration phase of swing. Because of the forces applied to the foot during sprinting, the height of the prosthetic limb is typically taller, accommodating the altered height that occurs with compression through the Cheetah foot. The goal is to have the pelvis level during stance and to eliminate any trunk or head movement.

The Flex-Run (Ossur) (**Fig. 6**) is designed for long distance running or jogging. Because of the foot's exaggerated posterior bow shape, the vertical compliance is much greater than in any other running foot design. The Flex-Run can be fabricated for unilateral transtibial, transfemoral, and bilateral amputees who want to run longer distances. To take full advantage of this foot, the athlete lands on the prosthetic toe, extending the hip throughout the support phase, and achieving maximal deflection of the foot. As the prosthetic limb is about to enter the acceleration or swing phase, the effort of jogging is minimized by allowing the foot to initiate the upward motion and, as the spring effect reaches a peak, continuing the upward acceleration by flexing the hip as the limb moves into the float phase. There is no evidence to support reduced work of running with the Flex-Run; however, the "bouncy" sensation that amputee runners experience allows for a more rhythmic running pattern, helping to achieve a physiologic steady state.

The 3 preferred knee systems for transfemoral amputee athletes are the Mauch Swing'N'Stance (SNS)-type hydraulic knee, the S-type swing-only hydraulic knee, or the Otto Bock Modular Polycentric Axis Joint (3R55) with hydraulic swing phase control. The Mauch hydraulic cylinder uses a single-axis frame and offers athletes a wide range of resistance adjustment and stance control with the SNS-Type; however, most competitive athletes use the S-type swing only hydraulic unit because stance control is no longer necessary with athletes who are successful runners. The

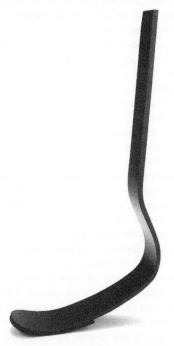

Fig. 6. The Flex-Run. (*Courtesy of* Ossur Americas, www.ossur.com, Foothill Ranch, CA; with permission.)

Otto Bock 3R55 Polycentric Axis Joint is a favorite for knee disarticulation athletes because of the instantaneous center-of-rotation capabilities of a 4-bar design providing increased toe clearance and greater stride symmetry.

Another accessory component that may be added to the prosthesis, or incorporated by the manufacturer into the foot design, is a shock absorber or rotator. These shock absorbers and rotators can be coupled with various foot designs to provide vertical shock absorption or long-axis rotation, respectively. Shock absorbers can help in reducing ground reaction forces during high impact activities. This reduction is of tremendous benefit for athletes who run long distances or participate in high-impact sports, and who would prefer to reduce the forces transmitted through the prosthesis. Conversely, they also absorb an undetermined amount energy that cannot be returned, thus reducing acceleration as the athlete moves into swing phase. As a result, many athletes who participate in high-speed sports may elect not to incorporate a shock absorber into their sport prosthesis.

Torsion adapters are often chosen by athletes who participate in multidirection sports such as tennis, or by individuals who generate rotation about the long axis, as with a golfer swinging a club. Theoretically, torsion adapters reduce the shear forces within the socket and permit greater rotation for improved performance. Once again, not all athletes who participate in tennis or golf find the added motion beneficial, because it can be difficult to control, or athletes may find the benefits not worth the additional weight and maintenance.

OUTCOMES

There is a dilemma with advanced prosthetic technology when trying to determine what the best prosthetic components are for each individual amputee. Common indictors such as materials, time of fabrication, complexity of design, and cost do not dictate the "best" components for each individual. Matching functional ability with the proper prosthetic components is the solution for optimizing physical performance. Most clinicians would suggest that coupling the correct prosthetic components for the appropriate level of function is one of the primary goals of the rehabilitation team. However, this goal is not easy to achieve.

At the root of the problem is the inability to define a successful prosthetic outcome. There are many interpretations for this common goal, from simply using the prosthesis "about an hour per day"[59] to "prosthetic use without external support on a daily basis."[60] There is no agreement about the threshold of "successful prosthetic outcome." The question is whether there is 1 threshold or many, as several investigators have advocated by virtue of offering multilevel functional scales and indices.

Currently in the United States, the only index of significant consequence to Medicare and managed care providers is the Durable Medial Equipment Regional Carrier (DMERC) K-levels or Medicare's Functional Classification Level (MFCL) index.[61] Its exceptional importance is solely because assignment to a particular level of function within this index determines the level of prosthetic care, and, consequently, the financial reimbursement a prosthetist will receive for the prosthetic services rendered. The functional level is determined by 3 determinants: (1) the patient's past medical history; (2) the patient's current condition, including the status of the residual limb and nature of other medical problems; and (3) the patient's desire to ambulate. In practice, the physician or prosthetist looks at health status or the number of comorbidities and asks the patient whether he or she wants to walk again. Currently, there is not 1 method of objective assessment used in determining the functional level of the lower-limb amputee; the traditional method of subjective clinical evaluation prevails.

There are 3 methods of outcomes measurement; self-report, professional report, and performance-based measures (**Table 2**). The preferred choice of assessment instrument is frequently a self-report, because of the ease of use and the ability to reflect the patient's perspective. In addition, there may be variances or inconsistencies with other methods of evaluation.[62] Professional report permits a rigid use of defined test item characteristics and can be performed quickly by the clinician, but the opportunity for subjectivity or bias is apparent if the evaluator is also the treating clinician. With these forms of assessment tools, the patient, family member, or clinician is asked to complete a questionnaire or similar type of survey, and a test score or descriptive profile is generated.

Physical performance can be the most objective measure, providing more accurate information of the patient's physical abilities. Weaknesses do apply, such as performance variation due to physical capacity on a given day, artificially created environments, and performance tasks that may illustrate only the patient's ability at a given point in their rehabilitation sequence, not at the base or final outcome. Few instruments in this category of testing have been designed specifically for the amputee. However, some have been applied to the amputee, with varying success.[45,63]

Although the K-level system for prescription remains a subjective exercise with no objective criterion, the 5-level index does adequately discriminate between the lower-limb amputee's levels of function. When performance-based measures such as 6-minute walk test, Amputee Mobility Predictor (AMP) or the self-report Amputee Activity Survey are applied statically, different scores were obtained between each of the K-levels.[45] As a result, the functional level of the amputee is well described and the ability to predict or determine the functional capabilities of the person with limb loss is possible. The AMP is the only functional assessment instrument that has demonstrated the ability to determine functional level or predict functional ability for amputees.[63,64,65]

The AMP has, however, been reported to have a ceiling effect for the highest level of amputee performance beyond the K-level classification. It seems that, when applied in the military amputee rehabilitation setting, where service members' physical performance is generally higher than that of civilians, the AMP has a ceiling effect.[66] As a result, there seems to be a need for a functional-outcomes measure for service members with limb loss or civilian amputees who are required to demonstrate a high level of physical functional ability for return to duty or employment, respectively.

The advantage of functional prediction tools is that higher-functioning prosthetic components could be prescribed before the start of prosthetic fabrication. The determination of the potential level of function would rest with the prescription decision makers, who would have much more objective data on which to base their decision. This determination would enable the value of each classification of prosthetic knee and foot component to be more easily depicted, and the ramifications to the amputee of the ultimate decision more easily understood in familiar terms. There would be a need to discriminate between the functional capabilities of the prosthetic components. To date, no means of objectively discriminating the functional values of different prosthetic feet or knees has been developed. Generally, it seems that the DMERC K-level classification of feet and knee components is based on cost or information provided by the manufacturers. Although this is most likely a flawed system, currently there is no objective measure to determine the functional value of a prosthetic component or to discriminate between components. The literature and evidence regarding the clinical use and prescription of prosthetic foot/ankle mechanisms was reviewed by clinical and scientific experts in April 2005. It was determined that prescription of prosthetic feet was a function

Table 2
The most notable self-report, professional report, and performance-based measures used with lower-limb amputees

Self-report	
Amputee activity survey	Day H. Amputee rehabilitation: finding a niche. Prosthet Orthot Int 1998;22:92–101
Sickness impact profile	Bergner M, Bobbitt R, Carter W, Gilson B. The Sickness Impact Profile: development and final revision of a health status measure. Med Care 1981;19:787–805
Reintegration to normal living	Wood-Dauphinee S, Opzoomer A, Williams J, et al. Assessment of global function: the reintegration to normal living index. Arch Phys Med Rehabil 1988;69:583–90
Prosthetic profile of the amputee	Gauthier-Gagnon C, Grise M. Prosthetic profile of the amputee: handbook of documents developed within the framework of a prosthetic follow-up study. Montreal Quebec, Canada: Ecole de Readaptation, Faculte de Medecine, Universite de Montreal, 1992
SF-36 health status profile	McHorney C, Ware J, Raczek A. The MOS 36-item short-form health survey (SF-36), II: psychometric and clinical tests of validity in measuring physical and mental health constructs. Med Care 1993;31:247–63
Prosthetic evaluation questionnaire	Legro M, Reiber G, Smith D, et al. Prosthetic evaluation questionnaire for persons with lower-limb amputations: assessing prosthesis-related quality of life. Arch Phys Med Rehabil 1998;79: 931–8
Orthotic Prosthetic User's Survey	Heinemann AW, Bode RK, O'Reilly C. Development and measurement properties of the Orthotics and Prosthetics Users' Survey (OPUS): a comprehensive set of clinical outcome measures. Prosthet Orthot Int 2003;27:191–206
Trinity Amputation and Prosthesis Experience Scales	Gallagher P, Maclachlan M. Development and psychometric evaluation of the Trinity Amputation and Prosthesis Experience Scales (TAPES). Rehabil Psychol 2000;45:130–55
Frenchay Activities Index	Franchignoni F, Brunelli S, Orlandini D, et al. Is the Rivermead Mobility Index a suitable outcome measure in lower-limb amputees? A psychometric validation study. J Rehabil Med 2003;35:141–4

Professional report	
Barthel Index	Mahoney F, Barthel D. Functional evaluation: the Barthel Index. Maryland State Med J 1965;14:61–5
Locomotor Capabilities Index	Gauthier-Gagnon C, Grise M-C, Lepage Y. The Locomotor Capabilities Index: content validity. J Rehabil Outcomes Measurement 1998;2(4):40–6
Functional Independence Measure	Davidoff G, Roth E, Haughton J, Ardner M. Cognitive dysfunction in spinal cord injury patients: sensitivity of functional independence measure subscales versus neuropsychologic assessment. Arch Phys Med Rehabil 1990;71:326–9
Physical performance instruments	
Six-minute walk	Cooper K. A means of assessing maximal oxygen uptake. JAMA 1968;203:201–4
Functional Ambulation Profile	Nelson R, Dm G, Everhart J, et al. Lower-extremity amputation in NIDDM: 12 year follow-up study in Pima Indians. Diabetes Care 1988;11:8–16
Two-minute walk	Butland R. Two-, six-, 12-minute walking tests in respiratory disease. Br Med J 1982;284:283–284
Timed get-up and go	Mathias S, Nayak USL, Isaacs B. Balance in elderly patients: the "get-up and go" test. Arch Phys Med Rehabil 1986;67:387–9
Berg Balance Measurement	Berg KO, Maki BE, Williams JI, et al. Clinical and laboratory measures of postural balance in an elderly population. Arch Phys Med Rehabil 1992;73:1073–80
Amputee Mobility Predictor	Gailey R, Roach K, Applegate B, Nash M. The Amputee Mobility Predictor (AMP): an instrument to assess determinants of the lower-limb amputee's ability to ambulate. Arch Phys Med Rehabil 2002;83:613–27

of clinical experience and subjective preference, rather than being based on the limited scientific evidence in support of energy storage and return prosthetic devices. The reviewers and experts agreed that there were promising examples of applicable and relevant research, but that there was simply insufficient evidence to use these results as drivers in the clinical decision-making process.[67]

In summary, the ability to define the functional abilities of the lower-limb amputee has been established with current K-level descriptors. There are currently performance-based functional-outcomes measures to assist clinicians in the prediction or determination of the functional capability of the lower-limb amputee. One self-report instrument has been found to predict and discriminate between functional K-levels. There is, however, a need for an instrument to determine the highest levels of physical performance of people with limb loss. There is no instrument or method of measure to discriminate the functional values of prosthetic feet and knees. Until such an objective measure is developed the ability to correctly match prosthetic components with the functional capabilities of the amputee will be a matter of subjective clinical judgment.

FUTURE DIRECTIONS

Research is being conducted across multiple disciplines to improve functionality of residual limb and lower-limb prosthetics. The CRRM is actively conducting research in several areas to improve the human-prosthesis interface. Options are being explored for augmentation of limb-lengthening techniques by using physical agents, such as electromagnetic fields (EMFs), to reduce distal bone loss to decrease the risk of fracture, and ultrasound to speed callus formation and decrease rehabilitation time. Work focused on improving the soft-tissue interface for osseointegration is being conducted to improve cell adhesion to the titanium implant, thereby creating an environmental seal restricting contamination of the bone and prosthesis in hopes of preventing infection, loosening, and subsequent bone loss.[18] Research is being conducted on sensors embedded in socket liners that will automatically adapt to fluctuations in body volume. The leg socket will adjust to the changing diameter of the wearer's residual limb during the course of a day, improving total contact and decreasing pain, pressure, and shear. Self-adjusting sockets could make the device more comfortable and prevent sores, bruises, and other complications.

Work is being conducted to investigate and improve the thermodynamics of the sock, liner, and socket layers. Elevated stump skin temperatures, and the accompanying thermal discomfort, are side effects of prosthesis use that may reduce amputee quality of life, particularly in hot or humid surroundings.[68] A study by Klute and colleagues[68] reported that the prescription of typical multilayer prostheses, constructed with the higher thermal conductivity materials, might reduce temperature-related discomfort in patients.

One of the main issues with most prosthetics is that they work as a passive system and do not replicate concentric muscle action. One possible solution to this problem may be found with artificial muscle technology (AMT). AMT refers to any device that expands or contracts with stimulation, performing functions similar to a biologic muscle. SRI International developed an electroactive polymer (EAP) that contracts like a muscle when voltage is applied. This electroactive polymer artificial muscle (EPAM) technology functions with high voltage at a low current, but there are also pneumatic muscles that operate with the force of pressurized air, and synthetic muscles that are powered by hydraulics.

SUMMARY

The boundaries once faced by individuals with amputations are quickly being overcome through biotechnology. Although there are currently no prosthetics capable of replicating anatomic function, there have been radical advancements in prosthetic technology, medical science, and rehabilitation in the past 30 years, vastly improving functional mobility and quality of life for individuals with lower-limb amputations. What once seemed impossible is rapidly becoming reality. The future seems limitless, and the replication of anatomic function now seems possible.

REFERENCES

1. Gailey R. As history repeats itself, unexpected developments move us forward: guest editorial. J Rehabil Res Dev 2007;44(4):7–14.
2. Eastridge BJ, Jenkins D, Flaherty S, et al. Trauma system development in a theater of war: experiences from Operation Iraqi Freedom and Operation Enduring Freedom. J Trauma 2006;61(6):1366–73.
3. Owens BD, Kragh JF Jr, Macaitis J, et al. Characterization of extremity wounds in Operation Iraqi Freedom and Operation Enduring Freedom. J Orthop Trauma 2007;21(4):254–7.
4. Zouris JM, Wade AL, Magno CP. Injury and illness casualty distributions among U.S. Army and Marine Corps personnel during Operation Iraqi Freedom. Mil Med 2008;173(3):247–52.
5. Pasquina P. Optimizing care for combat amputees: experiences at Walter Reed Army Medical Center. J Rehabil Res Dev 2004;3a:7–12.
6. Nerlich AG, Zink A. Ancient Egyptian prosthesis of the big toe. Lancet 2000; 356(9248):2176–9.
7. Thurston AJ. Pare and prosthetics: the early history of artificial limbs. ANZ J Surg 2007;77(12):1114–9.
8. Coco GA. A strange and blighted land: Gettysburg, the aftermath of a battle. Gettysburgh (PA): Thomas Publications; 1995.
9. Noe A. Extremity injury in war: a brief history. J Am Acad Orthop Surg 2006;14: S1–6.
10. US Armed Forces Amputee Patient Care Program. Walter Reed Army Medical Center Public Affairs Office. Available at: www.wramc.amedd.mil. Accessed June 01, 2009.
11. Gajewski D, Granville R. The United States Armed Forces Amputee Patient Care Program. J Am Acad Orthop Surg 2006;14:S183–7.
12. Branemark P-I, Hannson BO, Adell R, et al. Osseointegrated implants in the treatment of the edentulous jaw. Stockholm: Almqvist and Wiksell; 1977. p. 132.
13. Branemark P-I. Osseointegration and its experimental studies. J Prosthet Dent 1983;50:399–410.
14. Jacobs R, Branemark R, Olmarker K, et al. Evaluation of the psychophysical detection threshold level for vibrotactile and pressure stimulation of prosthetic limbs using bone anchorage or soft tissue support. Prosthet Orthot Int 2000;4: 133–42.
15. Codivilla A. On the means of lengthening in the lower limbs, the muscles, and tissues which are shortened through deformity. Am J Orthop Surg 2005;2:353.
16. Paley D. Problems, obstacles, and complications of limb lengthening by the Ilizarov technique. Clin Orthop Relat Res 1990;250:81–104.
17. Paley D. Current techniques of limb lengthening. J Pediatr Orthop 1988;8:73–92.

18. Aaron RK, Herr H, Ciombor D, et al. Horizons in prosthesis development for the restoration of limb function. J Am Acad Orthop Surg 2006;14(10):S198–204.
19. Wetz H, Gisbertz D. History of artificial limbs for the leg. Orthopade 2000;29(12): 1018–32.
20. Sonck WA, Cockrell JL, Koepke GH. Effect of liner materials on interface pressures in below-knees prostheses. Arch Phys Med Rehabil 1970;51:666–9.
21. Chino N, Pearson JR, Mikishko HA, et al. Negative pressures during swing phase in below-knee prostheses with rubber sleeve suspension. Arch Phys Med Rehabil 1975;56:22–6.
22. Dasgupta AK, McCluskie PJA, Patel VS, et al. The performance of the ICEROSS prosthesis amongst trans-tibial amputees with a special reference to the workplace- a preliminary study. Occup Med 1997;47:228–36.
23. Datta D, Vaidya SK, Howitt J, et al. Outcome of fitting an ICEROSS prosthesis: views of trans-tibial amputees. Prosthet Orthot Int 1996;20:111–5.
24. Sanders JE, Nicholson BS, Zachariah SG, et al. Testing of elastomeric liners used in limb prosthetics: classification of 15 products by mechanical performance. J Rehabil Res Dev 2004;41(2):175–86.
25. Silicone gel breast implants: the report of the independent review group. Cambridge: Jill Rodgers; c1998 July. Available at: http//www.silicone-review.gov.uk/silicone/. Accessed March 1, 2009.
26. Mak AF, Zhang M, Boone DA. State-of-the-art research in lower-limb biomechanics-socket interface: a review. J Rehabil Res Dev 2001;38(2):161–74.
27. Commean PK, Brunsden BS, Smith KE, et al. Below-knee residual limb shape change measurement and visualization. Arch Phys Med Rehabil 1998;79:772–82.
28. Commean PK, Smith KE, Cheverud JM, et al. Precision of surface measurements for below-knee residua. Arch Phys Med Rehabil 1996;77:477–86.
29. Fernie GR, Holliday PJ. Volume fluctuations in the residual limbs of lower limb amputees. Arch Phys Med Rehabil 1982;63:162–5.
30. Convery P, Buis AWP. Conventional patellar-tendon-bearing socket/stump interface dynamic pressure distributions recorded during the prosthetic stance phase of gait of a trans-tibial amputee. Prosthet Orthot Int 1998;22(3):193–8.
31. Sanders JE, Daly CH. Interface pressures and shear stresses: sagittal plane angular alignment effects in three trans-tibial amputee case studies. Prosthet Orthot Int 1999;23:21–9.
32. Board WJ, Street GM, Caspers C. A comparison of trans-tibial amputee suction and vacuum socket conditions. Prosthet Orthot Int 2001;25:202–9.
33. Goldstein B, Sanders JE. Skin response to repetitive mechanical stress: a new experimental model in pig. Arch Phys Med Rehabil 1998;79:265–72.
34. Kosiak M. Etiology of decubitus ulcers. Arch Phys Med Rehabil 1961;42:19–29.
35. Beil TL, Street GM, Covey SJ. Interface pressures during ambulation using suction and vacuum-assisted prosthetic sockets. J Rehabil Res Dev 2002; 39(6):693–700.
36. Segal AD, Orendurff MS, Klute GK, et al. Kinematic and kinetic comparisons of transfemoral amputee gait using C-Leg and Mauch SNS prosthetic knees. J Rehabil Res Dev 2006;43(7):857–70.
37. Orendurff MS, Segal AD, Klute GK, et al. Gait efficiency using the C-Leg. J Rehabil Res Dev 2006;43(2):239–46.
38. Williams RM, Turner AP, Orendurff M, et al. Does having a computerized prosthetic knee influence cognitive performance during amputee walking? Arch Phys Med Rehabil 2006;87(7):989–94.

39. Chin T, Machida K, Sawamura S, et al. Comparison of different microprocessor controlled knee joints on the energy consumption during walking in trans-femoral amputees: intelligent knee prosthesis (IP) versus C-leg. Prosthet Orthot Int 2006; 30(1):73–80.

40. Johansson JL, Sherrill DM, Riley PO, et al. A clinical comparison of variable-damping and mechanically passive prosthetic knee devices. Am J Phys Med Rehabil 2005;84(8):563–75.

41. Hafner BJ, Willingham LL, Buell NC, et al. Evaluation of function, performance, and preference as transfemoral amputees transition from mechanical to microprocessor control of the prosthetic knee. Arch Phys Med Rehabil 2007;88(2): 207–17.

42. Furman B. Progress in prosthetics. Washington, DC: Office of Vocational Research; 1962.

43. Torburn L, Perry J, Ayyappa E, et al. Below-knee amputee gait with dynamic elastic response prosthetic feet: a pilot study. J Rehabil Res Dev 1990;27:369–84.

44. Nielsen DH, Shurr DG, Golden JC, et al. Comparison of energy cost and gait efficiency during ambulation in below-knee amputees using different prosthetic feet. J Prosthet Orthot 1988;1:24–31.

45. Gailey R. Predictive outcome measures versus functional outcome measures in the lower limb amputee. J Prosthet Orthot 2006;15(1S):2–7.

46. Hafner B. Overview of outcome measures for the assessment of prosthetic foot and ankle components. J Prosthet Orthot 2006;18:105–12.

47. Barth DG, Schumacher L, Thomas SS. Gait analysis and energy cost of below-knee amputees wearing six different prosthetic feet. J Prosthet Orthot 1992;4: 63–75.

48. Lehmann JF, Price R, Boswell-Bessette S, et al. Comprehensive analysis of energy storing prosthetic feet: Flex-Foot and Seattle Foot Versus Standard SACH foot. Arch Phys Med Rehabil 1993;74:1225–31.

49. Schneider K, Hart T, Zernicke RF, et al. Dynamics of below-knee child amputee gait: SACH foot versus Flex Foot. J Biomech 1993;26:1191–204.

50. Macfarlane PA, Nielsen DH, Shurr DG, et al. Gait comparisons for below-knee amputees using a Flex-Foot versus a conventional prosthetic foot. J Prosthet Orthot 1991;3:150–61.

51. Wing DC, Hittenberger DA. Energy-storing prosthetic feet. Arch Phys Med Rehabil 1989;70:330–5.

52. Hansen AH, Childress DS, Knox EH. Prosthetic foot roll-over shapes with implications for alignment of trans-tibial prostheses. Prosthet Orthot Int 2000;24: 205–15.

53. Gailey R, Allen K, Castles J, et al. Review of secondary physical conditions associated with lower-limb amputation and long-term prosthetic use. J Rehabil Res Dev 2008;45(1):15–29.

54. Powers CM, Tourbum L, Perry J, et al. Influence of prosthetic foot design on sound limb loading in adults with unilateral below-knee amputations. Arch Phys Med Rehabil 1994;75:825–9.

55. Agrawal V, Gailey R, O'Toole C, et al. Symmetry in external work "SEW": a novel method of quantifying gait differences between prosthetic feet. Prosthet Orthot Int 2009;33(2):148–56.

56. Au SK, Herr H, Weber J, et al. Powered ankle-foot prosthesis for the improvement of amputee ambulation. Proceedings of the 29th Annual International Conference of the IEEE EMBS Cité Internationale, Lyon, France. August 23–26, 2007.

57. Hitt JK, Bellman R, Holgate M, et al. THE SPARKy (Spring Ankle with Regenerative Kinetics) Project: design and analysis of a robotic transtibial prosthesis with regenerative kinetics. Proceedings of the ASME 2007 International Design Engineering Technical Conferences & Computers and Information in Engineering Conference IDETC/CIE 2007. Las Vegas, Nevada, September 4–7, 2007.
58. Nolan L. Carbon fibre prostheses and running in amputees: a review. Foot Ankle Surg 2008;14:125–9.
59. Anderson A, Cummings V, Levine S, et al. The use of lower extremity prosthetic limbs by elderly patients. Arch Phys Med Rehabil 1967;48:533–8.
60. Moore T, Barron J, Hutchinson F, et al. Prosthetic usage following major lower extremity amputation. Clin Orthop 1989;238:219–24.
61. HCFA common procedure coding system HCPCS 2001. Washington, DC: US Government Printing Office; 2001. ch 5.3.
62. Siu A, Reuben D. Hierarchical measures of physical function in ambulatory geriatrics. J Am Geriatr Soc 1990;38:1113–9.
63. Condie E, Scott H, Treweek S. Lower limb prosthetic outcome measures: a review of the literature 1995 to 2005. J Prosthet Orthot 2006;18:13–45.
64. Gailey R, Roach K, Applegate B, et al. The amputee mobility predictor (AMP): an instrument to assess determinants of the lower limb amputee's ability to ambulate. Arch Phys Med Rehabil 2002;83:613–27.
65. Miller L, McCay J. Summary and conclusions from the Academy's Sixth State-of-the-Science Conference on lower limb prosthetic outcome measures. J Prosthet Orthot 2006;15(1S):51–60.
66. Pasquina P, Fitzpatrick K. The Walter Reed experience: current issues in the care of the traumatic amputee. J Prosthet Orthot 2006;15(1S):119–22.
67. Cummings DR, Kapp S. Prosthetic foot/ankle mechanisms. J Prosthet Orthot 2005;15(1S):2–7.
68. Klute GK, Rowe GI, Mamishev AV, et al. The thermal conductivity of prosthetic sockets and liners. Prosthet Orthot Int 2007;31(3):292–9.

Quality of Life Technology: The State of Personal Transportation

Linda van Roosmalen, PhD[a],*, Gregory J. Paquin, BSc[b],
Aaron M. Steinfeld, PhD[c]

KEYWORDS

- Transportation • Safety • Independence • Wheelchair
- Driving • Controls

For most of the United States population, community participation and basic activities of daily living depend on access to personal vehicular transportation. This culture of "automobility"[1] is likely to continue, and it seems that older persons will need to drive more in the future.[2] This trend is complicated by license loss among older drivers. The total drop in licenses among individuals between ages 60 and 84 years, for reasons other than death, was 1.8 million in 2000.[3,4]

As with the aging population, a related trend is seen in wheeled mobility use (eg, wheelchairs, scooters). In the past 30 years, a sixfold increase of wheeled mobility users has occurred among the United States population, and the total number is expected to reach 4.3 million by 2010.[5] Particularly relevant is that this "growth far exceeds the growth in the older population."[5] (p. 15)

Among individuals within this population, approximately a quarter drive and almost a third do not live in areas with public transit services. The Americans with Disabilities Act (ADA) requires that public transportation vehicles be accessible to the public, and requires demand responsive systems to be in place to serve individuals who have disabilities who are unable to use regular public transportation.[6] Lack of access to

Work presented in this manuscript is partially supported by Grant No. H133E060064 from the Department of Education and the National Institutes for Disability and Rehabilitation Research and the National Science Foundation under Grant No. EEC-0540865 and Grant No. EEC-0552351.

[a] Department of Rehabilitation Science and Technology, University of Pittsburgh, 2310 Jane Street, Suite 1300, Pittsburgh, PA 15203, USA
[b] California Department of Rehabilitation, 9720 South Norwalk Boulevard, Santa Fe Spring, CA 90670, USA
[c] Robotics Institute, Carnegie Mellon University, 5000 Forbes Avenue, Pittsburgh, PA 15213, USA
* Corresponding author.
E-mail address: Lvanroos@pitt.edu (L. van Roosmalen).

Phys Med Rehabil Clin N Am 21 (2010) 111–125
doi:10.1016/j.pmr.2009.07.009
1047-9651/09/$ – see front matter © 2010 Elsevier Inc. All rights reserved.

pmr.theclinics.com

transportation is one of the most frequently cited problems for rural residents.[7] For individuals who have mobility limitations living in remote areas or areas that are not along the route of fixed route transit services, special arrangements must be made, such as with para transit services for which eligibility criteria exist.

For all individuals, including those who have disabilities and those who are elderly, access to the community is important for employment, socialization, health services, and the operation of households and businesses. A study by Gray and colleagues[8,9] indicates that transportation is a key barrier to community participation among individuals who have disabilities. The infrastructure in the United States is built around the widespread use of motor vehicles and public transportation systems. These include commuter rail systems and metro, fixed, and demand route transportation services that are commonly in place for those who cannot afford, are unable to operate, or choose not to use a personal motor vehicle. Projects are underway to produce autonomous vehicle that can drive themselves. Until these technologies are perfected, persons who have disabilities choosing to drive themselves in a personal vehicle will have to rely on their own abilities to control a vehicle.

Equipment and modifications currently available allow vehicle drivers to compensate for many physical limitations. Devices to assist disabled drivers have steadily improved since the time of President Roosevelt.

As with all changes in technology, the ability to produce and profit from sales of devices is paramount. The driving mobility industry is unique in that the volume of sales is significantly low, causing small businesses to be the major developing sector of the industry and resulting in the development of product concepts that only address a particular functional disability. The device or product to support the device may have worked well, but a change in the way a disability is treated, new materials to lessen the weight of a product, the availability of colors, or other technology changes may have made some company's product undesirable.

PRACTICES TO PROMOTE SAFE AND INDEPENDENT DRIVING
Clinical Considerations in Driving

In the United States, approximately 11,000 individuals experience a new spinal cord injury (SCI) per year and have varying numbers of disabilities from stroke, muscular dystrophy, ataxia, spina bifida, amputations, reduced upper extremities (traumatic and congenital absence), amyotropic lateral sclerosis (ALS), multiple sclerosis, spinal muscular atrophy, polio, arthrogryposis, osteogenesis imperfecta, rheumatoid arthritis, and various other illnesses.[10,11]

Each injury, ailment, disease, or disorder has a unique set of motor, sensory, and cognitive issues to be addressed for the person to be considered a safe and independent driver. Each condition may have some expected limitation, but the degree of disability generally varies among individuals.[12] For example, the difference in physical ability of a person who has an SCI can vary significantly depending on the level and complexity of the injury. Further complications can arise if the event that caused the SCI created a secondary effect through a traumatic brain injury (TBI). This impairment may not be noticed until the interactive cognitive skills of driving are required.[13]

The question that must be answered for any potential driver (teen/adult/mature) during a clinical evaluation is whether the driver processes pertinent, environmental traffic information in a timely manner, and executes appropriate and timely responses based on the perceptions of situations encountered. The best person to answer this question is a trained and Certified Driver Rehabilitation Specialist (CDRS). A CDRS is knowledgeable in the selection, use, and application of devices and methods to aid drivers who have disabilities. An unbiased perspective about what type of equipment will work best for a driver can have a huge impact on driver safety, the longevity of their driving career, the cost of the modifications, and the ability to maintain the equipment.

The paths to obtain a referral to a driving evaluation can vary. If the potential driver is a private payer, the vehicle modifier would recommend a local driver evaluation program. If a third-party payer is involved, the CDRS would recommend a driver evaluation program; if the third party is a government entity, the CDRS may have an evaluation program or a contract within one. Various government agencies, such as Veterans Administration, State offices of Vocational Rehabilitation, Workers Compensation Fund, Victims of Crime, Department of Aging, and other health-related departments, may help provide funding for the driver evaluation.

Often a team approach is used to best understand all the details involved in determining the appropriate equipment and training for a safe and independent driver. An occupational therapist will establish the physical and cognitive baseline of a potential driver and a driving instructor will safely guide the driver through basic vehicle functions and an on-the-road evaluation. A rehabilitation engineer will provide equipment and methods for the driver to compensate for any physical limitations. All team members may participate in each portion of the evaluation and in the selection of appropriate assistive driving devices, and in some cases these roles are performed by the same individual.

Most clinicians involved with driving assessments, equipment selection, and driver evaluations are members of the Association for Driver Rehabilitation Specialists (ADED).[14] In 2008, the ADED had approximately 576 members, of which 229 were CDRSs.[14] This number is small compared with the increased need for services to enable older individuals and those who have disabilities to drive. As part of the Quality of Life Technology Engineering Research Center Safe Driving Project, the University of South Florida and University of Pittsburgh are currently evaluating the use of a driving simulator to train individuals who have disabilities to use adaptive driving equipment in a simulated driving environment. Driving simulators have potential to assist in driving assessments because of their relatively low cost, ability to track driver learning, and ability to make instrumentation adjustments on the fly. Obviously, actual road driving remains a key component in the assessment process and when learning safe driving in the community.[14]

Functional Abilities

A battery of tests and assessments are administered to create a baseline from which the CDRS team can appraise safe driving potential. These tests do not necessarily conclude the client's driving potential; they establish which functional abilities the person has and the limitations that could pose a problem when driving. The client's ability to compensate for any deficit while behind the wheel is the true test of a driver's potential.[15] The standardized and nonstandardized tests and assessments to determine safe driving potential address the following factors[16]:

- *Vision and perception:* The client is administered standardized test to determine visual acuity and visual fields, color vision, depth perception, contrast sensitivity, processing time, visual tracking, and the ability to multitask. These tests help determine how well the client sees objects and if their perception of the location is correct.
- *Strength and range of motion:* Physical characteristics of the client are measured. For each limb, strength and active range of motion are determined for the ability to operate the primary controls of the vehicle. Head rotation for scanning traffic is

observed and documented. Other areas assessed include joint restrictions in neck and limbs, motor control, dexterity, and balance.

- *Reaction time to determine eye–limb coordination:* Several tests are given to gather information on the potential driver's ability to process visual information and react to it properly. Characteristics about the client's disability are noted to determine factors such as the progressive nature of the disability and if it will impact the choice of driving equipment.
- *Cognitive issues and confidence:* Other tests will provide information about the potential driver's understanding of road signs, ability to engage in more complex driving situations, and ability to multitask. Areas observed include memory, visual processing, visual perception, visual special skills, selective and divided attention, and executive skills.
- *Driving assessment process:* Once the clinical details of the driver have been established, the evaluation progresses to the vehicle assessment. Access to the vehicle is investigated, ranging from whether the driver is able to transfer from the outside of the vehicle to the driver seat, to how the driver adjusts to sitting in the wheelchair at the driver station. Numerous arrangements and adjustments within these extremes dictate the final scenario for access. Once access has been established and safety systems are in place (shoulder/lap belt), the driving controls are considered. The dominant hand is usually chosen for steering, but this may deviate if other factors or equipment are presented.
- *Driver evaluation:* The potential driver is progressively given control of the vehicle. Depending on the situation, the CDRS or driving instructor may begin with the client steering in a safe environment, such as a parking lot. Eventually, the evaluation will progress to have the client also operate the gas/brake controls. They will gradually proceed onto the streets and then to even greater traffic interaction. The potential driver will be exposed to turns, controlled intersections, light and heavy traffic, and confusing situations to test their ability to respond appropriately.
- *Flexibility to test suspected capabilities:* Occasionally the CDRS or driving instructor may observe a characteristic of the potential driver that indicates a lacking driving skill or a cognitive limitation. This deficiency may be the result of the client being a new driver with little experience on the road, or could indicate a larger issue that will require substantial understanding of the client's disability and the mobility equipment used to compensate for the disability.
- *Endurance issues:* Persons who have certain disabilities frequently have limitations caused by fatigue (eg, from muscular dystrophy, multiple sclerosis, or post-polio syndrome). A CDRS and driving instructor who understand a person's disability can observe if the driver is showing signs of tiredness or lack of concentration from fatigue or extreme temperature changes. Startle responses can also impact the client's safe driving and also should be evaluated, for example by traversing rumble strips and speed bumps.

VEHICLE SELECTION AND MODIFICATION

Vehicle modifications should preferably be done by vehicle modifiers who follow guidelines established by the National Mobility Equipment Dealers Association (NMEDA).[12] This organization is dedicated to broadening the opportunities for people who have disabilities to drive or be transported in vehicles modified with mobility equipment.[12] Many vehicles are available to drivers who have disabilities, and the array of types and sizes of cars and vans is almost unlimited. When minivans and full size vans are modified with a lowered floor, the accessibility to vehicles for a wheelchair user has an even greater application. Although the main purpose of lowering the minivan floor is to position the eyes of a driver in a wheelchair at the correct height relative to the windshield, another benefit is that an access ramp can be at a lesser slope for ease of ingress.

Depending on whether the driver uses a wheelchair and the type of vehicle (sedan, SUV, truck, van, or minivan) there are several ways and assistive technologies available to help individuals who have disabilities enter and exit the vehicle. For individuals who have minor limitations, a simple grab bar may be adequate. A swivel seat can be used for individuals who are unable to maintain balance while stepping into the vehicle.

When individuals are unable to independently and safely transfer from a wheelchair into a motor vehicle seat, a ramp or lift must be installed to help with boarding and exiting to allow the wheelchair to be positioned in the driver station. Ramp systems are becoming popular and are made to slide out from under the floor and fold out from the doorway.

Wheelchair lifts have been used for more than 30 years and have drastically changed the mobility of individuals who have disabilities, allowing wheelchair users to be independent and mobile. The impact of mobility on a person's well-being, including the ability to get out and about, interact with the community, and be gainfully employed are some of the major desires of a complete life and should not be underestimated. As one wheelchair lift customer in 1979 stated, "Without what you do...I wouldn't have a life."

Major changes have occurred recently in the national standards applied to the manufacturing and installation of wheelchair lifts for individual use. These changes address safety concerns by adding warning devices and vehicle interlocks to prevent the lift from improper and unsafe use.[17,18] Wheelchair users may encounter space constraints in their vehicle. A transfer seat base can be used to position the original equipment manufacturer (OEM) seat at a desired location to best facilitate a transfer. The transfer seat base typically mounts to the floor in the driver location and the OEM seat is bolted to a top plate. The device allows the seat to move forward and backward, up and down, and rotate to the right through the use of control switches.

Drivers who have disabilities would dock the wheelchair behind the seat and transfer. After the transfer is complete, users would operate the switches to position the seat for driving. Some makers of transfer seat bases have successfully crash tested their product, so the OEM seat belts can be attached to the seat (B&D Independence Inc., Mt. Carmel, Illinois). Technology developed by Freedom Sciences (Freedom Sciences LLC, Philadelphia, Pennsylvania) allows wheelchair-seated drivers to pull up to the side of the vehicle and transfer into a power seat that extends from the vehicle so that it is level with the driver's wheelchair seat. After the individual has transferred into the power seat, the wheelchair is (remotely) parked in a docking system at the back of the vehicle. This system can be useful for individuals using powered mobility devices and who have the ability to perform independent side-to-side transfers.

DRIVING CONTROLS
Primary Controls

Primary controls refer to the steering, accelerator, and brake controls of the vehicle. For a disabled driver, the wheel and pedals may need to be modified to allow for weakness or limited range of motion. The control inputs may need to be relocated to a position where they can be reached. Various interfaces are used to allow a driver to have a secure connection with the vehicle. These control interfaces range from a simple spinner knob, to a yoke and T-shaped device for drivers who have grip strength, to tri-pin arrangements to allow a secure hold for drivers who have minimal grip strength.

If a driver has sufficient upper-extremity range of motion and strength, they may be able to use mechanical devices to operate the gas/brake controls. Rods and levers can be positioned so the driver's hand can operate the pedals. Controls that use a motor to move the pedals are referred to as *powered controls*. The driver would operate a lever that would cause a motor to move the OEM pedals.

Another example of powered controls can be found in reduced-effort steering. The strength required to turn the steering wheel is generally reduced by 50% or 75%, which can help a driver who lacks strength in steering. In the event of engine failure (such as caused by a fan belt coming off), the steering pump would stop providing power steering and the driver would require substantial strength to turn the steering wheel. A separate pump used for backup would turn on when it senses low hydraulic pressure in the steering system. This pump would allow steering to remain operational at reduced effort long enough for the driver to pull over to a safe location. A steering backup system is also advisable for standard power steering systems for drivers who have enough strength for the OEM power steering but not enough to turn the steering wheel when the engine is off. Most devices that reduce the force needed to operate primary controls incorporate a backup system that would allow for continued reduced effort on vehicle controls when the engine fails to operate.

New advances in vehicle controls have allowed for electronic or computer interfaces to control the steering, gas, and brake. This approach can be accomplished with a two-handed system or, at the most extreme level, a joystick input. At this "drive-by-wire" stage, the operator and the vehicle have no direct link. This method incurs some degree of risk from the possibility of electrical system failure. If designed correctly, this is not as big of a concern as one might think. In fact, many commercial jets are "fly-by-wire" and have performed well. Drive-by-wire provides an opportunity to select from a wide array of control choices, including joysticks, levers, and small-diameter rotary inputs, thus permitting custom control designs appropriate for a driver's specific needs.

This drive-by-wire technology has not been fully optimized for use in mainstream vehicles, and inherent control issues with electronic interfaces and computer controls remain. The main areas are the lag or delay in response time and the absence of sensory feedback from the road from the lack of a closed-loop system. Because of these limitations, drivers must possess above-average cognitive skills, and the training requirements to use drive-by-wire are extensive.

Secondary Controls

The primary controls are used to drive the vehicle. The secondary controls are used to manage the vehicle and interact with the elements and other drivers on the road. Operating the turn signals or shifting the transmission are some of the necessities when driving, and are examples of secondary control functions. Secondary controls are classified into three modes: A, B, and C. Turn signals, the horn, high-beam headlights, and wash/wipe functions fall into the mode A control category that is used when the vehicle is moving. Mode B controls can be operated when the vehicle is stopped and under driver control. Examples of mode B controls include transmission shifting, ignition, and vehicle startup. Mode C controls are used when the vehicle is stopped and includes the door locks, radio, hazard flashers, heater/vent/air conditioner (HVAC), light controls, mirrors, parking brake, power seats, rear accessories (defogger), and child safety window locks. Many devices are available to accommodate disabled drivers, and controls can be positioned to be operated by the elbow, by a free finger, by a mouth stick, or through voice input.

Early vehicle conversions used existing OEM switches, and attached levers and extensions to allow drivers to reach the secondary controls. These adaptations can still be used reliably, but the design of the newer vehicles precludes some previously used applications. Currently, individuals who have higher levels of disabilities are on the road, requiring a more sophisticated system to allow independent control of secondary vehicle functions. Operating a single switch with the touch of a finger or bump of the elbow can trigger a microcomputer to signal the driver to select a function, and a second action of the switch will operate the selected function. The system must match the driver's ability and comfort level so it can be used reliably.[19]

WHEELCHAIRS USED AS SEATS IN MOTOR VEHICLES
Drivers Using Original Equipment Manufacturer Seating

If a person's disability has caused a minimal loss of strength and limited range of motion in only one or two limbs, many simple methods of vehicle controls can be used. These drivers can often use the existing (OEM) vehicle seat. The seat may be accessed from the driver door or from the inside area of a van or minivan. If a mobility device is used, such as a wheelchair, scooter, crutch, or walker, the driver must stow and secure the aid in a safe location. Driving from the OEM seat is a preferred method because the seat is designed and tested to meet Federal Motor Vehicle Safety Standards (FMVSS).[20] The seat also provides a stable platform to drive from and it is designed to work with the vehicle-mounted safety systems, such as the head and backrest, seatbelt system, and airbag system designed to protect drivers in the event of a motor vehicle accident.

Drivers Seated in Wheelchairs

Individuals who remain in their wheelchairs while driving can often not use the OEM seats because of their postural needs or inability to independently transfer in a safe and timely manner from their wheelchair seat onto the OEM seat surface. Because OEM seats are designed to withstand crash-level loading and are positioned to function optimally with the airbag system and the three-point safety restraint (seatbelt), individuals who stay seated in their wheelchairs are disadvantaged in several ways. First, their wheelchair may not be designed to function as a seat in a motor vehicle. Second, the occupant restraint system or seatbelt system does not always fit optimally around the driver's pelvis and upper torso because belts interfere with the wheelchair frame and armrests. Third, the airbag may be disconnected because of the selection and placement of primary vehicle controls.[21,22]

Furthermore, a wheelchair must have sufficient rigidity to provide a stable driving platform and have a way to be tightly secured in the driving position during normal driving conditions but also during a vehicle impact. Individuals who use a power wheelchair with tilt-in-space features may encounter additional issues when using their tilt system in the tight driver station or while driving.

Depending on the level of disability, a wheelchair-seated driver's primary control system may range from a highly sensitized to a simple mechanical lever. In a highly sensitized system, even a small movement of the secured wheelchair or seating system may translate into significant alterations in driving control positioning, causing difficulty in maintaining lane position.

When selecting a wheelchair to use as a seat in a motor vehicle, experts recommend choosing one that complies with RESNA WC4: 2009, Section 19.[23] Section 19 establishes design and performance requirements and test methods for complete wheelchairs that are used as seats in motor vehicles. Recently, RESNA WC-4: 2009, Section 20 was added to include design and performance requirements and test methods for seating systems that are designed to retrofit various wheelchair base frames.[24] The so-called WC19-compliant wheelchairs feature appropriate wheelchair battery retention during vehicle impact (powered wheelchairs only), a crashworthy seat surface, four easily identifiable anchor points to secure the wheelchair with a four-point tiedown system, and an attachment point on the wheelchair frame to anchor a crash-safe wheelchair-mounted pelvic belt.[23] Awareness of WC19-compliant wheelchairs among CDRSs is important for providing wheelchair-seated drivers with optimal (transit-safe) wheelchair seating while driving in a motor vehicles.[22]

Although a four-point belt-type tiedown system is the standard system to secure wheelchairs in motor vehicles,[25] these systems are primarily designed to be used by an assistant. Wheelchair users are typically unable to independently secure their wheelchair with a four-point tiedown system. Therefore, wheelchairs used by drivers in private vehicles are commonly secured with an automated lock-down system that allows for independent and automatic docking of the wheelchair to the vehicle floor. This docking-type securement secures the wheelchair in a specific position and prevents the wheelchair from moving more than a nominal distance in and around three axes. Several wheelchair tiedown and occupant restraint (WTORS) manufacturers (EZ-Lock, Permobil, Q'Straint, and Sure-Lock) have developed docking systems and matching brackets that attach to the bottom of a wheelchair. To ensure safe driving, docking-type securement systems must be dynamically tested to meet performance criteria described in SAE J2249 and ISO-10542 standards.[25,26]

To minimize excessive rider movement and limit a wheelchair-seated driver from impacting driving controls, the windshield, or other interior structures, the driver must be able to use the safety belt system (shoulder and lap belt) independently. For this system to be effective, belts should fit snugly across the pelvis, chest, and shoulder.[27–29] The van modifier and CDRS must communicate to make sure that the safety belt system is placed so that the wheelchair-seated driver can easily and independently enter the driver station, and that belts fit snugly across the driver's pelvis and upper torso.

Q'Straint, in collaboration with the Rehabilitation Engineering Research Center on Wheelchair Transportation Safety, is currently developing a system that provides wheelchair-seated drivers with independent and easier access to the seatbelt system. And for individuals whose armrests interfere with proper belt routing, the lap belt can be disengaged from the shoulder belt and positioned through the armrest for a more optimal fit. Easy belt positioning and proper fit are best achieved if the wheelchair chosen has an open-style armrest that allows the pelvic belt to lie close to the body for optimal positioning and fit. A closed or T-shaped armrest prevents an optimal pelvic belt fit and forces the belt over or against the armrests structure,[22] allowing the lap belt to slide over the abdomen, causing internal injury during a frontal impact.[30,31]

If the muscles supporting the lower or upper torso are not adequate to maintain proper body position during severe driving maneuvers, additional (lateral) supports should be used, such as a chest harness, lateral stabilizers, pelvic supports, or shoulder pads. These postural supports should be used in addition to, rather than instead of, the seatbelt system because most wheelchair-mounted belts have not been crash tested and some are even designed to break away from the wheelchair during a vehicle crash.

Research further indicates that wheelchair-seated drivers are often positioned close to the steering wheel to reach the vehicle's adaptive equipment.[21,22] In vehicle accidents in which the air bag deploys, severe injuries can occur, especially if the driver is not using a properly positioned seatbelt system. The National Highway Traffic Safety Administration, which sets standards for motor vehicles, allows certain exemptions and alterations to air bags for vehicles used by disabled drivers. Air bags may be disconnected depending on the make and model of the vehicle. However, when disconnecting or removing an airbag, the driver should use a well-fitted and well-positioned safety belt for protection.

Finally, OEM vehicle seats are equipped with a headrest to limit head movement, reducing the risk for neck injury during frontal and rear impact.[32–34] Guidelines for using postural support devices by wheelchair users during motor vehicle travel state that excessive rearward head and neck movement can be reduced with a wheelchair-mounted headrest. Although headrests may not be designed to withstand crash-level loading,[35–37] they can provide partial protection (against whiplash) if positioned close to the back of the head.[38]

SAFETY AND INFORMATION SYSTEMS

Risk for occupant injury can be directly minimized through the use of safety and informational systems onboard a vehicle. Several technologies are on the market and the horizon for individuals who have disabilities and those who are elderly to help them drive safely.

Navigation

For drivers who do not have difficulty with divided attention, the value of in-vehicle navigation may be an important feature because of reductions in confidence or ability to navigate in unfamiliar territory. If drivers acknowledge this difficulty, they only drive on familiar routes. Thus, in-vehicle navigation systems are becoming attractive to drivers as a means to compensate for poor or impaired way-finding abilities. This interest includes nondisabled drivers in a new or confusing area who are impaired by the unfamiliarity of the environment.

Collision Warning Systems

Collision warning systems (CWS) warn for potential collisions and have obvious benefit in the form of early warnings for drivers who have difficulty perceiving the road scene or have slow response times. The desire to reduce rear-end crashes is the motivation for these systems, because approximately 30% of all crashes, injuries, and property damage are of this type.[39] CWS and blind-spot detectors have been on the market but have mostly been installed on commercial vehicles, such as tractor-trailers.

Blind-spot detectors can benefit individuals who have limited head or neck range of motion. Most sensors only watch ahead of the car, but some include side-looking presence sensors to help with lane change maneuvers. Research systems capable of more complex side warning have been tested,[40] but these are far from getting to market because of the difficulty of tracking vehicles in two dimensions. In all of these cases, a user interface indicates to the driver when a collision is imminent, thus prompting corrective action by the driver.

Adaptive Cruise Control

When CWS is tied to the automobile's cruise control, the vehicle can automatically respond to front obstacles by releasing the accelerator, shifting to a lower gear, or activating the brakes. This system is referred to as *adaptive cruise control* (ACC).

This feature has the potential to help drivers who have a tendency to stop too late or have trouble maintaining an appropriate following distance. Currently, ACC is an option on some luxury cars and is available in some modern commercial trucks. Most of these systems are designed for highway speeds but systems are also available that operate all the way down to stop-and-go traffic. Although CWS and ACC will likely improve safety for the general public, certain design concerns exist regarding ease of use and legal liability. Therefore, most consumers in the United States will encounter ACC before CWS.

Proximity Sensors and Obstacle Avoidance

One technology that is particularly attractive to drivers who have limited neck motion is the parking aid. Parking aids include rear proximity sensors and other parking collision avoidance systems.[41] These systems typically use audible alerts or iconic displays on the dashboard to indicate that the driver is about to back into an object. Anecdotal evidence also shows that these systems reduce the use of mirrors and direct visual inspection among the general public, which is further complicated by the rather poor performance of some of these systems.[42] Nevertheless, rear camera systems are becoming increasingly common. More recently, automated parallel parking and docking alongside curbs[43] is becoming a market reality; drivers can now purchase a semi-autonomous parallel parking option for certain vehicles.

Driving Behavior and Feedback

Opportunities also exist to observe driver behavior and provide feedback. This system is already being done in fleet vehicles[44] and is starting to be used by the regular public. This monitoring and coaching is a delicate process; drivers may consider the loss of privacy to outweigh the benefits. Systems with poor user interaction models run the risk of being perceived as a nuisance. Research in drowsy-driver monitoring[45] suggests that driver coaching systems that use a "trusted advisor" interaction model can provide effective information in a manner that drivers will accept. Research on this that is specific to drivers with disabilities is underway.[46] Current technologies, such as OnStar, provide a means for drivers in need to obtain remote road assistance. This type of direct communication can be especially helpful to individuals who have disabilities who are in need of emergency assistance.

THE FUTURE IN PERSONAL TRANSPORTATION
Paradigm Shift

Two major technologic paradigm shifts will occur in the foreseeable future. First, the automotive industry is starting to see market penetration by intelligent transportation systems (ITS). A decade ago, experts believed it would be possible to move directly from vehicles operated by humans to fully automated vehicles. After initial successes,[47,48] it became clear that the technical, institutional, and societal barriers are too difficult to overcome all at once. Instead, an incremental approach became the new paradigm, and the incorporation of new vehicle capability is occurring at the component level. ITS has steadily evolved from research prototypes to successful commercial products. Examples include automatic crash notification, collision warning and avoidance, lane-keeping assistance, vision enhancement systems, driver monitoring, and in-vehicle navigation systems.

The Defense Advanced Research Projects Agency (DARPA) Urban Grand Challenge[49] showed that automated driving in non-highway settings is considerably closer to reality, thus prompting renewed calls for more rapid progress toward fully automated cars.[50] This, of course, would provide significant value to drivers who have significant disabilities.

The second major technologic paradigm shift is in response to the aging of the population, which is leading to a greater awareness within the automotive industry that improvements must be made in various areas.[51] The industry is also interested in quicker production cycles and reusable components. A component designed to support the needs of older drivers in one model line may also be used in a model line targeted at younger drivers. These factors combine to present incentives to embrace universal design, and this is supported by a recent "wish list" of research initiatives, applications, and system changes presented by the American Medical Association, which includes a call for improvements in vehicle design on this function: "Age-related changes in vision, cognition, and motor ability may affect an individual's ability to enter/egress a motor vehicle with ease...We encourage vehicle manufacturers to explore and implement enhancements in vehicle design that address and compensate for these physiologic changes"[52]

ITS and the trend toward reusable components are fundamentally changing the way cars work. Multifunction displays on the dashboard are now common, and factory-installed drive-by-wire is on the horizon. Vehicles are already on the market with no mechanical link between the accelerator and the engine. These trends provide key opportunities to reduce the cost of vehicle modification through standardized communication protocols.[53-55]

The research community has already started merging adaptive driving with ITS. For example, drive-by-wire products designed for the vehicle modification market were used by competitors in DARPA's recent automated vehicle competitions.[56]

Universal design is a system design approach that can minimize the cost of conversion vans. Vehicles designed for a wide range of users who have (or do not have) disabilities will provide easier means for modification. For example, some van companies are introducing vans that feature low floors in their base models. This low floor design allows for easy conversion for someone who uses a wheelchair and needs a lift or ramp.

Finally, the cost of modified vans and equipment range between $200 and $90,000 for a fully equipped vehicle. These adaptation costs are normally absorbed by third-party payers, such as insurance or State offices of Vocational Rehabilitation. Alternative funding sources (for individuals that may not work) also exist to get driving systems paid. Examples of these would be Workers Compensation Fund, The National Center for Victims of Crime, and the Department of Aging. Some nongovernment organizations also provide assistance to persons who have disabilities, such as Make-a-Wish Foundation of America, Polio Survivors Association, church groups, and private fundraisers.

SUMMARY

To ride safely in a vehicle, disabled drivers must use adaptive equipment and technology that is specific to their functional abilities. Furthermore, to minimize passenger and driver injury and damage from driving controls in the case of an accident, they must wear a well-positioned shoulder and lap belt that they can independently secure. For individuals who ride while seated in their wheelchair (and for unoccupied wheelchairs), the wheelchair must be safely secured to the vehicle floor during transportation to maintain a safe distance to driving controls during the ride and to ensure the wheelchair does not move during vehicle maneuvers.

Several aspects of driving and preparing for driving can cause a disabled driver discomfort or present unsafe conditions. These instances include difficulty boarding or exiting the vehicle; maneuvering inside the vehicle into the driver area; securing the wheelchair in the docking system; positioning, securing, or releasing the seatbelt; wearing the seatbelt; reaching or using the primary and secondary controls; and loss of balance while making a turn. A CDRS and NMEDA equipment dealer must be consulted to help adjust controls, replace components, and select alternative devices that meet the user's needs. Although personal vehicles may soon be standard equipped with drive-by-wire controls and safety information systems to enhance safe driving for all, communication among drivers and passengers, a CDRS evaluator, and a NMEDA equipment dealer remain key in assuring the safety and independence of individuals who have disabilities when riding motor vehicles.

REFERENCES

1. Edsworth R. Class conflict and cultural consensus: the making of a mass consumer society in Flint Michigan. New Brunswick, NJ: Rutgers University Press; 1987.
2. Schieber F. Beyond TRB 218: Older driver research since 1988 [report]. Transportation Research Board 1999.
3. Office of Highway Policy Information. Highway statistics 2000. Available at: http://www.fhwa.dot.gov/ohim/hs00. Accessed August 20, 2009.
4. US Census Bureau. Census 2000 gateway. Available at: http://www.census.gov/main/www/cen2000.html. Accessed February 25, 2009.
5. LaPlante MP. Demographics of wheeled mobility device users. In: Space requirements for wheeled mobility [workshop]. Center for Inclusive Design and Environmental Access. Buffalo, New York, October 9–11, 2003.
6. Americans with Disabilities Act of 1990 (PL 101-336), 104 United States Statutes at Large. Washington, DC: Government Printing Office; 1990. p. 327–8.
7. RTC: Rural. Ruralfacts: inequities in rural transportation. Available at: http://rtc.ruralinstitute.umt.edu/Trn/TrnInequitiesFact.htm. Accessed March 20, 2008.
8. Chaves E, Boninger M, Cooper R, et al. Assessing the influence of wheelchair technology on perception of participation in spinal cord injury. Arch Phys Med Rehabil 2004;85(11):1854–8.
9. Gray D, Hollingsworth H, Stark S, et al. Participation survey/mobility: psychometric properties of a measure of participation for people with mobility impairments and limitations. Arch Phys Med Rehabil 2006;87(2):189–97.
10. Harvard AB. Disabilities and their implications for driving. Long Beach, (CA): NMEDA; 2006.
11. DeVivo MJ, Go BK, Jackson AB. Overview of the national spinal cord injury statistical center database. J Spinal Cord Med 2002, Winter;25(4):335–8.
12. National Mobility Equipment Dealers Association. National Mobility Equipment Dealers Association Guidelines. Available at: http://www.nmeda.org/members/members-pdfs/nmeda_guidelines.pdf. Accessed August 4, 2009.
13. Davidoff GN, Roth EJ, Richards JS. Cognitive deficits in spinal cord injury: epidemiology and outcome. Arch Phys Med Rehabil 1992;72:275–84.
14. Association of Driver Rehabilitation Specialists. Available at: http://www.driver-ed.org/i4a/pages/index.cfm?pageid=1. Accessed August 4, 2009.
15. Simoes NF, Lindblom L. Driving with a spinal cord disorder. In: Lin VW, Cardenas DD, Cutter NC, et al, editors. Spinal cord medicine: principles and practice. 1st edition. New York: Demos Medical Publishing; 2003. p. 723–31.

16. French D, Hanson CS. Survey of driver rehabilitation programs. Am J Occup Ther 1999;53(4):394–7.
17. Department of Transportation. FMVSS 403: platform lift systems for motor vehicles. Available at: http://www.carsafetylawyer.com/resources/federal-motor-vehicle-safety-standards-fmvss. Accessed August 4, 2009.
18. Department of Transportation. FMVSS 404: platform lift installations in motor vehicles. Available at: http://www.carsafetylawyer.com/resources/federal-motor-vehicle-safety-standards-fmvss. Accessed August 4, 2009.
19. Society of Automotive Engineers. SAE J2388: secondary control modifications. Warrendale (PA): Society of Automotive Engineers; 2002.
20. Department of Transportation. FMVSS 207: seating systems. Available at: http://www.carsafetylawyer.com/resources/federal-motor-vehicle-safety-standards-fmvss. Accessed August 4, 2009.
21. van Roosmalen L, de Jongh I, Ritchie N, et al. Safety system and usability issues for wheelchair-seated drivers and passengers of private vehicles: a pilot study. In: RESNA annual conference. Washington, DC, June 29, 2008.
22. van Roosmalen, Lane LA. Driving with a disability—clinical and technical perspectives. In: International Seating Symposium. Orlando, FL, March 12, 2009.
23. RESNA. RESNA WC-4: 2009, Section 19: wheelchairs used as seats in motor vehicles—draft. Arlington, VA: American National Standards Institute (ANSI)/Rehabilitation Engineering Society of North America (RESNA); 2009.
24. RESNA. RESNA WC-4: 2009, Section 20: wheelchair seating systems for use in motor vehicles—draft. Arlington, VA: American National Standards Institute (ANSI)/Rehabilitation Engineering Society of North America (RESNA); 2009.
25. Society of Automotive Engineers. SAE J2249: wheelchair tiedowns and occupant restraint systems—surface vehicle recommended practice. Warrendale, PA: SAE; 1999.
26. International Standards Organization. ISO/DIS 10542-1: wheelchair tiedowns and occupant restraint systems: part 1-requirements and test methods. Geneva, Switzerland: International Standards Organization; 2001.
27. van Roosmalen L. Wheelchair integrated occupant restraint system feasibility in frontal impact. Rehabilitation Science and Technology. Pittsburgh, PA: University of Pittsburgh; 2001.
28. van Roosmalen L, Bertocci GE, Karg P, et al. Belt fit evaluation of fixed vehicle mounted shoulder restraint anchors across mixed occupant populations. RESNA annual conference. Minneapolis, MN: RESNA Press; June 26, 1998.
29. van Roosmalen L, de Jongh I. Potential solutions to improve the safety of wheelchair seated drivers and passengers in private vehicles. Baltimore, MD: IASTED; 2008.
30. Bertocci GE, Souza AL, Szobota S. The effects of wheelchair-seating stiffness and energy absorption on occupant frontal impact kinematics and submarining risk using computer simulation. J Rehabil Res Dev 2003;40(2):125–30.
31. Adomeit D, Heger A, SAE International Web site. Motion sequence criteria and design proposals for restraint devices in order to avoid unfavorable biomechanic conditions and submarining. Available at: http://www.sae.org/technical/papers/751146. Accessed August 3, 2009.
32. States JD, Balcerak JC, Williams JS, et al. SAE International Web site. Injury frequency and head restraint effectiveness in rear-end impact accidents. Available at: http://www.sae.org/technical/papers/720967. Accessed August 3, 2009.
33. Svensson MY, Lovsund P, Haland Y, et al. SAE International Web site. Rear-end collisions—a study of the influence of backrest properties on head-neck motion

using a new dummy neck. Available at: http://www.sae.org/technical/papers/930343. Accessed August 3, 2009.

34. Maher J. Report investigating the importance of head restraint positioning in reducing neck injury in rear impact. Accid Anal Prev 2000;32:299–305.

35. Fuhrman S. Pediatric wheelchair and headrest design guidelines and the effect of headrests on relative injury risk under rear impact conditions [dissertation]. Pittsburgh, PA: University of Pittsburgh; 2008.

36. Fuhrman S, Karg P, Bertocci G. Effect of wheelchair headrest use on pediatric head and neck injury risk outcomes during rear impact. Accid Anal Prev 2008; 40(4):1595–603.

37. Karg P, Sprigle S. Development of test methodologies for determining the safety of wheelchair headrest systems during vehicle transport. Development 1996; 33(3):290–304.

38. RERC on Wheelchair Transportation Safety. Guidelines for use of secondary postural support devices by wheelchair users during travel in motor vehicles. Pittsburgh, (PA): Rehabilitation Engineering Research Center on Wheelchair Transportation Safety; 2006.

39. Singh S. Driver attributes and rear-end crash involvement propensity [NHTSA report]. US Dept. of Transportation, National Highway Traffic Safety Administration, National Center for Statistics and Analysis, Advanced Research and Analysis. No. DOT HS 809 540. March 2003.

40. Steinfeld A, Duggins D, Gowdy J, et al. Development of the side component of the transit integrated collision warning system. Presented at the IEEE Intelligent Transportation Systems Conference. Washington, DC, October 3–6, 2004.

41. Ward N, Hirst S. An exploratory investigation of display information attributes of reverse/parking aids. International Journal of Vehicle Design 1998;19(1):41–9.

42. National Highway Traffic Safety Administration. Vehicle backover avoidance technology study, report to congress. Washington, DC: US Department of Transportation; 2006.

43. Langer D, Thorpe C. Range sensor based outdoor vehicle navigation, collision avoidance and parallel parking. Auton Robots 1995;2(2):147–61.

44. Eisenberg A. These back-seat drivers are moving up front. Available at: http://www.nytimes.com/2007/02/04/business/yourmoney/04novel.html?scp=2&sq=carchip&st=cse. Accessed February 25, 2009.

45. Ayoob E, Steinfeld A, Grace R. Identification of an "appropriate" drowsy driver detection interface for commercial vehicle operations. Proceedings of the Human Factors and Ergonomics Society 47th Annual Meeting, Santa Monica, California, October 13–17, 2003. Santa Monica, California: Human Factors and Ergonomics Society; 2003.

46. Quality of Life Technology Center. DriveCap. Available at: http://www.cmu.edu/qolt/Research/projects/drivecap.html. Accessed February 25, 2009.

47. Shlodover S. AHS Demo '97 "Complete Success." Available at: http://www.path.berkeley.edu/PATH/Intellimotion/intel63.pdf. Accessed August 3, 2009.

48. Thorpe C, Jochem T, Pomerleau D. The 1997 automated highway free agent demonstration. Available at: http://www.ri.cmu.edu/pub_files/pub2/thorpe_charles_1997_2/thorpe_charles_1997_2.pdf. Accessed August 3, 2009.

49. Defense Advanced Research Projects Agency. Urban challenge. Available at: http://www.darpa.mil/grandchallenge. Accessed February 25, 2009.

50. Bunkley. GM to show a vehicle that drives by itself. Available at: http://www.nytimes.com/2008/01/07/automobiles/07auto.html?_r=1. Accessed February 25, 2009.

51. Waller P. The older driver. Hum Factors 1991;33(5):499–505.
52. Wang CC, Konsinski CJ, Schwartzberg JG, et al. Physician's guide to assessing and counseling older drivers. Available at: http://www.nhtsa.dot.gov/people/injury/olddrive/physician_guide/PhysiciansGuide.pdf. Accessed August 3, 2009.
53. Steinfeld A. Accessibility and intelligent transportation systems. U.S. Department of Education, Interagency Committee on Disability Research (ICDR). Washington, DC, July 22, 2006.
54. Steinfeld A. Smart systems in personal transportation. In: Helal A, Mokhtari M, Abdulrazak B, editors. Technology for aging, disability, and independence (Volume II):computing and engineering design and applications. Hoboken, (NJ): John Wiley & Sons; 2008.
55. Steinfeld A, Steinfeld E. Universal design in automobiles. In: Preiser WFE, Ostroff E, editors. Universal design handbook. New York: McGraw-Hill; 2001.
56. Olsen S. The pit crews behind DARPA's robot race. Available at: http://news.cnet.com/The-pit-crews-behind-DARPAs-robot-race/2100-11389_3-6188813.html. Accessed February 25, 2009.

Hand-Cycling: An Active Form of Wheeled Mobility, Recreation, and Sports

F.J. Hettinga, PhD[a],*, L. Valent, PhD[b], W. Groen, MSc[c],
S. van Drongelen, PhD[d], S. de Groot, PdD[a,e], L.H.V. van der Woude, PhD[a]

KEYWORDS

- Optimal performance • Paralympics • Power balance
- Clinical performance • Mobility • Spinal cord injury

Given the limited work capacity of wheelchair users in general, the stress of hand-rim wheelchair mobility results in fatigue and local discomfort of the upper extremities with the possible risk of repetitive strain injuries.[1–3] Different experiments on lever- and crank-propelled wheelchairs have shown that alternative propulsion mechanisms (levers, hub cranks) are less straining and more efficient than hand rims.[4–8] Hand-cycling (or hand-biking) has been found to be especially efficient, as well as less straining, and has become very popular over the last decades both in industrialized[4,5,9,10] and developing countries[11,12] in daily life and sports. Physiologic benefits of hand-cycling have been demonstrated in people with a chronic disability and even in early rehabilitation.[4,9,13–20]

Both in daily life and Paralympic sports performance, hand-biking is an interesting mode of training and exercise with many practical benefits. For example, hand-biking is recommended to maintain physical fitness and prevent arteriosclerotic diseases.[9,17,18,21,22] Also, hand-bikers can easily take part in training sessions together with participants in such able-bodied cyclic sports as cycling and roller-skating. Crank-propelled tricycle wheelchairs (ie, hand cycles) have in particular demonstrated

[a] Centre for Human Movement Sciences, University Medical Centre Groningen, University of Groningen, Antonius Deusinglaan 1, Sector F; Building 3215, Room 0330, 9713AV Groningen, The Netherlands
[b] Heliomare Rehabilitation Research and Development, Wijk aan Zee, The Netherlands
[c] Faculty of Human Movement Sciences, Research Institute MOVE, VU University, Amsterdam, The Netherlands
[d] Swiss Paraplegic Research, Nottwil, Switzerland
[e] Duyvensz-Nagel Research Laboratory, Rehabilitation Centre Amsterdam, The Netherlands
* Corresponding author.
E-mail address: f.j.hettinga@med.umcg.nl (F.J. Hettinga).

Phys Med Rehabil Clin N Am 21 (2010) 127–140
doi:10.1016/j.pmr.2009.07.010
1047-9651/09/$ – see front matter © 2010 Elsevier Inc. All rights reserved.

pmr.theclinics.com

their important role in more extreme environmental conditions in daily life in many non-Western countries.[8,11] Such wheelchairs enable greater physiologic responses—expressed in higher peak power production, mechanical efficiency, and, thus, endurance capacity—compared with those from hand-rim propulsion.[4,7] Lower muscular strain in terms of muscle activation was seen[23] compared with hand-rim wheelchair propulsion. In addition, biomechanical studies—still few in number—have generated some understanding of the underlying mechanisms of the improved performance in hand-cycling, again compared with hand-rim wheelchair propulsion.[21,24–27] Compared to hand-rim wheelchairs, hand-cycle wheelchairs enable higher velocities over a longer duration at the same or even a lower physical strain due to the following factors: (1) a natural grip of the hands to a well-formed handle bar, with the arms moving within the visual field, mostly making a fully circular motion and without the need for coupling-uncoupling actions in hand-rim propulsion; (2) the use of cranks and levers that allow the use of all flexor and extensor muscles around the arm-shoulder joints to actively contribute to external work over the full motion cycle; the latter in contrast to hand-rim propulsion where the discontinuous motion allows active work only during 30% to 40% of the cycle.[4,7,9,13–15,20,24,27–30] The continuous power generation over the full cycle in hand-cycling is suggested to result in an increased gross mechanical efficiency for hand-cycling, which may be almost twice as high as that in hand-rim propulsion.[31–33] This leads to a larger range of mobility, making hand-cycling a suitable mode of transportation and exercise mode at the recreational level in daily life as well as in fascinating high-level sports. Hand-cycling is interesting for persons with disabilities ranging from single-leg amputation/paralysis to complete spinal cord injuries.

HISTORY AND HAND-CYCLE TECHNOLOGY

Already in 1655, Stephen Farfler (http://de.wikipedia.org/wiki/Stephan_Farfler), a watchmaker with paraplegia, built his own, mainly wooden, self-propelled three-wheeled arm-crank wheelchair. In the 1900s and particularly halfway into the twentieth century, solid, yet large and heavy asynchronous hand bikes without gears were used in Europe as transportation modes for persons with disabilities.[7,29,34] In the late 1980s, the first modern hand bikes for persons with lower-limb disabilities were developed for recreation and sports.[5,35] The development of lightweight ergonomic and efficient hand cycles was motivated by the increasing popularity of using the hand bike in a sports setting. Over the last decade, hand-biking in sports gained even more popularity, and was added as an event to the World Championships for the first time in 1998. In 2004, hand-biking appeared for the first time at the Paralympics in Athens (www.paralympics.org). Nowadays, Paralympics are closely associated with the "regular" Olympics and receive the accompanying media attention. It is thus expected that hand-biking and other Paralympic sports will increase even more in popularity in the coming years.

   A strong ergonomics approach and thus the use of modern technology and lightweight and innovative materials has led to the reintroduction of the synchronous hand cycle in the mid-1980s for outdoor recreational use,[5,9,10,15,16,25] where earlier types used asynchronous propulsion.[7,34] These early hand cycles not only followed rules of bicycle technology, but also mimicked the existing arm-crank systems that became common for upper-body exercise testing in exercise physiology and rehabilitation and showed the first physiologic benefits (higher efficiency and peak power output and lower submaximal physical strain) of full cyclic upper body exercise of asynchronous arm cranking as opposed to hand-rim propulsion.[36–40]

Disadvantages of the early hand cycles, such as weight, size, and limited maneuverability, have partly been overcome. The use of tracker or attach-unit systems (**Fig. 1**A), an add-on front-wheel crank unit fitted onto a conventional daily hand-rim wheelchair, has made the crank-propulsion mechanism more practical for mobility in daily outdoor life.

With the use of the "fifth wheel", the hand-rim wheelchair can be converted into a multigear-based hand cycle for daily use (www.doubleperformance.nl). Here, persons sit in a supine position, comparable to a hand-rim wheelchair seating position. As was shown in different experiments,[4] these hand cycles must be preferred in outdoor wheeling for longer distances over the hand-rim wheelchair. According to DoublePerformance, a hand-bike expertise center in the Netherlands and Belgium, hand bikes can be classified as shown in **Fig. 2**. All existing types of (three-wheeled) hand bikes are shown, classified according to whether they are powered by arms alone or by both arms and the trunk. Also, values for frontal area are given, which are important

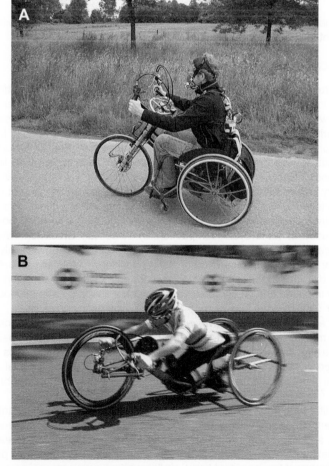

Fig.1. Different types of hand bikes. (A) A tracker system where an attach-unit with multiple gears and brakes is fixed to the common hand-rim wheelchair. (B) A Paralympic racing hand bike with the athlete in a kneeling position.

Classificationscheme Handbikes HEC							
AP	AP1	AP2	AP3	ATP	ATP1	ATP2	ATP3
Arm-Power				Arm-Trunk-Power			
wheelchair-sit	recumbent 60°	recumbent 30°	recumbent 0°	wheelchair-sit	car-seat	long-seat	knee-seat
upright	reclined	reclined	reclined	forward	forward	forward	forward
attach-unit	rigid frame	rigid frame	rigid frame	attach-unit	rigid frame	rigid frame	rigid frame
100%	62,6%	39,6%	33,3%	96,8%	82,8%	60,9%	60,3%
tour	tour	competition	competition	tour	tour	competition	competition
		HC-A,-B,-C1	HC-A,-B,-C1			HC-C1	HC-C2

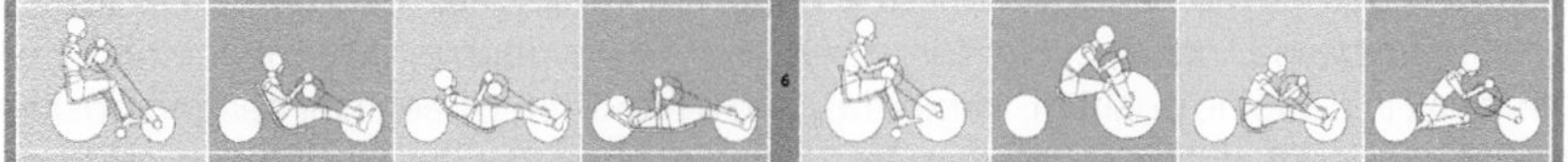

1=class handbike 2=propulsion-type 3=sitting-type 4=trunkposture 5=handbike-type 6=illustration 7=frontal area 8=handbike-use 9=competition-division © Double Performance • Handbike Expertise Centrum

Fig. 2. Classification of hand bikes according to whether they are powered by the arms alone or by the arms and trunk. Classification developed by Double Performance, a hand-bike expertise center in the Netherlands and Belgium. (*Data from* Double Performance BV, Gouda, The Netherlands; with permission.)

for aerodynamics as is described below. Two-wheeled hand cycles also exist today,[41] but have not been subject of experimental studies so far.

HAND-BIKE CONFIGURATION

In sports, frames with a low center of gravity have been developed to optimize aerodynamics in performance. In Paralympics, hand cycles are rigid-frame, three-wheeled (two rear and one front wheel) and propelled by the arms using pedals and a gearing system in front of the athlete (see **Fig. 1**B). Different hand-cycle configurations with different sitting postures are used (see **Fig. 2**), including those in which subjects lie completely supine (with low air friction, but with limited use of upper-body muscles), as well as those where subjects are in a kneeling position and actively involve the trunk function in propulsion (obviously at the cost of a higher air friction) (see **Fig. 2**). Those are all tricycle systems. A two-wheeled racer is also available (www.doubleperformance.nl). In the year 2000, the kneeling position was first introduced in hand-cycle competition by Kees van Breukelen (www.double performance.nl) and today competitors are classified in arm power–only or arm--trunk power competition, depending on sitting position.[33] Athletes compete in three functional divisions, men and women separated: lower-limb function partly or completely impaired and (1) complete loss of trunk stability, (2) a limited loss of trunk stability, or (3) a minimal loss of trunk stability (www.paralympics.org).

From an ergonomics perspective, wheeling and hand-cycle performance depends on vehicle mechanics, the hand-cycle–user interface, and the work capacity of the user/athlete (**Fig. 3**). Each of these components has different characteristics that affect performance in sports and daily life. Such a systematic ergonomics evaluation and subsequent optimization affect performance, freedom of mobility, and endurance.[7,34,42]

In daily life, where rolling resistance and internal friction are dominant resisting forces, maintenance and vehicle mechanics (mass, mass distribution, wheel/tire characteristics, and alignment) are critical. The flowchart (see **Fig. 3**) illustrates elegantly this complexity of performance-influencing factors within a combined physiologic and biomechanical framework of hand-cycling performance.

As stated above, in wheeled sports, different hand-cycle designs are used; important performance criteria include speed and time, but also performance capacity and

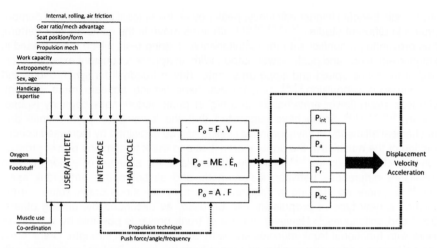

Fig. 3. Flowchart summarizing the ergonomics of the "hand-cycle–user combination," (ie, factors affecting performance and the subsequent constituents of performance). (*Adapted from* van der Woude LH, de Groot G, Hollander AP, et al. Wheelchair ergonomics and physiologic testing of prototypes. Ergonomics 1986;29(12):1561–73.)

ability level. With increasing velocity, good aerodynamics is increasingly important given the high velocities and their direct nonlinear effect on power requirement. Minimization of frontal area therefore is critical.[32] In such Olympic sports as cycling and speed skating, minimizing frontal plane area and thus lowering frictional losses are equally important.[43,44] Yet, aerodynamic design will affect the functional use of upper-body muscles.

In addition to aerodynamics and associated upper-body functions, other factors need to be considered when building a hand cycle for a specific user to improve comfort and mechanical efficiency. Zipfel and colleagues[31] mention crank alignment, seat angle and position relative to cranks, crank handle type, footrest alignment, wheel camber, wheel-base length, gear ratios, seat-to-floor height, materials, and components. Zipfel and colleagues[31] also mention current design problems of commercially available hand cycles: limited adjustability, poor trailing, poor aerodynamics, cables that get in the way of pedaling, minimal shock absorption, noncompatible components, gearing problems (which make it difficult to pedal uphill), difficulty with transfers, heaviness and bulkiness with transportation, and finally footrests dragging on the ground when making sharp turns. Developers have addressed most of these problems with a second-generation hand bike. In developing a third-generation hand bike, more advanced materials, finite element analysis software, and continued incorporation of bicycle technology and overall design innovation are necessary.[31] Further advancements clearly also require continued biomechanical and physiologic study to obtain evidence-based design guidelines.

SYNCHRONOUS VERSUS ASYNCHRONOUS

One of the issues that has received some research attention in hand-cycling is the propulsion mode. In contrast to hand cycles in the middle of the twentieth century, which were mainly based on mere bicycle technology, today's hand cycles all use a synchronous arm mode (ie, both hands propel in phase). This has considerable physiologic benefits (higher efficiency, peak power, lower local strain) as was demonstrated in different studies.[14,15,21,28,45] Both arms move in the same angular pattern, thus preventing a conflict with the simultaneous steering task, which is expressed in a higher-efficiency and peak-power output. With an apparent constant external workload at the same speed and slope on a motor-driven treadmill for synchronous and asynchronous propulsion,[21,45] synchronous hand-cycling appears more efficient, with less strain (lower arms/hands) and higher peak performance capacity (speed, power).[14,15,21,28,45] Some have suggested that the lower peak performance and mechanical efficiency in asynchronous cycling can be explained by increased cocontraction of the muscles in the upper extremities and trunk to combine power production with stable steering.[21,45] Indirectly, this explains the absence of systematic and consistent differences between synchronous and asynchronous arm-crank exercise,[46,47] where no steering is required. With a synchronous crank setup, "trunk power," a new type of propulsion, can be used, as described by, among others, Zipfel and colleagues.[31] However, he use of trunk power is possible by athletes or users with functional trunk muscles and with good abdominal strength. Crank arms can be longer, wider, and positioned further from the body. By leaning forward with each push, the mass of the upper body is used to add power to the stroke. Thus, not only arm, chest, and upper-back muscles are used, but also the abdominal muscles and the lower back contribute to propulsion.

CRANK LENGTH AND GEAR RATIO

Several aspects of the hand bike can be optimally adjusted to the athlete. The optimal crank length for arm-power hand cycles seems to be relatively short: Mechanical efficiency was found to be affected by crank length; a shorter crank (180 mm) was found to be more efficient than a longer crank (220 mm) at the same power output and cadence in well-trained hand-cyclists.[33] It is suggested that shorter cranks result in lower mechanical advantage and, consequently, require higher muscular forces, and that lower muscle contraction speeds result in a higher mechanical efficiency. The associated lower linear hand speed and smaller net displacement of the upper limb reduced internal work associated with movement while maintaining the constant external work. Furthermore, at submaximal exercise intensities, lower gear ratios are more efficient compared with higher gear ratios.[15,28,33]

GROSS EFFICIENCY AND FORCE EFFECTIVENESS

Gross mechanical efficiency is an important outcome measure of submaximal steady-state cyclic exercise, such as hand-cycling or hand-rim wheelchair propulsion/racing. It expresses task proficiency and is suggested to be sensitive to changes in the hand-cycle–user interface (gear ratio, seat orientation, crank orientation and length, hand bar design), but also expertise, training status, disability, and technique. Gross mechanical efficiency is defined as the ratio between external power output over total energy cost. Power output is often measured through a separate drag test when testing on a motor-driven treadmill,[4,15] but can also be measured under ambulant conditions with power sensors in the front-wheel axle (eg, Powertap[32]) or at the interface between the chain wheel and the cranks (eg, SRM[45]), which are both commercially available and can be used for monitoring training intensity. Power output has also been measured at the handle bar with a three-dimensional force sensing unit.[21] Total energy cost can be calculated by multiplying oxygen consumption, which is measured with stationary or ambulant units, with the oxygen equivalent, according to Garby and Astrup.[48]

The gross mechanical efficiency of a 27-year-old male athlete with paraplegia (a complete traumatic spinal cord injury) during marathon competition was 15.2% at a mean crank frequency of 78.6 rpm, with a maximum of 105 rpm.[9] Groen and colleagues[32] showed mean efficiencies of 16.0% ± 2.1% on treadmill and 18.8% ± 2.6% on track in elite hand-cyclists.[32] Values measured under laboratory conditions by Goosey-Tolfrey and colleagues[33] in trained athletes, with disabilities ranging from a single-leg amputation to a complete spinal cord injury (T4), were markedly higher (21.4% ± 3%) measured at 90 W compared with previous work (13.2% at 60 W and 14.4% at 80 W),[27] which is probably attributable to the level of experience and hand-bike configuration and optimization of the interface. Exercise intensity has also been found to influence gross and net efficiency in hand-cycling.[4,15,28,35,45] Also in cycling, exercise intensity influenced gross mechanical efficiency. This influence was partly due to higher relative cost of basal metabolism at lower intensities.[49,50] Other factors affecting gross efficiency in cycling, and thus possibly also in hand biking, are temperature,[51] pedal frequency,[49] and volume and intensity of training.[52] These are important enough to be taken into account.

In addition to the mechanical efficiency of hand-bike propulsion, the effectiveness of force application is an interesting factor to evaluate while measuring the technique benefits of synchronous hand-biking, expertise, or changes in the interfacing. Veeger and colleagues[53] introduced the fraction of effective force (FEF) to describe how effective the forces are applied to the hand rim in wheelchair propulsion. In hand-rim propulsion, FEF is relatively low, but optimal in terms of mechanical efficiency, despite the fact that it is close to 50% to 80%.[54] Previous research has shown that an effective force is applied only for a limited time during cycling.[55] Hand-cycling is also a cyclic movement but little is known about the force application. It is apparent that force is produced over the major part of the cycle using a push-and-pull phase of the arms and trunk, although initial research shows that the FEF may be relatively low.[21] This low FEF may be due to the same functional-anatomic constraints that apply in wheelchair propulsion.

The effectiveness of force application during submaximal synchronous hand-cycling was recently evaluated using an instrumented handle bar with six degrees of freedom to measure forces and torques in three dimensions (**Fig. 4**). For six subjects, a pattern of FEF was found showing an average FEF above 80% between −7° and 100° and between 205° and 310° of the crank rotation. Mean FEF was between 79% and 83% and significantly influenced by velocity (**Fig. 5**). The decline in FEF with velocity was also found in wheelchair propulsion and was probably related to less optimal coordination and direction of forces. Overall FEF was relatively high compared with wheelchair propulsion, and the effect of gravity should be taken into account to be able to judge the applied forces and joint torques. The latter can be done with a linked segment analysis. Besides gross mechanical efficiency and force effectiveness, other technique-related variables can be investigated to understand, evaluate, and optimize athletic performance and health benefits.

THE PARALYMPIC ATHLETE

In hand-bike athletes, only about 30% to 65% of the body muscle mass is involved in exercise compared with cycling, resulting in a significantly lower energy expenditure at the same percentage of peak VO_2. Peak VO_2 values can be as high as 30 to 40 mL/min/kg. Highly trained hand-cycle athletes can reach values of 50 mL/min/kg, where well-trained cyclists can reach values as high as 75–85 mL/min/kg.[16] Not much is known on values reached during competition, in real competitive settings.

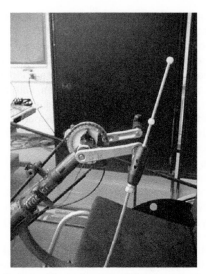

Fig. 4. Instrumented handle bar with six degrees of freedom to measure forces and torques in three dimensions.

Though limited to only one athlete, one study has been performed that gave insight into possibilities and dangers of a Paralympic athlete during competition.[9] Exercise-induced metabolic, pulmonary, cardiovascular, and energetic responses of a 27-year-old male athlete with a complete traumatic spinal cord injury at the level of the fourth thoracic vertebra (T4) were examined during a marathon. Mean oxygen uptake was 1580 mL/min, with a peak value of 2535 mL/min. Mean load during the marathon was 84.1 W, with a maximum of 211 W. Lactate accumulation (2.9 mmol during the race) was limited because of the lesion level and reduced muscle mass. If

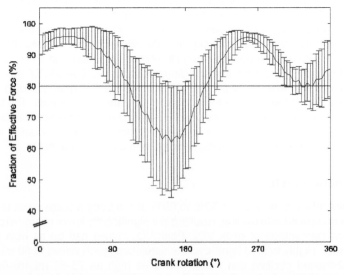

Fig. 5. Mean and standard deviation of fraction of effective force for hand-biking at 1.39 ms^{-1}.

hand-bike training is performed daily, current values for energy expenditure should conform to American College of Sports Medicine (ACSM) guidelines, which are aimed at reducing the risk for arteriosclerotic disease. Individuals with a spinal cord lesion are not able to sweat below the level of the lesion and have therefore a disturbed thermoregulation. Because of the disturbed thermoregulation, core temperature values were high since environmental temperature was not higher than 20°C to 22°C. In cycling, it was shown that time to exhaustion in a hot environment was inversely related to initial body temperature and rate of heat storage,[56] and the use of precooling strategies to postpone high body temperatures and optimize performance in the heat is advised. In arm-cranking exercise, wearing an ice vest before or during exercise has been shown to improve intermittent sprint performance in the heat for athletes with tetraplegia,[57] but the use of precooling methods might be particularly effective in hand-cycling endurance performance with a spinal cord injury.

The study by Abel and colleagues[9] examined physiologic variables, but did not take kinematic parameters into account. Though hand bikes have many benefits and are considered more efficient and less constraining than hand-rim wheelchairs, kinematic parameters during sprint performance (8-second sprints) in inexperienced handbikers suggest that high amplitudes and fast angular joint accelerations of the upper extremity were near or superior to the ergonomic recommendations generally advised.[25] To prevent overuse injuries, this suggestion should be taken into account in training schedules.

POWER BALANCE AND THE USE OF MODELS TO PREDICT PERFORMANCE

One way to study cyclic human (sports) performance is with the use of the power balance model (PBM) proposed by Van Ingen Schenau.[58] This model has enabled predictions of performance in various cyclic activities, such as cycling, running, and speed skating. Furthermore, the model has proven to be an effective tool for uncovering the performance-determining factors in speed skating,[45] as well as for finding optimal pacing strategies in track cycling.[44] The approach of the PBM appears to be highly appropriate in the study of hand-rim wheelchair propulsion,[7,30] although limited data on the applicability of the PBM to hand-cycling are available. Groen and colleagues[32] modeled performance in elite hand-cyclists under laboratory as well as track conditions using the PBM.

This would provide indicators of mechanical constraints (air friction, rolling friction) of submaximal as well as peak-performance hand-cycling and generate a better understanding of the concomitant metabolic cost and mechanical efficiency in elite hand-cycling in the laboratory but also on the racing track. To apply the PBM to elite hand-cycling, realistic values for power output and power losses on a range of regular velocities must be obtained on a treadmill and on a track in association to the physiologic responses under these conditions. Four elite Dutch hand-cyclists rode at three intensities (70%, 85%, and 100% of estimated peak race-power output) in a standardized instrumented hand cycle, both on a treadmill and on an indoor cycling track (250 m). Biomechanical and physiologic data were obtained:[32] VO_2 on the treadmill ranged from 1661 to 2825 mL·min^{-1} at 98 and 167 W respectively. VO_2 on the track ranged from 1356 to 2555 mL·min^{-1} at 102 and 168 W respectively. The empirically derived relationship between velocity (v) and power output (PO) (ie, the PBM) on the track was: $PO = 0.20v3 + 2.90v$ ($R^2 = 0.95$), where PO represents power output, v represent velocity, 0.20 represents the air friction constant, 2.90 represents the rolling friction force, and R^2 represents the multivariate coefficient of determination (**Fig. 6**).

The estimated power output by the model was replicated nicely on the treadmill with the help of a pulley system that provided an external force. This is illustrated by the linear regression $y = 0.97x - 2.4$ ($R^2 = 0.85$).

Mean gross mechanical efficiency during submaximal performance was 16.0% $\pm$ 2.1% on the treadmill and 18.8% $\pm$ 2.6% on the track ($P = .12$). It can be concluded that hand-cycling is a relatively efficient mode of propulsion with associated high metabolic demand at race velocities. The PBM enabled simulation of realistic power conditions on a treadmill. In addition, it proved useful in offering insight into the magnitude of power dissipation during elite hand-cycling.[32]

HAND-CYCLING IN CLINICAL REHABILITATION

During clinical rehabilitation, various aerobic exercise modes are available to improve the physical capacity of patients with spinal cord injury. In the past decade, the add-on hand cycle has become popular for mobility in the Netherlands and hand-cycling has become an integrated part of the rehabilitation program. Valent and colleagues[17,18] evaluated the effects of a structured hand-cycle training program on physical capacity in subjects with spinal cord injury. Twenty subjects followed hand-cycle training in addition to usual clinical rehabilitation and were compared with matched control subjects. The primary outcome was hand-rim wheelchair capacity as measured by peak power output (PO_{peak}), peak oxygen uptake (VO_{2peak}) and oxygen pulse. Secondary outcomes were arm muscle strength, pulmonary function, and hand-cycle capacity. Strong tendencies for improvement attributed to hand-cycle training were found in wheelchair capacity, reflected by PO_{peak} and oxygen pulse.[17,18] Shoulder exo- and endorotation and unilateral elbow flexion strength improved but pulmonary function did not. Hand-cycle capacity (PO_{peak}) improved, as evident in comparing pre- and posttest results **(Fig. 7)**. Additional hand-cycle training during clinical rehabilitation seems to show similar or slightly favorable results on fitness and muscle strength compared with regular care.[18]

Hand-cycling seems to be a safe exercise mode for persons with a spinal cord injury to build up fitness and muscle strength, showing similar or superior results over those associated with usual rehabilitation care. The small heterogeneous subject group and large variation in length of the training period may have affected the statistical power of this study and future research on hand-cycle training protocols is recommended.[17,18]

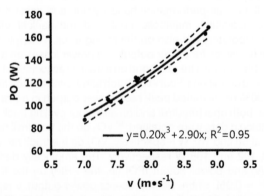

Fig. 6. The empirically derived relationship between velocity (v) and power output (PO) for hand-cycling.

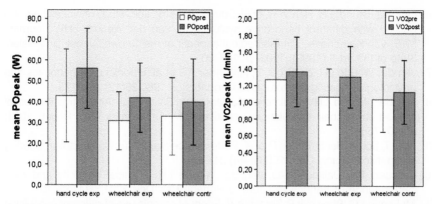

Fig. 7. Mean PO$_{peak}$ (*left*) and VO$_{2peak}$ (*right*) of the pretest (*white bars*) and the posttest (*gray bars*) for the hand-cycle test (experimental group only) and the wheelchair test experimental (exp) and control (contr) group.

Other problems associated with disability-associated inactivity are obesity and the higher risk of atherosclerosis due to obesity.[22] These should also be taken into account in the rehabilitation program. Knechtle and colleagues[16] studied the intensity levels at which hand-bike training reached the highest rate of fat oxidation. Well-trained hand-bike athletes have their highest fat oxidation at 55% VO$_{2peak\ hand-bike\ cycling}$ at a heart rate of 135 bpm $\pm$ 6 bpm compared with, for example, well-trained cyclists at 75% VO$_{2\ peak\ cycling}$ at a heart rate of 147 bpm $\pm$ 14 bpm.[16]

SUMMARY

Hand-cycling is a quickly growing sports discipline, an increasingly important recreational activity, and a means of daily transportation for persons with lower-limb impairment. Even in early rehabilitation, hand-cycle exercise appears profitable. Limited research has been conducted to date, although research interest is growing. In addition to evidence-based technological innovation, combined biomechanical and (psycho) physiologic research may lead to a further understanding of hand-cycling in both activities of daily living and sports performance.

REFERENCES

1. Boninger ML, Robertson RN, Wolff M, et al. Upper limb nerve entrapments in elite wheelchair racers. Am J Phys Med Rehabil 1996;75(3):170–6.
2. Nichols PJ, Norman PA, Ennis JR. Wheelchair user's shoulder? Shoulder pain in patients with spinal cord lesions. Scand J Rehabil Med 1979;11(1):29–32.
3. Boninger ML, Cooper RA, Shimada SD, et al. Shoulder and elbow motion during two speeds of wheelchair propulsion: a description using a local coordinate system. Spinal Cord 1998;36(6):418–26.
4. Dallmeijer AJ, Zentgraaff ID, Zijp NI, et al. Submaximal physical strain and peak performance in handcycling versus handrim wheelchair propulsion. Spinal Cord 2004;42(2):91–8.
5. Maki KC, Langbein WE, Reid-Lokos C. Energy cost and locomotive economy of handbike and rowcycle propulsion by persons with spinal cord injury. J Rehabil Res Dev 1995;32(2):170–8.

6. Oertel J, Brundig B, Henze W, et al. Spiroergometric field-study of wheelchair propulsion with different hand-drive systems. In: van der Woude, LHV, Hopman, MTE, van Kemenade, CH Biomedical aspects of manual wheelchair propulsion: State of the art II (1999). 1999. p. 187–90.

7. van der Woude LH, de Groot G, Hollander AP, et al. Wheelchair ergonomics and physiological testing of prototypes. Ergonomics 1986;29(12):1561–73.

8. van der Woude LHV, Dallmeijer AJ, Janssen TWJ, et al. Alternative modes of manual wheelchair ambulation - an overview. Am J Phys Med Rehab 2001; 80(10):765–77.

9. Abel T, Schneider S, Platen P, et al. Performance diagnostics in handbiking during competition. Spinal Cord 2006;44(4):211–6.

10. Janssen TW, Dallmeijer AJ, van der Woude LH. Physical capacity and race performance of handcycle users. J Rehabil Res Dev 2001;38(1):33–40.

11. Mukherjee G, Bhowmik P, Samanta A. Effect of chronic use of different propulsion systems in wheelchair design on the aerobic capacity of Indian users. Indian J Med Res 2005;121(6):747–58.

12. Mukherjee G, Samanta A. Arm-crank propelled three-wheeled chair: physiological evaluation of the propulsion using one arm and both arm patterns. Int J Rehabil Res 2004;27(4):321–4.

13. Abel T, Kroner M, Rojas Vega S, et al. Energy expenditure in wheelchair racing and handbiking - a basis for prevention of cardiovascular diseases in those with disabilities. Eur J Cardiovasc Prev Rehabil 2003;10(5):371–6.

14. Abel T, Rojas Vega S, Bleicher I, et al. Handbikin: Physiological responses to synchronous and asynchronous crank montage. Eur J Appl Physiol Occup Physiol 2003;3(4):1–9.

15. Dallmeijer AJ, Ottjes L, de Waardt E, et al. A physiological comparison of synchronous and asynchronous hand cycling. Int J Sports Med 2004;25(8): 622–6.

16. Knechtle B, Muller G, Knecht H. Optimal exercise intensities for fat metabolism in handbike cycling and cycling. Spinal Cord 2004;42(10):564–72.

17. Valent L, Dallmeijer A, Houdijk H, et al. The effects of upper body exercise on the physical capacity of people with a spinal cord injury: a systematic review. Clin Rehabil 2007;21(4):315–30.

18. Valent LJ, Dallmeijer AJ, Houdijk H, et al. Influence of hand cycling on physical capacity in the rehabilitation of persons with a spinal cord injury: a longitudinal cohort study. Arch Phys Med Rehabil 2008;89(6):1016–22.

19. Valent LJ, Dallmeijer AJ, Houdijk H, et al. The individual relationship between heart rate and oxygen uptake in people with a tetraplegia during exercise. Spinal Cord 2007;45(1):104–11.

20. Verellen J, Brent G, Van de Vliet P, et al. Consistency of the within cycle torque distribution pattern during handcycling: a pilot study. Eur Bull APA; www.bulletin-apacom. 2004;3(2).

21. Bafghi HA, de Haan A, Horstman A, et al. Biophysical aspects of submaximal hand cycling. Int J Sports Med 2008;29(8):630–8.

22. Nash MS. Exercise as a health-promoting activity following spinal cord injury. J Neurol Phys Ther 2005;29(2):87–103, 6.

23. DeCoster A Van Laero M, Blonde W. Electromyographic activity of shoulder girdle muscles during handbiking. In: Van der Woude LHV, et al, editors. Biomedical aspects of manual wheelchair propulsion Amsterdam IOS Press 1999. p. 138–142.

24. Bressel E, Bressel M, Marquez M, et al. The effect of handgrip position on upper extremity neuromuscular responses to arm cranking exercise. J Electromyogr Kinesiol 2001;11(4):291–8.
25. Faupin A, Gorce P, Campillo P, et al. Kinematic analysis of handbike propulsion in various gear ratios: implications for joint pain. Clin Biomech (Bristol, Avon) 2006; 21(6):560–6.
26. Faupin A, Gorce P, Meyer C, et al. Effects of backrest positioning and gear ratio on nondisabled subjects' handcycling sprinting performance and kinematics. J Rehabil Res Dev 2008;45(1):109–16.
27. Verellen J, Theisen D, Vanlandewijck Y. Influence of crank rate in hand cycling. Med Sci Sports Exerc 2004;36(10):1826–31.
28. van der Woude LH, Bosmans I, Bervoets B, et al. Handcycling: different modes and gear ratios. J Med Eng Technol 2000;24(6):242–9.
29. van der Woude LH, Dallmeijer AJ, Janssen TW, et al. Alternative modes of manual wheelchair ambulation: an overview. Am J Phys Med Rehabil 2001;80(10): 765–77.
30. van der Woude LH, Veeger HE, Dallmeijer AJ, et al. Biomechanics and physiology in active manual wheelchair propulsion. Med Eng Phys 2001;23(10):713–33.
31. Zipfel E, Olson J, Puhlman J. Design of a custom racing hand-cycle: review and analysis. Disabil Rehabil Assist Technol 2009;4(2):119–28.
32. Groen WM, van der Woude LHV, de Koning JJ. The power balance model applied to handcycling. Med Sci Sports, Excerc, Submitted for 2009.
33. Goosey-Tolfrey VL, Alfano H, Fowler N. The influence of crank length and cadence on mechanical efficiency in hand cycling. Eur J Appl Physiol 2008; 102(2):189–94.
34. Bennedik K, Engel P, Hildebrandt G. Der Rollstuhl. Rheinstetten: Schindele Verlag; 1978.
35. Gangelhoff J, Cordain L, Tucker A, et al. Metabolic and heart rate responses to submaximal arm lever and arm crank ergometry. Arch Phys Med Rehabil 1988; 69(2):101–5.
36. Gass GC, Camp EM. The maximum physiological responses during incremental wheelchair and arm cranking exercise in male paraplegics. Med Sci Sports Exerc 1984;16(4):355–9.
37. Hintzy F, Tordi N, Perrey S. Muscular efficiency during arm cranking and wheelchair exercise: a comparison. Int J Sports Med 2002;23(6):408–14.
38. Martel G, Noreau L, Jobin J. Physiological responses to maximal exercise on arm cranking and wheelchair ergometer with paraplegics. Paraplegia 1991;29(7): 447–56.
39. Sawka MN. Physiology of upper body exercise. Exercise and Sport Sciences 1986;14:175–211.
40. Sawka MN, Glaser RM, Wilde SW, et al. Metabolic and circulatory responses to wheelchair and arm crank exercise. J Appl Physiol 1980;49(5):784–8.
41. Cooper R. An arm-powered racing bicycle. Assist Technol 1989;1(3):71–4.
42. Brubaker CE, McLaurin CA. Ergonomics of wheelchair propulsion. In: Golbranson FL, Wirta RW, editors. Wheelchair III; report of a wheelchair on specially adapted wheelchairs and sports wheelchairs 1982. p. 22–37.
43. de Koning JJ, Bobbert MF, Foster C. Determination of optimal pacing strategy in track cycling with an energy flow model. J Sci Med Sport 1999;2(3):266–77.
44. de Koning JJ, Foster C, Lampen J, et al. Experimental evaluation of the power balance model of speed skating. J Appl Physiol 2005;98(1):227–33.

45. van der Woude LH, Horstman A, Faas P, et al. Power output and metabolic cost of synchronous and asynchronous submaximal and peak level hand cycling on a motor driven treadmill in able-bodied male subjects. Med Eng Phys 2008; 30(5):574–80.

46. Hopman MT, van Teeffelen WM, Brouwer J, et al. Physiological responses to asynchronous and synchronous arm-cranking exercise. Eur J Appl Physiol Occup Physiol 1995;72(1–2):111–4.

47. Mossberg K, Willman C, Topor MA, et al. Comparison of asynchronous versus synchronous arm crank ergometry. Spinal Cord 1999;37:569–74.

48. Garby L, Astrup A. The relationship between the respiratory quotient and the energy equivalent of oxygen during simultaneous glucose and lipid oxidation and lipogenesis. Acta Physiol Scand 1987;129(3):443–4.

49. Ettema G, Loras HW. Efficiency in cycling: a review. Eur J Appl Physiol 2009; 106(1):1–14.

50. Moseley L, Jeukendrup AE. The reliability of cycling efficiency. Med Sci Sports Exerc 2001;33(4):621–7.

51. Hettinga FJ, De Koning JJ, de Vrijer A, et al. The effect of ambient temperature on gross-efficiency in cycling. Eur J Appl Physiol 2007;101(4):465–71.

52. Hopker J, Coleman D, Passfield L. Changes in cycling efficiency during a competitive season. Med Sci Sports Exerc 2009;41(4):912–9.

53. Veeger HE, van der Woude LH, Rozendal RH. Effect of handrim velocity on mechanical efficiency in wheelchair propulsion. Med Sci Sports Exerc 1992; 24(1):100–7.

54. de Groot S, Veeger HE, Hollander AP, et al. Consequence of feedback-based learning of an effective hand rim wheelchair force production on mechanical efficiency. Clin Biomech (Bristol, Avon) 2002;17(3):219–26.

55. Ericson MO, Nisell R. Efficiency of pedal forces during ergometer cycling. Int J Sports Med 1988;9(2):118–22.

56. Gonzalez-Alonso J, Teller C, Andersen SL, et al. Influence of body temperature on the development of fatigue during prolonged exercise in the heat. J Appl Physiol 1999;86(3):1032–9.

57. Webborn N, Price MJ, Castle P, et al. Cooling strategies improve intermittent sprint performance in the heat of athletes with tetraplegia. Br J Sports Med 2008 Jun 14 [Epub ahead of print].

58. van Ingen Schenau GJ. Cycle power: a predictive model. Endeavour 1988;12(1): 44–7.

Wheelchair Basketball Quantification

Angel Gil-Agudo, PhD[a],*, Antonio Del Ama-Espinosa[b],
Beatriz Crespo-Ruiz[b]

KEYWORDS

- Wheelchair • Basketball • Propulsion • Classification
- Biomechanics

Since the work of Sir Ludwig Guttmann in the National Spinal Injuries Centre (Stoke Mandeville, Aylesbury, UK) during the second half of the 1940s after World War II, there have been many developments in sports for athletes with physical disabilities. Initially, sports activities were considered a therapeutic tool and introduced in rehabilitation treatment programs. However, objectives have expanded and sports for athletes with disabilities attract increasing numbers of spectators, establish the professional prestige of athletes, and earn the recognition of the mass media. In the first Paralympic Games held in Rome in 1960, 400 athletes participated, and in the most recent Paralympic Games held in Beijing in 2008, 4000 athletes from 150 countries competed.

One of the most debated aspects of disability sports is sport classifications. Classifications arise from the need to guarantee the fairness of results and ensure equal opportunities for athletes with different types and grades of disability. For some, this constitutes the essence of disability sport and is the area where research is most needed.[1] A basic goal of classification is to ensure that winning or losing an event depends on talent, training, skill, fitness, and motivation rather than unevenness of disability-related variables among competitors.[2] A classification system should adequately reflect a player's abilities and distinguish fairly between different classes of athlete.[3]

Classification systems have adapted to the circumstances of sports for athletes with disabilities. No classification system existed when wheelchair sports were introduced. It soon became evident that open competitions favored the less disabled. More severely disabled athletes were noncompetitive in individual sports or found it difficult

[a] Department of Physical Medicine and Rehabilitation, National Hospital for Spinal Cord Injury, SESCAM, Toledo, Spain
[b] Department of Biomechanics and Technical Aids, National Hospital for Spinal Cord Injury, SESCAM, Toledo, Spain
* Corresponding author. Department of Biomechanics and Technical Aids, National Hospital for Spinal Cord Injury, SESCAM, Finca la Peraleda s/n. 45071, Toledo, Spain.
E-mail address: amgila@sescam.jccm.es (A. Gil-Agudo).

Phys Med Rehabil Clin N Am 21 (2010) 141–156
doi:10.1016/j.pmr.2009.07.002
1047-9651/09/$ – see front matter © 2010 Elsevier Inc. All rights reserved.

pmr.theclinics.com

to participate in team sports.[4] As disability sports grew in popularity with people with spinal cord injuries, the first attempt at classification established one class for paraplegics and another for tetraplegics. This initial division led to a subdivision into various classes using as a constant reference the level of the spinal cord lesion. The classification was determined by manual muscle testing of the upper and lower extremities and trunk balance. Consequently, the initial classification systems were based on the level of the metameric spinal cord injury.[5]

When athletes with different physical impairments (such as amputees and people with poliomyelitis sequelae or cerebral palsy) began to participate, classification systems were developed that were based on the anatomic injury. Each group competed separately using the different classification systems. The introduction of a functional classification system in the 1980s allowed athletes with different physical impairments to compete with each other. Using this system, people from various impairment groups were included in the same class and classification became sport and event specific. International classifiers define functional classification in disability sports as the ordering of competitors into classes according to their performance potential, based on the relation between impairment and sport activity.[6] The purpose of the classification is to minimize the influence of impairment on the outcome of competition.[6] Accordingly, classification criteria should be based on the relation between the functional potential of the athlete and the determinants of sport-specific performance.[7] The only object of classification should be to classify the physical potential of the athlete.

Introduction of the functional system has stimulated debate and research. Some authors maintain that this model increases the scale of competition by reducing the number of classes, thus ensuring a significant number of athletes to create credible competition within each class.[8] Other authors emphasize that the functional classification system is now sport specific and understandable.[2] This has allowed athletes and technicians to become classifiers as the system is based on observation and medical knowledge is not needed.

In contrast, other authors question the suitability of functional classification systems.[9,10] For them, the classification process can best be described as a medical and functional evaluation used to place athletes with disabilities at the most appropriate level of competition.[9,10] Moreover, the functional system may be more difficult for classifiers because of the large number of impairments that are considered simultaneously.[10] Functional classification may penalize the best athletes and improperly classify new athletes who have not yet achieved their functional potential.[10] The same authors point out that this system has never been statistically validated.[10]

Classification of athletes with disabilities in most competitions is difficult and designing a perfect system is complicated. Advances in equipment design have contributed to the discussion about sports involving wheelchair propulsion. For these reasons and given the importance of developing classification systems that are as exact as possible, classification has become the topic on which most of the research into the sports of people with disabilities has focused. Published studies have focused on various topics, but few have raised objections to using data based on objective methods to characterize and validate each of the groups defined in the classification systems.[11,12] The literature on this topic is sparse and classification is rarely scrutinized in an expressly critical and systematic manner, not even by the research community.[2,13]

There are different approaches to the problem. Analyses have been made of each of the classes from the perspectives of physiology,[14,15] athletic performance,[7,11,16] and biomechanics.[17,18] This article discusses these questions more closely with special attention to wheelchair basketball.

CLASSIFICATION SYSTEMS IN WHEELCHAIR BASKETBALL

Wheelchair basketball is probably the most popular sport for the disabled. According to the estimates of the International Wheelchair Basketball Federation (IWBF), the number of players worldwide is approximately 30,000. Wheelchair basketball is one of the sports with the best-developed functional classification system.[19] Before 1983, all classification systems were based solely on the athlete's neurologic level of disability. Previous studies of various types of disabilities categorized by medical rather than functional parameters found that a classification system based on evaluations of the neurologic level often favors athletes with amputations and postpolio paralysis, placing athletes with spinal cord injuries at a disadvantage.[4]

In 1982, wheelchair basketball changed from a medical classification system to a functional classification system. The current Player Classification System (PCS) adopted by the IWBF was used for the first time in international competition in July 1984 at the VIIth World Paralympic Games in Aylesbury, UK.[20] Under this system, the players were tested on their ability to play the game, not on their medical disability. The current wheelchair basketball classification is based on players' functional capacity in terms of playing skills: pushing, pivoting, shooting, rebounding, dribbling, passing, and catching. It is not an assessment of a player's skill level, only of the player's functional capacity to complete the task.[19]

In basketball players with different functional limitations, the players' level of trunk function directly affects performance of the different skills. In particular, trunk movement and stability during basketball are the basis for assigning a player to a particular class. Therefore, the level of sitting balance and trunk movement of wheelchair basketball players have become the fundamental elements used in defining the classes and in developing a testing procedure fair to all.[20] Classes are defined according to players' "volume of action." Each class has a clearly defined maximal volume of action that the players in that class must exhibit. The volume of action refers to the extremes at which a player's trunk stability allows him or her to reach, without gripping the wheelchair, before tipping.[19] Players are now classified in their playing environment, on the basketball court, and in their playing wheelchair. This system made wheelchair basketball the first sport to include athletes with different disabilities on teams.

This system considers four main classes (from 1 to 4). Corresponding with the class, each player is assigned a sport classification from 1 to 4 (**Table 1**), with intermediate 0.5 classes for exceptional cases that do not fit exactly into one class. Class 4.5

Table 1
Description of classes in the functional classification system of wheelchair basketball in relation to trunk movement

Class	Description
Class I	No functional sitting balance when in a wheelchair without back support. The trunk cannot be moved in any plane without the help of at least one arm
Class II	Fair to good sitting balance. Players can rotate the trunk to the right or left when sitting upright without the support of the backrest
Class III	Optimal sitting balance and optimal trunk movements in the horizontal and sagittal planes without using the arm to hold any part of the wheelchair
Class IV	Optimal sitting balance and optimal trunk movements in all planes

From Strohkendl H. The new classification system for wheelchair basketball. In: Sherrill C, editor. Sport and disabled athletes. Proceedings of the 1984 Olympic Scientific Congress. Champaign (IL): Human Kinetics Publisher; 1986. p. 101–12; with permission.

players have minimal disability. The classification assigned to each player is important because the total number of player points for any given team configuration, that is, the sum of the points of all 5 players on the court, is 14.0.

The IWBF applies the functional classification system at all international events.[19] This system is used in most national competitions. In the United States, however, the National Wheelchair Basketball Association (NWBA) uses a system that identifies 3 classes based on a medically oriented model[7]: class 1, T7 injuries and higher; class 2, T8 to L2 and some amputees (bilateral hip disarticulation); and class 3, L3 and lower injuries and all other amputees.[3,21]

In the initial version of the PCS, the classification procedure included 3 parts that increased the possibility of reaching a fair determination, especially in the case of athletes on the borderline of the class.[20] These 3 parts include the following:

1) A medical part, which provides an approximate determination of the level of trunk function while seated in a wheelchair. This procedure entails evaluating muscle force, level of sensation, and presence of other impairments, such as vertebral fusion, spasticity, or contracture.
2) A functional part, which entails testing the athlete's level of trunk movement and sitting balance while seated in the wheelchair.
3) Observation during the game when testing does not yield a clear decision.

However, the procedure has evolved and the medical part has now almost disappeared, except for especially complex cases. In most cases, the classification centers on observation during the game. Players are observed in their competition wheelchairs, complete with the strapping they will use, in a training situation before the tournament commences. Based on this initial observation, a player is assigned to the class with which he or she begins the tournament. The player is then observed in a competition game. At this time the classification is confirmed or modified if the classification panel feels that it is necessary.[19]

Classifiers are trained to observe and analyze trunk movement according to protocol during the execution of basketball skills such as wheelchair propulsion, dribbling, passing, shooting, and rebounding the ball. Consequently, the PCS relies on the skill of the classifiers to recognize the player's physical ability in executing these fundamental movements in wheelchair basketball.[7]

One proof of the acceptance of this classification system is that it has remained in use for more than 20 years with only small modifications. The last 20 years have been the period of greatest expansion and professionalization of wheelchair basketball. Acceptance of the PCS is based on the recognition of this system by the people most closely involved in wheelchair basketball: the trainers and players. The PCS is based on an observation of movements that requires no medical or anatomic knowledge. This not only makes the system comprehensible to most trainers and players, but also allows those who are particularly interested to become classifiers.

Despite the successful implementation of the system, the basis of the classification is less consistent than would be desirable. The player classification assigned can be the key factor in deciding relevant issues, such as whether or not a player can be included in a certain team, obtain financial backing, be selected by the national team, participate in a Paralympic Games, or have to abandon the practice of wheelchair basketball.

There have been many advances in wheelchair design since the IWBF and NWBA classification systems were developed and approved in 1982 and 1984, respectively.[3] Like the track athlete's shoes or the cyclist's bicycle, a wheelchair is a piece of equipment used in competition. It has evolved with the sport to accommodate players and enhance their playing skills.[22] Sport wheelchairs that differ substantially from traditional wheelchairs help to bridge the gap between players with different disabilities. Experienced athletes learn how to use and customize their wheelchairs to enhance their abilities.[3] Altering the seat design can improve stability or expand the volume of action. Wheelchair design is customized for each player, considering such elements as the player's classification and functional situation and the position he or she is going to play (**Fig. 1**). The wheelchair becomes a key element when the classification is assigned. Consequently, elements that objectively validate the present system of classification are needed, given the importance of the decisions, their subjectivity, and the fact that the classification systems were initially conceived when wheelchair basketball was played with traditional wheelchairs.

VALIDATION OF CLASSIFICATION SYSTEMS IN WHEELCHAIR BASKETBALL

The validation of classification systems is under consideration in most disability sports. In swimming, researchers have taken different approaches to the classification of swimmers. First, the race performance of well-defined groups of swimmers in the various classes has been compared. Based on statistical criteria, suggestions were made concerning separation and combination of existing classes.[16,23] In a second approach, the results of biomechanical race analyses were used.[24] Aspects such as race performance and stroke rate and length were compared among functional classes at the 1995 European Swimming Championship for people with disabilities. It was concluded that the system was logical.[24] Using a third approach, other authors examined the chance of any impairment group attaining a medal or qualifying for the final in a major championship meet. They found that some impairment groups did win more medals than others.[16] The fourth approach involves comparing specific functional abilities among classes for physiologic capacity.[25] Because all the criteria presented some problems, Daly and Vanlandewijck[26] proposed 2 additional criteria based on methods used for individual technical diagnoses. Following this research, the present classification system appears to be approaching fairness for freestyle events, but the system may not yet have achieved its goal of fairness for breaststroke.[26]

Only a few studies to date have examined the viability of wheelchair basketball classification systems.[3,11,12,14,27–29] In the case of the NWBA classification system,

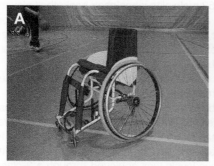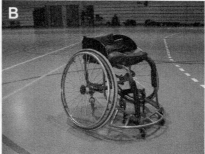

Fig.1. Differences in a single sport (wheelchair basketball) in the wheelchairs of players with different classifications. (*A*) The wheelchair of a class 1 player has a high backrest and a backward-tilted seat to improve the player's precarious stability. (*B*) The wheelchair belongs to a class 4 player who is trying to maximize the volume of action with a small backrest and the seat parallel to the floor.

Brasile[30] analyzed the performance evaluation of 79 male wheelchair basketball players using a wheelchair basketball skill test with 3 added measures: pass for accuracy with the nondominant hand; 1-minute shot with nondominant hand; and spot shot.[11] The conclusion was that level of disability, as indicated by NWBA class level, may influence performance level. However, it was also apparent that the amount of time spent practicing, previous experience in the sport, and age might influence overall performance in wheelchair basketball.[11] A final suggestion was to consider adopting a 2-class system that would combine class II and III participants into one class.[11] Following this suggestion, a group consisting of 46 men was tested during 2 NBWA summer basketball camps held in consecutive years. Their performance in a 20-m sprint using their own wheelchair was measured and evaluated.[3] Since no differences were found between class II and III, this study supported the claim that a 3-class system may not accurately reflect the skill level of the players.[3,12]

To clarify the influence of disability level on wheelchair propulsion performance, 40 highly trained male athletes classified into groups according to the International Stoke Mandeville Wheelchair Sports Federation (ISMWSF) classification system for wheelchair basketball[20] were analyzed.[14] The user-related parameters, approached from a biomechanical and physiologic point of view, were (1) the force applied to the hand rims at different velocities on a wheelchair ergometer, (2) maximal aerobic power during wheelchair propulsion on a treadmill, and (3) propulsion technique at different velocities on a treadmill at constant submaximal power output.[14] The authors found little impact of the level of functional disability on the application of isometric and dynamic force on hand rims, no differences in maximal power output, and maximal aerobic power between classes; propulsion technique could not be proven to be dependent on functional ability.[14] Subjects with remarkable differences in their class often demonstrate a comparable wheelchair propulsion style. The authors advised caution when proposing a reduction of classes in the ISMWSF wheelchair basketball classification system on the basis of their results because other important wheelchair basketball-specific parameters, such as the volume of action of the players and maneuverability with the wheelchair, were not examined.[14] The same research group analyzed the relation between the level of physical impairment and sports performance in elite wheelchair basketball players.[12] They evaluated the quality of individual game performance using the Comprehensive Basketball Grading System.[31] The force applied to wheelchair hand rims was measured with an ergodyn device and then the subjects in their wheelchairs performed a maximal exercise capacity test on a motor-driven treadmill. The study group included 52 male elite wheelchair basketball players classified into 4 functional ability classes according to the functional classification system devised for the IXth Paralympic Games in Barcelona in 1992.[32] They concluded that basic scientific measures of potential performance and visual observations of sport performance can contribute to a fair classification of players.[12] However, previous experience in the sport, motivation, tactical instructions, and other variables may also influence overall performance in wheelchair basketball.

In the case of the PCS, few studies have been made at a national level with field-test analysis[27,28] and field-performance analysis.[12,29] Brasile and Hedrick[27] made several multivariate analyses with different combinations of classes to discern differences in field-test performance across class levels. The best combination of classes with significant differences in scores across class levels was achieved through a 3-class system. However, in a game performance analysis, Molik and Kosmol[29] did not find any differences between 2-point and 3-point players.

At the international level, the only validation studies of this system found were made during the 1998 World Championship for Wheelchair Basketball (Gold Cup) in Sydney,

Australia. Vanlandewijck and colleagues[7,15] validated the classification system by studying the class dependency of field performance in elite male and female wheelchair basketball players in a similar way to how the classification system for swimmers was validated at the 1996 Paralympic Games in Atlanta, Georgia, USA.[16] In the first of the two studies, data were collected from 144 highly trained male wheelchair basketball players from 12 national teams participating in the championship. The authors found a clear relationship between the functional classification of elite wheelchair basketball players and their sport-specific performance at the highest international level. So, the PCS seems to reflect existing differences in the performance potential of elite players. Game performance was measured considering offensive and defensive moves such as rebounds, steals, blocked shots, assists, turnovers, fouls, free throws made, free throws missed, 2- and 3-point goals made and missed, forced turnovers on defense, and technical fouls.[7] On the other hand, taking into account that classification versus performance is strongly influenced by the position of the on-court player, it was concluded that the PCS in wheelchair basketball is based on an interval scale, although a slight underestimation of the potential of class II and II players was noted.[7] The same research group published a report using data derived from 95 highly trained female wheelchair basketball players from 8 national teams participating in the same event, the 1998 World Championship for Wheelchair Basketball (Gold Cup) in Sydney, Australia.[15] The parameters analyzed were the same as in the previous report. In the female wheelchair basketball players, a clear relation was demonstrated between the players' functional classification and sport-specific performance at the highest international standard. In this case, the PCS respects the absolute ratios between classes. This study indicated that the functional classification system slightly underestimates the contribution of female class II players and slightly overestimates the contribution of female class III players to the team's game performance.[15]

Although not directly related to classification validation, it is worth reviewing the contribution of the physiologic analysis of wheelchair basketball players in characterizing functional classes.[33,34] The overall drag and power requirements of propelling a sport-customized wheelchair for wheelchair basketball players and their maximal power output during a sprint effort under actual wheelchair use conditions have been reported.[33] In this study, although the class of each of the players is indicated, no relations are established between class and the physiologic data obtained.[33] In a later study, the objective was to develop a field-test battery that could be used by trainers and coaches to evaluate a player's overall wheelchair basketball performance. The authors stated that a full examination of wheelchair basketball players should include at least an assessment of aerobic capacity, anaerobic capacity, and specific wheelchair basketball skills.[34] Although this study was not made in a population of elite wheelchair basketball players, results were promising with respect to establishing a complete test battery for trainers and coaches in ordinary training sessions for evaluating overall wheelchair basketball potential considering the functional classification.[28]

In a more recent study, the results of the physiologic profiles of the national Great Britain male wheelchair basketball team in preparation for the 2000 Paralympic Games were analyzed.[35] Twelve players completed all sessions. The IWBF basketball classifications were recorded as other demographic data, but were not correlated with physiologic data because it would have required a larger sample covering the full range of classifications (1.0–4.5 IWBF classes).[35] The peak oxygen consumption (Vo_2 peak) before departure for the Paralympic Games was higher than obtained in 1998 and 1999 for the same athletes and also higher than found in previous studies.[36,37] It seems logical to assume that technical advances in wheelchair design and improvements in mechanical efficiency in conjunction with improved training regimes were largely responsible for these improvements in the peak oxygen uptake values.[38]

CONTRIBUTION OF BIOMECHANICS TO DISABILITY SPORTS

Biomechanics has been recently introduced in sports for athletes with disabilities and has generated discussion with respect to several issues. The initial purpose of most biomechanical studies in wheelchair sports was to prevent injuries related to propulsion.[39,40] This objective is common to biomechanical studies in the general population. Athletes in wheelchairs are not at any greater risk of presenting repetitive strain injuries such as shoulder impingement and carpal tunnel syndrome.[39,40]

The objective of preventing sport injuries was broadened to include optimizing athletic performance.[41] Sports performance optimization has been approached from the perspectives of ergonomics and skill proficiency. In earlier studies, biomechanical analysis techniques have been used to compare and examine the propulsion techniques of senior male, senior female, and junior male athletes and to determine the relationship between the kinematic variables and performance in an 800-m race.[42] Kinematic patterns were later analyzed for a range of wheelchair propulsion speeds (6.0, 6.5, and 7.0 m/s) and the relation between wheelchair propulsion and pushing economy was examined.[43] It was concluded that adaptations to speed changes occur, initially by decreasing cycle time and increasing cycle rate, and later by increasing elbow flexion.[43]

As indicated earlier in this discussion, one of the questions that require more quantitative information is classification systems. Biomechanical analysis techniques may be most appropriate for contributing scientific evidence to the validation of different methods of classification. Among the most significant examples are the studies by Chow and colleagues[17] of the application of kinematic analysis techniques to the movement characteristics of wheelchair field events, such as shot-putting and javelin throw, performed by wheelchair athletes of different functional classes.[18] In both studies, the different classes are described and characterized from a kinematic point of view.

A double research approach is warranted to obtain insight into the basic musculoskeletal mechanisms involved in hand rim wheelchair propulsion, combining dynamic simulation and optimization procedures in mathematical models with experimental data collection under realistic wheelchair propulsion conditions. Ideally, muscle activity patterns recorded with electromyograph (EMG) signals should be synchronized with three-dimensional recording of movement and force-generation patterns during hand rim wheelchair propulsion under realistic conditions.[41] These approaches are complementary, as the experimental data serve as input for the model, thereby allowing the model algorithms to be refined. The output of the model provides insight into the underlying mechanism of human movement.[41]

When conducting biomechanical analysis of wheelchair propulsion, the setup of the laboratory in which the experiments are made can affect results. The aim is to use a laboratory setup that closely approximates real-life wheelchair propulsion conditions. Stationary ergometer systems have been used extensively to study wheelchair propulsion technique.[44–49] As backward tilting is prevented on most stationary ergometers, the forces generated on hand rims are much higher compared with the same task under field conditions, especially during the acceleration phase of a sprint task.[41] Consequently, it can be assumed that the forces applied to the hand rim and upper limb trajectory are also altered. Furthermore, the inertial forces acting on the wheelchair as a result of acceleration and deceleration of the trunk and arms are neglected by stationary ergometers. Although some wheelchair simulators meet more realistic criteria, these remarks are still applicable.[50]

Authors such as Richter[51] claim that wheelchair propulsion on a treadmill produces propulsion typical of the real movement of wheelchairs in response to acceleration-deceleration during propulsion phases (**Fig. 2**). There is a deceleration phase during the second part of the recovery phase that is amplified by inertial forces acting on the wheelchair system, caused by an increased forward segmental velocity of the upper limbs to prepare for hand contact with the hand rims.[52] Based on these findings, some authors recommended the treadmill for a more realistic and accurate simulation of wheelchair propulsion.[52]

Data collection using EMG and kinematic equipment is the same as in sport activities for athletes without disabilities. However, differences are found in the kinetic equipment for manual wheelchair propulsion. Cooper and Cheda[53] described a force-sensing hand rim for dynamic measurement of wheelchair racing forces and torques. A later version of this force-measuring wheel, called SmartWheel (Three Rivers Holding LLC, Mesa, AZ, USA), allows measurement of three-dimensional hand rim forces and moments (**Fig. 3**).[54] This device can be mounted on the user's everyday or sports wheelchair and can also be used to study force-generation strategies under sport-specific conditions, thus making it possible to address all the movement dynamics components, such as starting, wheeling, braking, and turning.[41]

APPLICATIONS OF BIOMECHANICS IN WHEELCHAIR BASKETBALL

Studies based on biomechanical analysis techniques in wheelchair basketball have been useful in several ways. Biomechanical studies of wheelchair basketball aimed at optimizing sport performance also address wheelchair configuration. One example is the analysis of the effects of rear-wheel camber on the mechanical parameters produced during wheelchair sprinting of wheelchair basketball players. The effect of wheel camber on overall resistance has been a controversial issue in the literature and contradictory results have been published.[55] In a recent study, an ergometer was used to estimate the influence of wheelchair wheel camber on kinetic and kinematic parameters of wheelchair propulsion cycles.[56] Their results demonstrated an increase in residual torque proportional to the increase in wheel camber (from 9° to 12° to 15°). This increased rolling resistance may explain the slower mean velocity and higher power output in relation to wheel camber.[56]

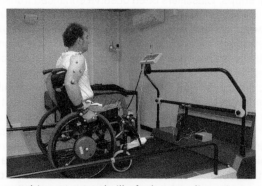

Fig. 2. Wheelchair propulsion on a treadmill of adequate dimensions.

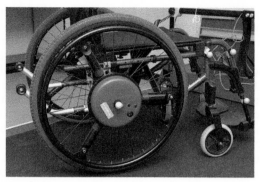

Fig. 3. The SmartWheel device for recording kinetic propulsion data. It can be adapted to the athlete's wheelchair.

One study used biomechanical analytical techniques to optimize the release conditions for free throws in wheelchair basketball. The purpose of this simulation study was to determine the optimal conditions and corresponding arm movement pattern for free throws by players classified as PCS 3 to 4.5 in wheelchair basketball.[57] In this case, as also occurs in able-bodied sports, biomechanical knowledge was used to propose adaptations in technique to improve performance. The aim was not to analyze how players in each class perform free throws. The right arm of the player holding a basketball was modeled as a two-dimensional, 3-segment linked system comprising the upper arm, forearm, and hand and ball. Torque actuators for the right arm were inserted at the proximal end of each segment, which gave the model the ability to add energy to the system. According to this study, the optimal release speed and angle of projection are greater for free throws made from a wheelchair than for free throws made from a standing position. Free-throw shooting from a wheelchair places more emphasis on a player's ability to generate the increased shoulder flexion torque required by the shot.[57]

Biomechanics can also contribute to optimizing wheelchair basketball in trunk and lower extremity stabilization. This is highly relevant because the player's action depends on trunk stability. In the current PCS, players are evaluated based on their observed trunk control in the wheelchair while using strapping or positioning that may improve their function. Technology is now available to alter sitting position to improve trunk stability, sitting posture by changing the seat height or the backrest-to-seat angle, and by attaching the trunk, pelvis, or lower extremities to the wheelchair with different straps. Classifiers often observe enhanced trunk control in players who use various wheelchair adaptations, such as trunk or lower-extremity fixation, and sometimes switch the player to a higher (more able) classification.[58] However, more objective evidence is needed to document the improvement in function observed and to justify reclassifying athletes who choose to use such strapping. Curtis and colleagues[58] described a methodology for the kinematic analysis of trunk mobility in wheelchair users. They compared the sitting trunk mobility of wheelchair users with various levels of spinal cord injury to able-bodied control subjects who performed similar movements and the influence of strapping different body parts on trunk mobility.[55] This study provided strong evidence that a chest strap increases functional reach in the sagittal plane, but functional reach does not appear to be enhanced by a thigh strap in subjects with high or low thoracic paraplegia.[58]

Another application of biomechanics to wheelchair basketball is the objective description of how certain movements are made, highlighting differences with other populations. Coutts[59] compared the kinematics of wheelchair propulsion between basketball and track athletes on a wheelchair ergometer. During the first 3 pushes, basketball players had a higher push rim velocity throughout effort, but a higher wheelchair velocity only at the end of the first push.[59] The kinematic aspects of the reduced shooting ability of tetraplegic wheelchair basketball players were compared with those of able-bodied basketball players.[60] Tetraplegic players showed significantly smaller values for the vertical component of ball release velocity and maximum wrist-flexion angular velocity than able-bodied players. For a specific shoulder horizontal adduction motion, a larger range of shoulder abduction motion was observed in tetraplegic wheelchair players.[60]

A novel use of biomechanics in wheelchair basketball is in the analysis of player classifications. Despite being generally accepted, the current wheelchair classification system is based on the observations of classifiers, which can be subjective. Objective knowledge of the characteristics of each of the classes is needed. In this field, biomechanical analysis may have much to offer. Little, if any, quantitative research has been completed to date on the mechanics of wheelchair basketball.[61] The available literature tends to be qualitative in nature, based on coaches' opinions and subjective analyses. However, an understanding of the mechanism of the movements in wheelchair basketball is essential. A further distinction must be made regarding objective differences in the mechanics of movement in each player classification group.[61]

One attempt to describe the characteristics of the different classes from a biomechanical point of view was a study, already mentioned earlier in this article,[14] that also examined physiologic differences. The user-related parameter from a biomechanical perspective was the force applied to the hand rim at different velocities on a wheelchair ergometer. The authors found little impact of the level of functional disability on the isometric and dynamic forces applied to hand rims between classes II and III (ISMWSF wheelchair basketball classification).

Nonetheless, it may be more appropriate to analyze the key movements on which classifiers focus when classifying players. Malone and colleagues[62] indicated the need for further study to determine the biomechanical characteristics of wheelchair basketball shooting so that comparisons could be made among classes and between individuals. As no previous research had yet compared shooting technique across classifications, Goosey-Tolfrey and colleagues[63] carried out a study to examine the differences in technique in the completion of a successful free throw by players of different functional classifications. Players were allocated to 2 different groups according to IWBF classification. Group 1 contained class 2 players and group 2 contained class 4 players. The study was restricted to class 2 and class 4 players because of the low number of elite, experienced players in the other classes.[63] Two video cameras were used to record the free throws. Despite the large variance between players, they appeared to use 2 different shooting strategies to generate the release velocity necessary for the ball to reach the basket.[63] Malone and colleagues[61] compared shooting mechanics by player classification. One of the purposes of the investigation was to identify differences in ball release parameters between classes.[61] Two video cameras were used for kinematic analysis in 67 right-handed free throws: 7 shots (class 1), 16 shots (class 2), 18 shots (class 3), and 26 shots (class 4). The results of this study demonstrated significant differences between wheelchair basketball classes in the free-throw shooting mechanics required for a clean shot. Apparently, different techniques are used by the upper classes (3 and 4) and lower classes (1 and 2), as demonstrated by several aspects of the shooting motion and ball trajectory.[61]

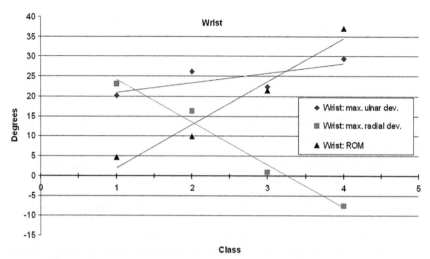

Fig. 4. Correlations between kinematic values and the classification of wheelchair propulsion in a group of 10 wheelchair basketball players.

Wheelchair propulsion is another element on which classification is based. Some preliminary attempts have been made to determine the biomechanical characteristics of wheelchair propulsion during sprinting so that comparisons can be made among classes and between individuals, as with shooting (Gil-Agudo, MD, personal communication, 2009). Ten wheelchair basketball players participated in this pilot study. All of them had been classified by European IWBF classifiers and were considered elite players because they had participated in international events. A treadmill of suitable dimensions for wheelchairs was used to simulate realistic propulsion conditions. The kinematic variables were recorded using 4 camcorders with infrared filter supported by infrared torches. A statistically significant negative correlation was found between the classification score and the following variables: push time; ratio of the duration of the push phase/recovery phase; contact angle; percentage of the cycle at which hand off occurs; percentage of the cycle at which follow-through occurs; maximum carpal radial deviation; and maximum carpal flexion. In contrast, as the class increased from 1 to 4, the value of carpal range of movement in ulnar-radial deviation increased (**Fig. 4**).

One controversy may be that functional classifications are made during actual games, because the setting of the biomechanical analysis laboratory is unrealistic in many ways. The authors recommend continuing this study with a larger sample and extending the analysis to the other key features of the classification (shooting, dribbling, rebound, and manual propulsion).

SUMMARY

Classification systems are a key element in sports for athletes with disabilities, specifically, wheelchair basketball. The fairness of competition depends largely on an adequate classification system. Early classification systems were based on anatomic considerations that were analyzed by doctors. The current classification systems are based on functional aspects related to the player's residual capacities and are applied by classifier observation. Studies to evaluate and validate the suitability of classification systems from a scientific perspective are needed. Biomechanical analysis of each of the essential movements of wheelchair basketball is a useful tool.

REFERENCES

1. Sherrill C. Disability sport and classification theory: a new era. Adapt Phys Act Quart 1999;16:206–15.
2. Vanlandewijck YC, Chappel RJ. Integration and classification issues in competitive sports for athletes with disabilities. Sport Sci Rev 1996;5:65–8.
3. Doyle T, Davis RW, Humphries B, et al. Further evidence to change the medical classification system of the National Wheelchair Basketball Association. Adapt Phys Act Quart 2004;21:63–70.
4. Weiss M, Curtis KA. Controversies in medical classification of wheelchair athletes. In: Sherrill C, editor. Sport and disabled athletes. Champaign (IL): Human Kinetics Publisher; 1986. p. 93–100.
5. International Stoke Mandeville Games Federation. Guide for doctors. Aylesbury (England): International Stoke Mandeville Games Federation; 1982.
6. Kruimer A. Classificatie in gehandicaptensport. [Classification in disability sports]. Geneeskunde en Sport 2000;33:31–5 [in Dutch].
7. Vanlandewijck YC, Evaggelinou C, Daly DD, et al. Proportionality in wheelchair basketball classification. Adapt Phys Act Quart 2003;20:369–80.
8. Higgs C, Babstock P, Buck J, et al. Wheelchair classification for track and field events: a performance approach. Adapt Phys Act Quart 1990;7:22–40.
9. McCann C. Sports for the disabled: the evolution from rehabilitation to competitive sport. Br J Sports Med 1996;30:279–80.
10. Richter KJ, Adams-Mushett, Ferrara MS, et al. Integrated swimming classification. A faulted system. Adapt Phys Act Quart 1992;9:5–13.
11. Brasile FM. Performance evaluation of wheelchair athletes: more than a disability classification level issue. Adapt Phys Act Quart 1990a;7:289–97.
12. Vanlandewijck YC, Spaepen AJ, Lysens RJ. Relationship between the level of physical impairment and sports performance in elite wheelchair basketball players. Adapt Phys Act Quart 1995;12:139–50.
13. DePauw KP. Research on sport for athletes with disabilities. Adapt Phys Act Quart 1986;3:292–9.
14. Vanlandewijck YC, Spaepen AJ, Lysens RJ. Wheelchair propulsion: functional ability dependent factors in wheelchair basketball players. Scand J Rehabil Med 1994;26:37–48.
15. Vanlandewijck YC, Evaggelinou C, Daly DD, et al. The relationship between functional potential and field performance in elite female wheelchair basketball players. J Sports Sci 2004;22:668–75.
16. Sheng KW, Williams T. Paralympic swimming performance, impairment and the functional classification system. Adapt Phys Act Quart 1999;16:251–70.
17. Chow JW, Chae WS, Crawford MJ. Kinematic analysis of shot-putting performed by wheelchair athletes of different medical classes. J Sports Sci 2000;18:321–30.
18. Chow JW, Kuenster AF, Young-tae L. Kinematic analysis of javelin throw performed by wheelchair athletes of different functional classes. J Sports Sci Med 2003;2:36–46.
19. International Wheelchair Basketball Federation (IWBF). Player classification system wheelchair basketball. 2002. IWBF web site. Available at: www.iwbf.org/classification.

20. Strohkendl H. The new classification system for wheelchair basketball. In: Sherrill C, editor. Sport and disabled athletes. Proceedings of the 1984 Olympic Scientific Congress. Champaign (IL): Human Kinetics Publisher; 1986. p. 101–12.
21. National Wheelchair Basketball Association (NWBA). 2009. NWBA web site. Available at: http://www.nwba.org.
22. Madorsky JG, Curtis KA. Wheelchair sports medicine. Am J Sports Med 1984;12: 128–32.
23. Gehlsen GM, Karpuk J. Analysis of the NWAA swimming classification system. Adapt Phys Act Quart 1992;9:141–7.
24. Pelayo P, Sydney M, Wille F, et al. Stroking parameters in top level disabled swimmers. In: Macconnet P, Gaulard J, Margaritis I, et al, editors. Proceedings of the 1st Annual Congress of the European College of Sport Science: frontiers in sports science, the European perspective. Nice (France): University of Nice Sophia-Antipolis; 1996. p. 156–7.
25. Chatard JC, Lavoire JM, Ottez H, et al. Physiological aspects of swimming performance for persons with disabilities. Med Sci Sports Exerc 1992;24(11): 1276–82.
26. Daly DJ, Vanlandewicjk Y. Some criteria for evaluating the fairness of swimming classification. Adapt Phys Act Quart 1999;16:271–89.
27. Basile FM, Hedrick BN. The relationship of skills of elite wheelchair basketball competitors to the international functional classification system. Ther Recreation J 1996;30:114–27.
28. Vanlandewijck YC. Reliability of a 25 m shuttle run test, adapted for wheelchair basketball players. Communication to the 11th International Symposium for Adapted Physical Activity, 1997. Quebec, Canada.
29. Molik B, Kosmol A. In search of objective criteria in wheelchair basketball player classification. In: Doll-Tepper G, Kröner M, Sonnenschein W, editors. Vista '99 – new horizons in sports for athletes with a disability. Proceedings of the International Vista '99 Conference. Köln (Germany): Meyer & Meyer Sport; 2001. p. 355–68.
30. Brasile F. Wheelchair basketball skills proficiencies versus disability classification. Adapt Phys Act Quart 1986;3:6–13.
31. Byrnes D. Comprehensive basketball grading chart. In Hedrick B, Byrnes D, Shaver L editors. Wheelchair basketball. Washington, DC: Paralyzed Veterans of America. p. 146–53.
32. Paralympics Barcelona. General and functional classification guide. COOB '92. Paralympics Division: Barcelona, Spain; 1992. p. 27–32.
33. Coutts KD. Drag and sprint performance of wheelchair basketball players. J Rehabil Res Dev 1994;31:138–43.
34. Vanlandewijck YC, Daly DJ, Theisen DM. Field test evaluation of aerobic, anaerobic and wheelchair basketball skills performances. Int J Sports Med 1999;20: 548–54.
35. Goosey-Tolfrey VL. Physiological profiles of elite wheelchair basketball players in preparation for the 2000 Paralympic Games. Adapt Phys Act Quart 2005;22: 57–66.
36. Miles D, Sawka MN, Wilde SW, et al. Pulmonary function changes in wheelchair athletes subsequent to exercise training. Ergonomics 1982;25:239–46.
37. Rotstein AM, Sagiv D, Ben-Sira G, et al. Aerobic capacity and anaerobic threshold of wheelchair basketball players. Paraplegia 1994;32:196–201.
38. Cooper RA. Wheelchair racing sport science: a review. J Rehabil Res Dev 1990; 27:295–312.

39. Boninger ML, Robertson RN, Wolff M, et al. Upper limb nerve entrapments in elite wheelchair racers. Am J Phys Med Rehabil 1996;75:170–6.
40. Burham RS, Chan M, Hazlett C, et al. Acute median nerve dysfunction from wheelchair propulsion: the development of a model and study of the effect of hand protection. Arch Phys Med Rehabil 1994;75:513–8.
41. Vanlandewijck Y, Theisen D, Daly D. Wheelchair propulsion biomechanics. Implications for wheelchair sports. Sports Med 2001;31(5):339–67.
42. Goosey VL, Fowler NE, Campbell IG. A kinematic analysis of wheelchair propulsion techniques in senior male, senior female and junior male athletes. Adapt Phys Act Quart 1997;14:156–65.
43. Goosey VL, Campbell IG. Pushing economy and propulsion technique of wheelchair racers at three speeds. Adapt Phys Act Quart 1998;15:36–50.
44. Goosey VL, Campbell IG. Symmetry of the elbow kinematics during racing wheelchair propulsion. Ergonomics 1998;41(12):1810–20.
45. Koontz, Cooper RA, Boninger ML, et al. Shoulder kinematics and kinetics during two speeds of wheelchair propulsion. J Rehabil Res Dev 2002;39:635–50.
46. Collinger JL, Boninger ML, Koontz AM, et al. Shoulder biomechanics during the push phase of wheelchair propulsion: a multisite study of persons with paraplegia. Arch Phys Med Rehabil 2008;89:667–76.
47. Kulig K, Newsam CJ, Mulroy SJ, et al. The effect of level spinal cord injury on shoulder joint kinetics during manual wheelchair propulsion. Clin Biomech 2001;16:744–51.
48. O'Connor TJ, Robertson RN, Coper RA. Three-dimensional kinematic analysis and physiologic assessment of racing wheelchair propulsion. Adapt Phys Act Quart 1998;15:1–14.
49. Boninger ML, Cooper RA, Shimada SD, et al. Shoulder and elbow motion during two speeds of wheelchair propulsion: a description using a local coordinate system. Spinal Cord 1998;36:418–26.
50. Niesing R, Eijskoot F, Kranse R, et al. Computer-controlled wheelchair ergometer. Med Biol Eng Comput 1990;28:329–38.
51. Richter WM, Rodriguez R, Woods KR, et al. Stroke pattern and handrim biomechanics for level and uphill wheelchair propulsion at self-selected speeds. Arch Phys Med Rehabil 2007;88:81–7.
52. Vanlandewijck YC, Spaepen AJ, Lysens RJ. Wheelchair propulsion efficiency: movement pattern adaptations to speed changes. Med Sci Sports Exerc 1994; 26(11):1373–81.
53. Cooper RA, Cheda A. Measurement of racing wheelchair propulsion torque. Proceedings of the 12th International Conference of the IEEE Engineering in Medicine and Biology Society. 1989;5:2311–22.
54. Asato KT, Cooper RA, Robertson RN, et al. SMART/sup wheels: development and testing of a system for measuring manual wheelchair propulsion dynamics. IEEE Trans Biomed Eng 1993;40:1320–4.
55. van der Woude LH, Veeger HE, Dallmeijer AJ, et al. Biomechanics and physiology in active manual wheelchair propulsion. Med Eng Phys 2001;23(10):713–33.
56. Faupin A, Campillo P, Weissland T, et al. The effects of rear-wheel camber on the mechanical parameters produced during the wheelchair sprinting of handibasketball athletes. J Rehabil Res Dev 2004;41(3B):421–8.
57. Schwark BN, Mackenzie SJ, Sprigings EJ. Optimizing the release conditions for a free throw in wheelchair basketball. J Appl Biomech 2004;20:153–66.
58. Curtis K, Kindlin CM, Reich KM, et al. Functional reach in wheelchair users: the effects of trunk and lower extremity stabilization. Arch Phys Med Rehabil 1995;76:360–7.

59. Coutts KD. Kinematics of sport wheelchair propulsion. J Rehabil Res Dev 1990; 27(1):21–6.
60. Nunome H, Doyo W, Sakurai S, et al. A kinematic study of the upper-limb motion of wheelchair basketball shooting in tetraplegic adults. J Rehabil Res Dev 2002; 39(1):63–71.
61. Malone LA, Gervais PL, Steadward RD. Shooting mechanics related to player classification and free throw success in wheelchair basketball. J Rehabil Res Dev 2002;39(6):701–10.
62. Malone LA, Nielsen AB, Steadward RD. Expanding the dichotomous outcome in wheelchair basketball shooting of elite male players. Adapt Phys Act Quart 2000; 17:437–9.
63. Goosey-Tolfrey V, Butterworth D, Morris C. Free throw shooting technique of male wheelchair basketball players. Adapt Phys Act Quart 2002;19:238–50.

Neural Interface Technology for Rehabilitation: Exploiting and Promoting Neuroplasticity

Wei Wang, MD, PhD[a,b,c], Jennifer L. Collinger, PhD[a,d],
Monica A. Perez, PhD, PT[a], Elizabeth C. Tyler-Kabara, MD, PhD[b,e],
Leonardo G. Cohen, MD[f], Niels Birbaumer, PhD[g], Steven W. Brose, DO[a],
Andrew B. Schwartz, PhD[b,h], Michael L. Boninger, MD[a,b,d],
Douglas J. Weber, PhD[a,b,c],*

KEYWORDS

• Brain-computer interface • Neural interface • Neuroplasticity
• Stimulation • Recording • Rehabilitation

This work was supported by the National Science Foundation under Cooperative Agreement EEC-0540865, Telemedicine and Advanced Technology Research Center (TATRC) of the US Army Medical Research and Material Command Agreement W81XWH-07-1-0716, a special grant from the Office of the Senior Vice Chancellor for the Health Sciences at the University of Pittsburgh, National Institutes of Health (NIH) grants from the NIBIB (1R01EB007749) and NINDS (1R21NS056136), and grant number 5 UL1 RR024153 from the National Center for Research Resources (NCRR), a component of the NIH and NIH Roadmap for Medical Research. Its contents are solely the responsibility of the authors and do not necessarily represent the official view of NCRR or NIH.

[a] Department of Physical Medicine and Rehabilitation, University of Pittsburgh, 3471 Fifth Ave., Suite 202, Pittsburgh, PA 15213, USA
[b] Department of Bioengineering, University of Pittsburgh, 300 Technology Drive, Pittsburgh, PA 15213, USA
[c] Quality of Life Technology (QoLT) Engineering Research Center, 417 South Craig Street, Room 303, Pittsburgh, PA 15213, USA
[d] Human Engineering Research Laboratories, VA Pittsburgh Healthcare System, 7180 Highland Drive, Building 4, 151R-1, Pittsburgh, PA 15206, USA
[e] Department of Neurological Surgery, University of Pittsburgh, Pittsburgh, PA 15213, USA
[f] Human Cortical Physiology Section and Stroke Neurorehabilitation Section, National Institute of Neurological Disorders and Stroke (NINDS), NIH, 10 Center Drive, MSC 1430, Bethesda, MD 20892, USA
[g] Institute of Medical Psychology and Behavioral Neurobiology, University of Tuebingen, Gartenstr 29, Room 210, D-72074, Tuebingen, Germany
[h] Department of Neurobiology, University of Pittsburgh, 200 Lothrop Street, E1440 BSTWR, Pittsburgh, PA 15213, USA
* Corresponding author. Department of Physical Medicine and Rehabilitation, Department of Bioengineering, University of Pittsburgh, 3471 Fifth Ave., Suite 202, Pittsburgh, PA 15213.
E-mail address: djw50@pitt.edu (D.J. Weber).

Phys Med Rehabil Clin N Am 21 (2010) 157–178
doi:10.1016/j.pmr.2009.07.003
1047-9651/09/$ – see front matter © 2010 Elsevier Inc. All rights reserved.

The primary goal of rehabilitation is to restore physical, psychological, and social functions and improve the quality of life for individuals with various motor, sensory, or cognitive impairments. Although treatment options vary from pharmacologic agents to physical exercise, this review article focuses on neural interface technology, also called neuroprosthetics, which functions by directly interacting with the nervous system either electrically or magnetically. More than 200 years ago, Luigi Galvani documented that leg muscle contraction can be elicited by electrical stimulation of the femoral nerve.[1,2] However, it is only in the last several decades that neural interface technology started to receive increasing attention from biomedical engineers, neuroscientists, and clinicians, largely due to great advances in electronic medical devices and system neuroscience research. The US Food and Drug Administration (FDA) approved cochlear implants (CIs) for treating hearing loss in 1984 and deep brain stimulators (DBS) for treating Parkinson disease in 2000.[3] The National Institutes of Health currently holds a biannual Neural Interface Conference with the goal of bringing industry partners, clinicians, and researchers together to discuss key issues and future directions related to neural interface technology.[4]

This review classifies neural interface devices and systems into 2 categories, neural recording systems and neural stimulation systems, based on the direction of information flow. Neural recording systems retrieve information from the nervous system through electrophysiological recording methods, such as electroencephalography (EEG) and microelectrode recording of single-neuron activities. Neural stimulation systems feed information into the nervous system by electrically or magnetically activating or inhibiting neural activity. These 2 categories represent a simplified classification scheme, as certain neural interface devices, such as implantable responsive neurostimulators for epilepsy treatment, are capable of neural recording and stimulation.[5,6] As the term neural interface technology covers a broad range of devices and systems, it is a daunting task to provide a detailed and informative discussion on each device and system in 1 review article. Many books, special journal issues, and review articles are excellent references for neural interface technology.[7–15] Hence, this article reviews neural interface technology from 3 unique perspectives: (1) neural interface systems that are currently under active research but have not yet reached clinical practice, to illustrate not only what has been accomplished but also what will be accomplished in the near future; (2) neural interface technology with systems that the authors have directly worked with in their rehabilitation research and clinical practice to provide a first-hand view of neural interface technology; (3) neural interface technology in association with neuroplasticity, a foundation for neurologic rehabilitation, demonstrating that those 2 concepts work symbiotically to improve the quality of life for individuals with disabilities (**Fig. 1**). Neuroplasticity will help those individuals to make better use of their neural interface devices,[16–19] and neural interface technology can also promote neuroplasticity for functional recovery.[7,20]

NEURAL INTERFACE TECHNOLOGY FOR NEURAL RECORDING

This section focuses on the application of neural interface technology to support brain-computer interface (BCI) devices. The primary goal of BCI technology is to establish a direct communication pathway between the brain and external devices enabling faster and more intuitive communication and control for individuals with motor disabilities caused by stroke, spinal cord injury (SCI), limb amputation, and degenerative neurologic disorders. In this sense, BCI is a type of assistive technology, and what differentiates it from traditional assistive devices is that user commands are extracted directly from brain activity without the need for users to exert any overt

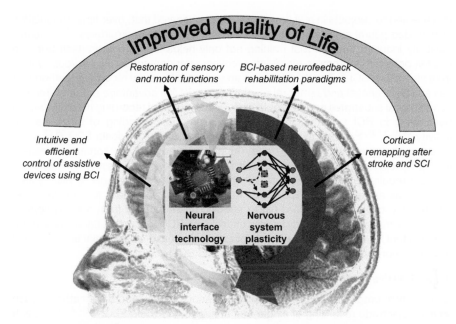

Improved Quality of Life

Restoration of sensory
and motor functions

BCI-based neurofeedback
rehabilitation paradigms

Intuitive and
efficient
control of assistive
devices using BCI

Cortical
remapping after
stroke and SCI

**Neural
interface
technology**

**Nervous
system
plasticity**

Fig. 1. The symbiotic relationship between neural interface technology and nervous system plasticity. Their close interaction leads to increased efficacy of neural interface devices and improved functional recovery of the nervous system, which eventually leads to better quality of life. The neural interface technology is exemplified by a photo of a microelectrode array for cortical surface recording. A schematic of a three-layer neural network models nervous system plasticity. When a group of neurons in the intermediate layer were damaged as a result of neurologic disorders (*red "×"*) such as stroke, the input layer neurons (*green dots*) develop or strengthen connections (*dashed lines*) with spared neurons (*blue dots*) in the intermediate layer promoting functional recovery. (*Courtesy of* Dr. Justin Williams, University of Wisconsin-Madison, Madison, WI, USA, and James A. Hokanson, University of Pittsburgh, Pittsburgh, PA, USA.)

movement. BCI systems, with the capability to provide real-time feedback of neural activity, have also received considerable attention as rehabilitation tools for stroke and SCI patients.[7,20] The goal is to induce neuroplasticity through the operation of BCI devices for functional recovery instead of using BCI systems permanently as assistive technology. In a typical BCI setup, multiple channels of neural signals are recorded simultaneously and fed into a decoding module. The decoding module then processes and decodes neural signals in real time to extract a BCI signal that can be used to control movement of a computer cursor or other external devices, such as a robotic arm or a communication aid.

Three factors are critical for the success of BCI applications. The first is the neural substrate (ie, neural activities), which encode a certain type of information that can be decoded as a BCI control signal. Many BCI applications were developed based on cortical representations of movement.[19,21,22] Motor system neurophysiology studies have shown that activity of motor cortical neurons is modulated by movement, and that firing rates of a population of motor cortical neurons can be used to predict hand movement direction, speed, and position.[23–30] This provides a neural substrate for extracting movement signals from the brain. The second factor for success is cortical plasticity induced by training through biofeedback. When subjects are trained to operate a BCI system, visual or other sensory feedback of the decoded movement is presented to subjects in real time. It has been observed that, over time, modulation of recorded neural signals is enhanced as user performance improves.[16–19] Neuroplasticity induced through BCI training not only helps BCI operation itself but also has the potential to promote functional recovery after damage to the nervous system from stroke and SCI.[31] The third factor is an appropriate neural recording method that has sufficient spatial and temporal resolution to take full advantage of the aforementioned neural substrates and neuroplasticity. Various neural recording modalities have been used in BCI systems, including microelectrode recording of single-neuron activity,[19,21,22,32,33] subdural electrocorticography (ECoG),[34,35] scalp EEG,[36,37] magnetoencephalography (MEG),[38] and functional magnetic resonance imaging (fMRI).[39] Depending on the targeted application, different BCI systems may have different requirements for the neural recording method. For example, a BCI system that acts as an assistive device needs to be portable, potentially fully implantable, and has the capability to record highly specific neural activity from a small cortical area. In contrast, portability may be less critical for a BCI system that serves as a rehabilitation tool if it can offer whole-head coverage with reasonable spatial and temporal resolution noninvasively, such as an MEG-based BCI system.

BCI as Assistive Technology

Considerable progress has been made using various neural recording methods, such as microelectrode recording of single-unit activities and scalp EEG.[19,21,22,33,40] Each recording modality has its own advantages and disadvantages. Single-unit recording requires craniotomy and surgical insertion of microelectrode arrays into the cortex, and it has been suggested that microelectrode recording may lack long-term reliability due to foreign body reaction.[15] In addition, single-unit recording typically requires sophisticated hardware and software systems. To capture the occurrence of spikes associated with action potentials, advanced data acquisition hardware with a high sampling rate (typically 25,000–50,000 Hz) is required. However, it offers the highest spatial and temporal resolution and can extract BCI control signals with multiple degrees of freedom with high accuracy. Researchers have demonstrated that nonhuman primates can achieve high-precision control of robotic arms to perform a self-feeding task,[22] and clinical trials in human subjects are currently underway to test the safety and efficacy of BCI systems based on microelectrode recording of neuronal activity.[21] At the other end of the spectrum, scalp EEG can be recorded noninvasively with much simpler recording systems (eg, sampling rate can be less than 1000 Hz), but it has a low spatial resolution (30 mm)[41] and a low signal-to-noise ratio, especially at higher frequencies (>60 Hz) due to signal attenuation caused by the skull. It has been demonstrated that subjects can control the movement of a two-dimensional cursor with EEG by modulating their sensorimotor rhythm (10–30 Hz),[40] but extensive training is often required.

In parallel with the work of other groups using microelectrode recording and scalp EEG, the authors have been developing BCI systems using ECoG and micro-ECoG. ECoG (sometimes also called intracranial EEG) recently received considerable attention as a promising modality for BCI application.[34,35] ECoG recordings are often performed for patients with intractable epilepsy for presurgical brain mapping and seizure foci localization. Patients' ECoG signals are recorded continuously for epilepsy monitoring, and those signals can be split off and fed into a second neural recording system for BCI research. Because its electrodes are placed inside the skull, ECoG preserves a wide range of high-frequency components (40–200 Hz) of the electrical field potential generated by neuronal activities. Several groups of researchers, including the authors, found that the power of high-frequency bands increases significantly during movement, and varies systematically with movement direction (**Fig. 2**).[34,42] The high-frequency band of ECoG signals encodes desired movement direction, similar to the high-frequency band of local field potential signals recorded in animal studies.[43] Thus, ECoG potentially contains rich information for extracting BCI control signals. Several studies have shown that human subjects can achieve effective control of cursor movement within a short period of time with ECoG (**Fig. 3**).[34,35,42]

Implantation of these standard subdural ECoG grids typically requires a craniotomy that exposes a large portion of cortical surface. For BCI applications, such an invasive craniotomy is impractical and can be avoided with a new technique called micro-ECoG. A micro-ECoG electrode grid can be described as a miniature version of the regular ECoG grids with smaller electrodes and closer spacing between electrodes. Micro-ECoG grids can record neural activity from a localized cortical volume with high spatial and temporal resolution, which makes it possible to extract even richer and more specific information from micro-ECoG signals for controlling BCI devices. Furthermore, a micro-ECoG grid can easily be implanted through a small burr hole in a minimally invasive surgery, and it can be placed on top of the dura mater. By leaving the dura intact, risks of various complications, such as infection, can be significantly reduced. Previously, the Cleveland Clinic Foundation group reported no serious complications from epilepsy monitoring using epidural electrodes, and there was zero instance of purulent wound infection from 500 epidural electrodes inserted.[44]

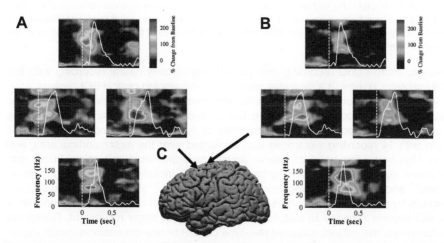

Fig. 2. Movement modulation of ECoG signals recorded from 2 representative subdural ECoG electrodes above the motor cortical area as the subject performed a center-out movement with a two-dimensional cursor controlled by a joystick. (*A, B*) Each panel shows 4 spectrograms arranged corresponding to cursor movement direction (up, down, left, and right). Time 0 represents movement onset (also marked with white vertical lines). Color represents percent change from baseline. Solid white curves are cursor velocity profiles. (*C*) Locations of subdural ECoG electrodes. A grid of 64 electrodes (*red dots*) covers the left frontal and parietal cortical areas. The 2 electrodes the responses of which are depicted in (*A*) and (*B*) are marked with blue "+" signs and black arrows. For the high-frequency band, there is a significant increase in power during movement. Furthermore, the high-frequency band power differs across 4 different movement directions, with a strong activation for rightward movement in (*A*) and downward movement in (*B*).

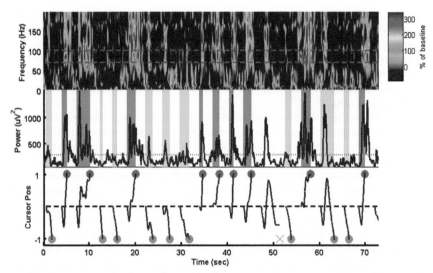

Fig. 3. Real-time control of one-dimensional computer cursor movement using an ECoG channel. (*Top*) The time-frequency plot of the ECoG signal. Color represents percentage change from baseline. The red dashed lines mark the frequency band used to control the cursor (70–100 Hz). (*Middle*) Instantaneous power of the 70 to 100 Hz band (*blue curve*) and its baseline power (*red line*). (*Bottom*) Vertical cursor position plotted as a function of time (*blue curve*). The cursor always started from the center of the screen at the beginning of each trial. The red and green dots indicate the time and cursor vertical position when a top or a bottom target was hit. "×" indicates an unsuccessful trial. For this subject, an accuracy of 73% was achieved within the first 10 minutes of the brain-control session; the chance level was 50%.

Hence, micro-ECoG recording may provide high-quality neural recording with low clinical risks, making it a desirable platform for developing clinical BCI devices.

With approval from the Institutional Review Board at the University of Pittsburgh, the authors recently conducted a micro-ECoG study in a human subject undergoing subdural ECoG recording for the purpose of epilepsy monitoring. A micro-ECoG grid with 14 recording electrodes was implanted over the motor cortical area, and the high-frequency band of neural signals recorded from this micro-ECoG grid showed significant modulation by hand movement, including individual finger movement[45] and grasping/pinching movement of the hand.[46] Modulation of micro-ECoG signals by hand movement offers a neural substrate that is critical to the success of a BCI system intended to restore volitional control of finger movement. During the experiment, the subject achieved real-time control of one-dimensional cursor movement within 30 minutes. Offline analysis showed that hand posture (open vs closed) can be predicted accurately using micro-ECoG signals and that individual finger movement can be decoded with an accuracy of 73% (chance level 20%).[45]

The capability to decode hand movement from micro-ECoG recording has great clinical significance. Loss of hand function leads to difficulties in simple daily tasks, such as grooming, feeding, and dressing, and it significantly affects quality of life. In addition to high-level SCI patients, many individuals with hand function impairments caused by other neurologic disorders, such as stroke,[47] may benefit from this technology. A large number of stroke patients have upper limb paresis on admission to hospital (60%–70%)[48] and 55% to 75% of stroke survivors have limited upper-extremity function.[49,50] Our study suggests that it is possible to develop a minimally invasive implantable BCI device based on micro-ECoG recording to provide control signals for prosthetic hands or functional electrical stimulators to reanimate paralyzed hands.

For all the BCI systems mentioned above, regardless of the neural signal (single-unit activity, EEG, ECoG, and so forth), when a subject operates a BCI system, neuroplasticity plays a critical role. Through closed-loop training with real-time feedback of cursor or robotic arm movement, BCI systems induce neuroplasticity that greatly facilitates BCI control.[16–19] Meanwhile, neuroplasticity induced by BCI not only benefits BCI operation itself, but may also potentially facilitate functional recovery. In the next 2 sections, the goal of using BCI devices changes from simply operating the device to serving as a tool for stroke and SCI rehabilitation.

BCI as a Rehabilitation Tool

In addition to controlling assistive devices that can replace or augment impaired functions, BCI technology can also facilitate the restoration of function through neuroplasticity.[7,20] Traditional therapies for restoring motor function focus on forced use of the impaired limb. Most notably, constraint-induced movement therapy and electromyogram (EMG)-based biofeedback have proven to be fairly successful strategies for improving muscle strength and performance of activities of daily living.[51–55] However, the success of these therapies depends on the patient having a moderate degree of residual function to start with. In the case of SCI or severe hemiplegia, alternative therapies for restoration of function need to be explored. In particular, this article focuses on research that seeks to engage neuroplasticity using BCI as a neurofeedback tool to elicit changes along the corticospinal pathway.

Neurofeedback is a technique in which an individual learns to voluntarily modulate, or change, his or her brain activity.[56,57] Current clinical applications of neurofeedback include the treatment of epilepsy, anxiety, and, more recently, attention deficit hyperactivity disorder (ADHD).[56–59] Users are provided with real-time feedback of some feature of their neural activity, often the amplitude of oscillatory signals originating within the cortex. Based on this feedback, the individual learns to control the neural signal of interest. Voluntary modulation of sensorimotor rhythm amplitude is often learned through neurofeedback to control a BCI device. It is well established that neuroplasticity can be induced, and that control of voluntary modulation can be improved, with BCI training.[16,17,19,21,31,38,60] In addition to improving brain control of external devices, such as computer cursors and robotic arms, neuroplasticity induced by BCI training may also directly facilitate motor function recovery. Many previous studies have shown that functional recovery is often associated with cortical activity returning to a state close to that of an unimpaired individual.[61–63] BCI training through neurofeedback can directly influence cortical activity and potentially restore a normal cortical activation pattern, which could have a positive effect on downstream neuromuscular systems.

A recent study investigated the feasibility of restoring movement using BCI training in chronic stroke patients.[20,31] In that study, subjects learned to modulate their brain activity to control an orthosis that opens and closes the hand. Eight participants with chronic hand weakness secondary to stroke underwent training focused on modulating sensorimotor rhythm amplitude as measured by MEG. MEG sensors over the sensorimotor region that were activated during imagery of movement of the paralyzed hand were selected as control channels for the MEG-based BCI. Motor imagery and observation, for example, of an individual performing the intended task, represent powerful inductors of cortical plasticity.[64–67] Sensorimotor rhythm amplitude controlled the vertical position of a computer cursor and the subjects tried to hit a top or bottom target. In addition, the same neural signals were coupled to control of the hand orthosis. The orthosis guided the hand into an open or closed position depending on the sensorimotor rhythm amplitude relative to a predetermined threshold. After 3 to 8 weeks of training, these 8 patients were able to achieve an average success rate of 72% for the 2-target task. Although this success rate may seem modest, it should be noted that most of these patients were able to achieve control with MEG sensors above the sensorimotor areas ipsilateral to their subcortical stroke lesions. No significant changes in gross hand motor function were measured for any of the patients. Hand function improvement was not expected in those patients, as they started the study with a 0/5 score on the Medical Research Council scale with completely paralyzed hands. To further improve the efficacy of this neurofeedback paradigm, particularly in patients who retain some level of hand motor function, BCI can be combined with functional neuromuscular stimulation to generate brain-controlled muscle contraction. The famous Hebb rule for neuroplasticity is often summarized as "the neurons that fire together, wire together".[68,69] Temporally coupled motor cortex activation, muscle contraction, and somatosensory feedback may promote neuroplasticity for motor functional recovery based on similar principles.

A Comprehensive Rehabilitation Approach Combining Action Observation, Motor Imagery, and BCI Neurofeedback

The authors believe that the feasibility and effectiveness of a BCI-based neurofeedback paradigm can be further enhanced by combining BCI-based neurofeedback with 2 additional training paradigms: action observation and motor imagery. Action observation training is based on the concept of a human mirror neuron system (MNS). Neurons in the human MNS fire when individuals act and when they observe the same action performed by another person.[70–73] These neurons "mirror" the behavior, as if the observers are themselves acting. The human MNS plays a critical role for motor learning, action imitation, action understanding, speech, and social interaction.[71,74] In addition to the classic human MNS, including the inferior parietal lobule, ventral premotor cortex, and the caudal part of the inferior frontal gyrus,[75,76] multiple human and animal studies have also shown that the motor cortex demonstrates congruent activities during action observation and action execution.[75,77–79] Just like action observation, motor imagery, or the imagined movement of a body part, can also activate multiple sensory and motor cortical areas. Motor imagery is believed to be a covert stage of action execution that draws on cortical areas that are typically involved in motor planning and execution, such as the supplemental motor area, premotor cortex, and the primary motor cortex (M1).[80,81]

Action observation and motor imagery can elicit a certain degree of motor cortical activity in the absence of overt movement. They offer clinicians opportunities to directly activate cortical areas that cannot be activated otherwise, such as cortical areas representing a paralyzed limb. They may be able to strengthen neural pathways that remain intact, and also facilitate activation of motor cortical areas. Multiple studies have demonstrated that action observation and motor imagery can elicit sensorimotor cortical activity and, at least temporarily improve motor functions of paralyzed limbs after stroke and SCI.[82–84] As discussed in the last section, a BCI-based neurofeedback training paradigm has the potential to promote neuroplasticity and functional recovery. A comprehensive rehabilitation approach that merges BCI neurofeedback, action observation, and motor imagery will bring even greater benefits to patients than using any of those paradigms alone. First, action observation and motor imagery will facilitate BCI training. They allow a BCI system to optimize its decoding algorithm to extract motor-related information from cortical activity without overt movement from patients. They also offer an intuitive way for patients to learn to voluntarily modulate their cortical activity to operate a BCI system. Enhanced performance in BCI operation will make the neurofeedback paradigm more effective, potentially improving motor function recovery. Second, BCI systems can at least partially provide real-time feedback of actions that a patient is imagining, making motor imagery training more engaging and effective than simple motor imagery without any feedback.

The authors are currently developing such a rehabilitation paradigm to enhance motor cortical modulation in individuals with tetraplegia. In the case of incomplete SCI, it is our goal to maximize the amount of information transferred through remaining corticospinal pathways to enhance residual function. For others, maximizing voluntary control of cortical modulation may increase the effectiveness of BCI technology and future spinal cord regeneration therapies. Preliminary studies investigated motor cortical activity in able-bodied volunteers and individuals with tetraplegia during action observation and action execution, with a primary focus on hand motor function. The study was approved by the Institutional Review Board at the University of Pittsburgh. Results from 2 participants are reported here. One participant was a 29-year-old man with no history of neuromuscular disease, and the other was a 34-year-old man with a C7-level complete SCI that occurred 15 years before his participation in this study. A whole-head 306-channel MEG system (Elekta Neuromag) was used to record cortical activity noninvasively while subjects performed simple hand movements under 4 different conditions:

1) Observed: participants watched a video of the movements while they remained resting.
2) Imitated: participants performed the movements along with the video presentation.
3) Imagined: participants imagined performing the movements in response to a visual cue.
4) Overt: participants overtly performed the specified movement in response to a visual cue.

The time sequence and visual feedback provided during the experimental paradigm are shown in **Fig. 4**. Two different hand movements were tested: (1) grasping an object; (2) tapping an object with the finger tips using wrist flexion and extension. A total of 40 repetitions were collected using a randomized block design for each "condition × movement" combination.

The power of sensorimotor rhythm (10–30 Hz) was used as an indicator of motor cortical activation. Time-frequency plots averaged over all repetitions from

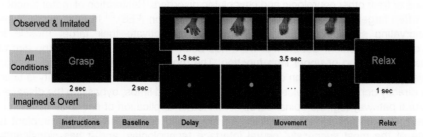

Fig. 4. The behavioral tasks used to study cortical activity during action observation, imitation, motor imagery, and overt movement. For all conditions an instruction slide specifies a "grasp" or "tapping" trial and is followed by a 2-second baseline period. For the observed and imitated conditions, a movie of the specified movement is shown following a brief delay period. For the imagined and overt conditions, movement time is indicated by the fixation dot turning from red to green. "Relax" signals the end of the trial.

a representative MEG channel above the motor cortex are shown in **Fig. 5**. In general, similar results were obtained from the able-bodied subjects and the subjects with SCI. For the overt and the imitated conditions, the power of sensorimotor rhythm decreased preceding movement, followed by a "rebound" (power increase). However, differences in cortical activation between those 2 subjects were noted, particularly in the imagined condition. The able-bodied subject showed a stronger decrease in sensorimotor rhythm power during the delay period and a clear post-movement rebound. A shortened period of power decrease was observed in the subject with tetraplegia, whereas the rebound occurred immediately at movement onset and was earlier than that seen in the able-bodied subject. For both subjects, the observed condition led to similar cortical activation as the overt condition, although to a lesser degree. These preliminary results provide strong support for pursuing a rehabilitation paradigm that combines MEG-based BCI and neurofeedback training with action observation and motor imagery. Future research is targeted to determining whether this new training paradigm can increase activation of the motor cortex and whether or not this translates to actual functional improvements.

NEURAL INTERFACE TECHNOLOGY FOR FUNCTIONAL NEURAL STIMULATION

Neural stimulation allows us to directly modulate activity of the nervous system. Compared with neural recording devices, to a certain degree, neural stimulation devices have had more success in being translated from basic research into clinical practice with a profitable market to support an active medical device industry in this domain.[85] Neural stimulation devices have benefited many patients with sensory, motor, and other neurologic disorders.[13,14] Just like BCI applications, successful neural stimulation applications also rely on 3 factors: neural substrate, neuroplasticity, and the appropriate neural stimulation technique. CIs are an example.[86] Their neural substrate is the tonotopic organization of the basal membrane and the auditory nerve. Stimulating electrodes are inserted along the auditory nerve to elicit neural activities that represent the different frequency components of sound. Neuroplasticity again plays a critical role, as even the most advanced CI devices currently being marketed only have about 16 electrodes to represent a limited number of frequency components of sound, but neuroplasticity induced by extensive training, especially in early childhood, allows CI users to learn to discriminate various sounds, understand speech, and even enjoy music.[87]

Neural stimulation technology can be used to replace specific sensorimotor functions or treat other neurologic and psychiatric disorders. Restoration of motor function is often targeted using functional electrical stimulation (FES).[88] In FES, nerve fibers innervating specific muscles are stimulated to activate their target muscle in a controlled fashion. Substantial work has been done in this area, with the aim of restoring walking or upper limb function. The most recent and exciting advance in this area is the combination of BCI with FES, whereby motor cortical activity is used to directly control FES devices to reanimate paralyzed limbs, bypassing the diseased neural pathway (eg, the spinal cord).[89,90] Another application of neural stimulation is the restoration of sensory function. As mentioned earlier, the cochlear implant is one of the most successful neural interface technologies, and it has significantly improved the quality of life for many individuals with deafness. Neural interface devices to restore vision are also being investigated in research laboratories and start-up medical device companies.[91–93] Neural stimulation targeted to modulate cortical and subcortical activities is being used to treat neurologic and psychiatric disorders such as epilepsy, Parkinson disease, and depression.[13,14]

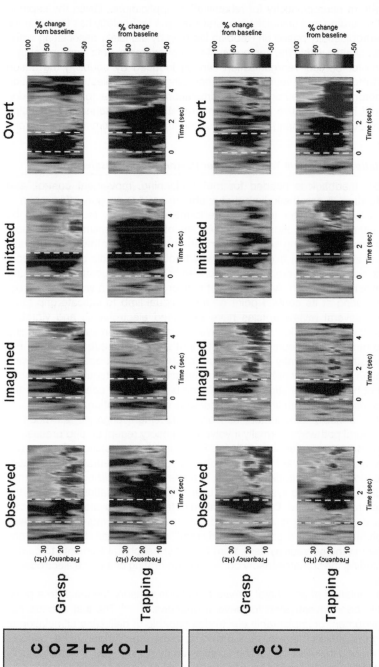

Fig. 5. Frequency band power modulation over time for 2 movements (grasp and tapping) under 4 conditions (observed, imagined, imitated, and overt) compared between a control subject (*top panel*) and a subject with tetraplegia (*bottom panel*). A single representative sensor over the contralateral sensorimotor cortex is pictured. Percent change in power from baseline (resting) is plotted for frequencies ranging from 4 to 40 Hz. The white dotted line at time = 0 seconds indicates the start of the delay period. The second white dotted line at time = 1.5 seconds indicates the start of the movement period. A characteristic decrease in power before movement followed by a "rebound" was observed for both subjects in the imitated and overt conditions. The same activation pattern was observed at a lower intensity for observed and imagined movements.

Just like BCI devices that can serve as assistive technology or as rehabilitation tools, neural stimulation technologies are being investigated for their potential to promote long-term neuroplasticity for rehabilitation applications. Given the capabilities of neural recording and stimulation, neural interface technology has the potential to promote neuroplasticity based on Hebbian learning by artificially associating activities of 2 separate sites within the nervous system. For example, Fetz's group demonstrated that motor cortical reorganization can be induced by coupling the action potentials of 1 motor cortical neuron (neural recording site) with electrical stimulation of another motor cortical neuron (neural stimulation site).[94] The following section provides a brief but informative sample of neural stimulation technology, focusing on neural stimulation for restoring somatosensation and cortical stimulation for stroke rehabilitation.

Neural Stimulation as Assistive Technology for Restoring Somatosensation

Somatosensory feedback is needed for motor planning, movement control, and activity modification. A prosthetic limb that is able to provide sensory information to its user may allow for greater functional performance. Sensory feedback can be provided as either a substitution or replacement of normal sensation.[15] Sensory substitution involves delivering sensory information through a pathway or modality (ie, eye, ear, or skin) different from the pathway through which this type of sensory information is normally delivered or experienced.[95] Sensory substitution typically takes a noninvasive approach. An example of sensory substitution would be a prosthetic hand vibrating at its contact point on the residual limb to indicate grip force being applied. Several review articles have examined electrotactile and vibration methods of sensory feedback.[96,97] Users have indicated that it may be challenging to respond to more than 1 source of sensory input using this feedback design. For example, a prosthetic hand may provide force feedback of hand opening or closing through vibration, but usually not both.[98] A drawback to electrotactile stimulation is pain induced at high levels of stimulation,[99] which is a particular concern due to the common presence of phantom limb pain in persons with amputation.

In contrast to sensory substitution, sensory replacement engages, as much as possible, the neural pathways normally involved in sensory reception and processing via somatosensory neural interfaces (SSNIs). SSNIs involve stimulation of an individual's nervous system to deliver information directly to a user's neural networks supporting perception and feedback control. A prosthetic hand utilizing an SSNI may directly stimulate the nervous system of the user to provide sensations of touch and position of the prosthetic hand. Direct stimulation of the nervous system more closely approximates sensation that is experienced by an unimpaired individual and also offers the potential to relay a greater "bandwidth" of information. Stimulation can occur anywhere in the nervous system, from the most peripheral elements to central structures including the somatosensory cortex via penetrating or surface electrodes of various types.

Electrical stimulation of peripheral nerves to provide sensory feedback to a prosthetic user has been investigated for several decades.[100,101] The last decade has seen the development of implantable electrodes capable of delivering stimulation to nerves through multiple channels, thus providing more specific and richer sensory feedback.[102] Among the electrode systems reviewed by Riso in 1999,[102] longitudinally inserted intrafascicular electrodes have since been refined and can be used for individual finger sensory input.[103] This system has been used to provide feedback of grip force and joint position to individuals with upper limb amputation at or below elbow level while controlling a robotic arm.[104] This system allows the user to adjust the position of the robot arm with no visual feedback from the unit. More investigation is needed to see if chronic systems based on this technology are feasible, because concerns regarding the stiffness of the implanted metal filaments relative to the surrounding nerve tissue have been raised.[102]

Central stimulation of neural elements is also a possibility to provide sensory feedback for prosthetic applications. Work by Weber and colleagues in cats indicates that penetrating electrodes inserted into the dorsal root ganglion (DRG) can be used for sensory recording and sensory stimulation.[105] Cortical responses seen from DRG stimulation are similar to those seen with physiologic motion. Given the access to neural architecture and large action potentials visualized when recording from it, the DRG is an excellent structure to consider for neural prosthetic applications. Spinal cord stimulation, although commonly performed for pain management,[106] may be another potential approach for providing neuroprosthetic sensory feedback. A similar scenario presents itself in the case of the thalamus, which, like the spinal cord, has been investigated for stimulation for pain control.[107] Cortical stimulation for sensory feedback has been investigated through a variety of methods including intracortical microstimulation,[108] transcranial magnetic stimulation,[109,110] and transcranial direct current stimulation (tDCS),[111] and are likely routes of continued research.

Neural Stimulation as a Rehabilitation Tool for Promoting Neuroplasticity

In addition to directly replacing or supplementing lost motor and sensory functions, neural stimulation may be able to promote neuroplasticity for rehabilitation by directly modulating activity of the nervous system.[112,113] Earlier studies have shown that motor cortical representation of limbs can be altered through intracortical microelectrical stimulation in animals[114] and in humans through direct noninvasive cortical stimulation.[115] Recent studies using animal stroke models have shown that upper limb function can be improved after cortical surface electrical stimulation.[116] These studies led to clinical trials of the first fully implantable cortical surface electrical stimulation device aiming to improve upper-extremity function.[113,117] Stimulating electrodes were implanted epidurally above M1, and the electrodes were tunneled underneath the skin to the chest and connected to a subclavicular pulse generator.[113] Focal high-frequency stimulation (eg, 50 or 100 Hz) was applied to the motor cortex. Several small-scale studies examined the changes in upper limb function, measured as the Fugel-Meyer score, following invasive cortical stimulation.[113] Subjects who received cortical stimulation along with motor training showed higher Fugel-Meyer scores than those who only received motor training at 12 weeks post-implant.[113] However, a larger-scale phase III clinical trial recently reported contradictory results, showing little difference in motor function improvement between motor training alone and combined motor training and cortical stimulation.[118] In their 2009 article,[118] Plow and colleagues discussed various factors that need to be further investigated and controlled for in future studies using invasive cortical stimulation, such as localization of cortical stimulation sites, descending pathway viability, and differences between animal and human studies. It was also suggested that noninvasive cortical stimulation will provide important insights into the efficacy of invasive cortical stimulation.

Noninvasive cortical stimulation can be performed using repetitive transcranial magnetic stimulation (rTMS) and tDCS.[112] At least 2 approaches have been explored using these noninvasive stimulation techniques.[112] One approach is to directly enhance motor cortical excitability of the stroke-affected hemisphere using ipsilesional cortical stimulation, which is also the approach taken by the implantable electrical cortical stimulators.[112] The other approach is to reduce interhemispheric inhibition from the intact to the affected hemisphere by stimulating the hemisphere contralateral to stroke lesion. Both approaches have been shown to improve motor performance for stroke survivors, and motor function improvement was greater when cortical stimulation was coupled with motor training than when using cortical stimulation alone.[113,119] Previously, it was reported that improvement in motor performance typically only lasts for a limited period of time after cortical stimulation (e.g., less than an hour).[113] However, a recent study demonstrated that anodal tDCS led to prolonged motor skill enhancement over multiple days by potentially acting on motor skill consolidation mechanisms.[120] Although clinical protocols of cortical stimulation, either invasive or noninvasive, still need to be refined and their efficacy needs to be further investigated, noninvasive cortical stimulation using rTMS has been applied to modulate the excitability of a targeted cortical area to study various sensorimotor and cognitive functions. The rest of this section reviews in detail the effects of rTMS on cortical excitability and the potential mechanisms underlying these effects, which will eventually guide clinical application of cortical stimulation.

rTMS is a novel and painless way to stimulate the human brain noninvasively with the purpose of modulating the functions of the stimulated cortical regions or interconnected areas. Several studies have examined the effects of rTMS on the excitability of the hand[121] and leg[122,123] motor representations in M1. The duration of aftereffects of rTMS over M1 is often between 15 and 60 minutes, and depends on stimulation parameters such as the number of pulses applied, rate of application, and intensity of each stimulus. In some cases, the stimulus intensity used is below the threshold for evoking a muscle twitch in relaxed muscles, so that any effects observed could not be attributed to sensory input produced by movement. In this regard, stimulation of M1 at a subthreshold intensity and at a frequency of 1 Hz for about 25 minutes (1500 total stimuli) reduced the size of the motor evoked potentials (MEPs) evoked in finger muscles for the next 30 minutes.[124] Stimulation at frequencies higher than 1 Hz tends to increase rather than decrease cortical excitability. The aftereffects of rTMS also depend on the pattern of the individual TMS pulses. For example, Huang and collaborators[125] used theta-burst stimulation (TBS), a protocol in which three 50-Hz pulses are applied regularly 5 times per second for 20 to 40 seconds. In this protocol, low intensities of stimulation produce suppression of MEP size and if each TBS burst is applied for only 2 seconds, followed by a pause of 8 seconds and then repeated, the aftereffect becomes facilitatory.

Several studies have documented that rTMS induces adaptations in cortical neuronal circuitries.[121,126–128] In this regard, high-frequency subthreshold rTMS can reduce short-interval intracortical inhibition in the stimulated M1.[121,129] Although the cellular mechanisms of aftereffects of rTMS are not yet understood, some hypotheses have been postulated. It has been proposed that operating mechanisms include changes in the effectiveness of synapses between cortical neurons (long-term depression [LTD] and long-term potentiation [LTP] of synaptic connections). Like LTP/LTD, there is evidence from pharmacologic interventions that the aftereffects of rTMS depend on the glutamatergic N-methyl-D-aspartate (NMDA) receptor, as they are blocked by a single dose of the NMDA-receptor antagonist dextromethorphan.[130] Another example is the use of an NMDA-receptor antagonist that can block the suppressive and facilitatory effect of some rTMS protocols.[131–133] Another study demonstrated that aftereffects of rTMS on M1 excitability disappear when MEPs are tested in actively contracting muscle rather than at rest.[134] In this study the investigators suggested that rTMS was to some extent changing the level of excitability of the resting corticospinal system, rather than changing the effectiveness of transmission at synapses within the cortex. It is possible that both effects occur to different degrees depending on the parameters of rTMS.

In humans and nonhuman primates, corticospinal cells exert modulation over a large group of spinal interneurons.[135] Therefore, it is possible that activating corticospinal neurons by rTMS may also induce changes in spinal neuronal circuitries. Perez and collaborators[122] applied 15 trains of 20 pulses at 5 Hz at intensities between 75% and 120% of the resting motor threshold of the tibialis anterior muscle and reported a decrease in the size of the soleus H-reflex at stimulus intensities ranging from 92% to 120% of the resting motor threshold. In this study the investigators demonstrated that rTMS increased the level of presynaptic inhibition at the terminals of Ia afferent fibers but did not change the level of disynaptic reciprocal Ia inhibition. At rTMS frequencies of 1 Hz, changes have also been reported in spinal cord reflexes. Valero-Cabré and collagues[136] applied 600 pulses of 1-Hz rTMS at 90% of the resting motor threshold of the flexor carpi radialis (FCR) muscle and reported a lasting decrease in threshold and an increase in size of the FCR H-reflex. It is possible that a different stimulation frequency will have a different effect on spinal cord excitability.

Studies on able-bodied volunteers and stroke survivors have demonstrated that rTMS can noninvasively modulate motor cortical excitability and influence motor functions in a controlled fashion. Furthermore, the other form of noninvasive cortical stimulation, tDCS, can also modulate motor and cognitive functions in a polarity-specific manner in health and disease, and facilitate the design of sham interventions.[137–139] However, better understanding of the effects and underlying mechanism of cortical stimulation techniques is needed to provide scientific guidance for future clinical trials aiming to promote neuroplasticity and functional recovery using invasive or noninvasive cortical stimulation.

SUMMARY

This article reviews neural interface technology and its relationship with neuroplasticity. Two types of neural interface technology are reviewed, highlighting specific technologies that the authors work with directly: (1) neural interface technology for neural recording, such as the micro-ECoG BCI system for hand prosthesis control, and the comprehensive rehabilitation paradigm combining MEG-BCI, action observation, and motor imagery training; (2) neural interface technology for functional neural stimulation, such as somatosensory neural stimulation for restoring somatosensation, and noninvasive cortical stimulation using rTMS and tDCS for modulating cortical excitability and stroke rehabilitation. The close interaction between neural interface devices and neuroplasticity leads to increased efficacy of neural interface devices and improved functional recovery of the nervous system. This symbiotic relationship between neural interface technology and the nervous system is expected to maximize functional gain for individuals with various sensory, motor, and cognitive impairments, eventually leading to better quality of life.

REFERENCES

1. Galvani L. De viribus electricitatis in motu musculari. Commentarius. (Commentary on the effects of electricity on muscular motion) De Bononiesi Scientarium et Ertium Instituto atque Academia Commentarii 1791;7:363–418.
2. Malmivuo J, Plonsey R. Bioelectromagnetism: principles and applications of bioelectric and biomagnetic fields. New York: Oxford University Press; 1995.
3. Pena C, Bowsher K, Costello A, et al. An overview of FDA medical device regulation as it relates to deep brain stimulation devices. IEEE Trans Neural Syst Rehabil Eng 2007;15:421–4.

4. Chen D, Fertig SJ, Kleitman N, et al. Advances in neural interfaces: report from the 2006 NIH Neural Interfaces Workshop. J Neural Eng 2007;4: S137–42.
5. Morrell M. Brain stimulation for epilepsy: can scheduled or responsive neurostimulation stop seizures? Curr Opin Neurol 2006;19:164–8.
6. Skarpaas TL, Morrell MJ. Intracranial stimulation therapy for epilepsy. Neurotherapeutics 2009;6:238–43.
7. Daly JJ, Wolpaw JR. Brain-computer interfaces in neurological rehabilitation. Lancet Neurol 2008;7:1032–43.
8. Donoghue JP. Bridging the brain to the world: a perspective on neural interface systems. Neuron 2008;60:511–21.
9. Donoghue JP, Nurmikko A, Black M, et al. Assistive technology and robotic control using motor cortex ensemble-based neural interface systems in humans with tetraplegia. J Physiol 2007;579:603–11.
10. Finn WE, LoPresti PG. Handbook of neuroprosthetic methods. Philadelphia: CRC; 2002.
11. Horch KW, Dhillon G. Neuroprosthetics: theory and practice. Hackensack, NJ: World Scientific Publishing Company; 2004.
12. Lebedev MA, Nicolelis MA. Brain-machine interfaces: past, present and future. Trends Neurosci 2006;29:536–46.
13. Sakas DE, Panourias IG, Simpson BA. An introduction to neural networks surgery, a field of neuromodulation which is based on advances in neural networks science and digitised brain imaging. Acta Neurochir Suppl 2007;97(2):3–13.
14. Sakas DE, Panourias IG, Simpson BA, et al. An introduction to operative neuromodulation and functional neuroprosthetics, the new frontiers of clinical neuroscience and biotechnology. Acta Neurochir Suppl 2007;97(1):3–10.
15. Schwartz AB, Cui XT, Weber DJ, et al. Brain-controlled interfaces: movement restoration with neural prosthetics. Neuron 2006;52:205–20.
16. Gage GJ, Ludwig KA, Otto KJ, et al. Naive coadaptive cortical control. J Neural Eng 2005;2:52–63.
17. Helms Tillery SI, Taylor DM, Schwartz AB. Training in cortical control of neuroprosthetic devices improves signal extraction from small neuronal ensembles. Rev Neurosci 2003;14:107–19.
18. Jarosiewicz B, Chase SM, Fraser GW, et al. Functional network reorganization during learning in a brain-computer interface paradigm. Proc Natl Acad Sci U S A 2008;105:19486–91.
19. Taylor DM, Tillery SI, Schwartz AB. Direct cortical control of 3D neuroprosthetic devices. Science 1829;296:2002–32.
20. Birbaumer N, Cohen LG. Brain-computer interfaces: communication and restoration of movement in paralysis. J Physiol 2007;579:621–36.
21. Hochberg LR, Serruya MD, Friehs GM, et al. Neuronal ensemble control of prosthetic devices by a human with tetraplegia. Nature 2006;442:164–71.
22. Velliste M, Perel S, Spalding MC, et al. Cortical control of a prosthetic arm for self-feeding. Nature 2008;453:1098–101.
23. Ashe J, Georgopoulos AP. Movement parameters and neural activity in motor cortex and area 5. Cereb Cortex 1994;4:590–600.
24. Georgopoulos AP, Kettner RE, Schwartz AB. Primate motor cortex and free arm movements to visual targets in three-dimensional space. II. Coding of the direction of movement by a neuronal population. J Neurosci 1988;8:2928–37.
25. Georgopoulos AP, Schwartz AB, Kettner RE. Neuronal population coding of movement direction. Science 1986;233:1416–9.

26. Kettner RE, Schwartz AB, Georgopoulos AP. Primate motor cortex and free arm movements to visual targets in three-dimensional space. III. Positional gradients and population coding of movement direction from various movement origins. J Neurosci 1988;8:2938–47.

27. Moran DW, Schwartz AB. Motor cortical representation of speed and direction during reaching. J Neurophysiol 1999;82:2676–92.

28. Paninski L, Fellows MR, Hatsopoulos NG, et al. Spatiotemporal tuning of motor cortical neurons for hand position and velocity. J Neurophysiol 2004;91:515–32.

29. Schwartz AB, Kettner RE, Georgopoulos AP. Primate motor cortex and free arm movements to visual targets in three-dimensional space. I. Relations between single cell discharge and direction of movement. J Neurosci 1988;8:2913–27.

30. Wang W, Chan SS, Heldman DA, et al. Motor cortical representation of position and velocity during reaching. J Neurophysiol 2007;97:4258–70.

31. Buch E, Weber C, Cohen LG, et al. Think to move: a neuromagnetic brain-computer interface (BCI) system for chronic stroke. Stroke 2008;39:910–7.

32. Serruya MD, Hatsopoulos NG, Paninski L, et al. Instant neural control of a movement signal. Nature 2002;416:141–2.

33. Wessberg J, Stambaugh CR, Kralik JD, et al. Real-time prediction of hand trajectory by ensembles of cortical neurons in primates. Nature 2000;408:361–5.

34. Leuthardt EC, Schalk G, Wolpaw JR, et al. A brain-computer interface using electrocorticographic signals in humans. J Neural Eng 2004;1:63–71.

35. Schalk G, Miller KJ, Anderson NR, et al. Two-dimensional movement control using electrocorticographic signals in humans. J Neural Eng 2008;5:75–84.

36. Fabiani GE, McFarland DJ, Wolpaw JR, et al. Conversion of EEG activity into cursor movement by a brain-computer interface (BCI). IEEE Trans Neural Syst Rehabil Eng 2004;12:331–8.

37. Sellers EW, Donchin E. A P300-based brain-computer interface: initial tests by ALS patients. Clin Neurophysiol 2006;117:538–48.

38. Mellinger J, Schalk G, Braun C, et al. An MEG-based brain-computer interface (BCI). Neuroimage 2007;36:581–93.

39. Lee JH, Ryu J, Jolesz FA, et al. Brain-machine interface via real-time fMRI: preliminary study on thought-controlled robotic arm. Neurosci Lett 2009;450:1–6.

40. Wolpaw JR, McFarland DJ. Control of a two-dimensional movement signal by a noninvasive brain-computer interface in humans. Proc Natl Acad Sci USA 2004;101:17849–54.

41. Freeman WJ, Holmes MD, Burke BC, et al. Spatial spectra of scalp EEG and EMG from awake humans. Clin Neurophysiol 2003;114:1053–68.

42. Degenhart AD, Sudre G, Collinger J, et al. Comparison of ECoG signal modulation between hand and brain-controlled cursor movement tasks. In: Society for Neuroscience, Washington, DC; 2008.

43. Heldman DA, Wang W, Chan SS, et al. Local field potential spectral tuning in motor cortex during reaching. IEEE Trans Neural Syst Rehabil Eng 2006;14:180–3.

44. Niedermeyer E, Silva FLd. Electroencephalography: basic principles, clinical applications, and related fields. 5th edition. Philadelphia: Lippincott Williams & Wilkins; 2004.

45. Wang W, Degenhart AD, Collinger JL, et al. Human motor cortical activity recorded with micro-ECoG electrodes during individual finger movements. In IEEE EMBS, Minneapolis (MN); 2009.

46. Vinjamuri R, Weber DJ, Degenhart AD, et al. A fuzzy logic model for hand posture control using human cortical activity recorded by micro-ECoG electrodes. In IEEE EMBS, Minneapolis (MN); 2009.

47. Wisneski KJ, Anderson N, Schalk G, et al. Unique cortical physiology associated with ipsilateral hand movements and neuroprosthetic implications. Stroke 2008;39: 3351–9.
48. Hunter S, Crome P. Hand function and stroke. Rev Clin Gerontol 2002;12:68–81.
49. Nakayama H, Jorgensen HS, Pedersen PM, et al. Prevalence and risk factors of incontinence after stroke. The Copenhagen Stroke Study. Stroke 1997;28:58–62.
50. Olsen TS. Arm and leg paresis as outcome predictors in stroke rehabilitation. Stroke 1990;21:247–51.
51. Brucker BS, Bulaeva NV. Biofeedback effect on electromyography responses in patients with spinal cord injury. Arch Phys Med Rehabil 1996;77:133–7.
52. Kohlmeyer KM, Hill JP, Yarkony GM, et al. Electrical stimulation and biofeedback effect on recovery of tenodesis grasp: a controlled study. Arch Phys Med Rehabil 1996;77:702–6.
53. Lin KC, Wu CY, Liu JS, et al. Constraint-induced therapy versus dose-matched control intervention to improve motor ability, basic/extended daily functions, and quality of life in stroke. Neurorehabil Neural Repair 2009;23: 160–5.
54. Petrofsky JS. The use of electromyogram biofeedback to reduce Trendelenburg gait. Eur J Appl Physiol 2001;85:491–5.
55. Wolf SL, Winstein CJ, Miller JP, et al. Retention of upper limb function in stroke survivors who have received constraint-induced movement therapy: the EXCITE randomised trial. Lancet Neurol 2008;7:33–40.
56. Angelakis E, Stathopoulou S, Frymiare JL, et al. EEG neurofeedback: a brief overview and an example of peak alpha frequency training for cognitive enhancement in the elderly. Clin Neuropsychol 2007;21:110–29.
57. Heinrich H, Gevensleben H, Strehl U. Annotation: neurofeedback – train your brain to train behaviour. J Child Psychol Psychiatry 2007;48:3–16.
58. Monderer RS, Harrison DM, Haut SR. Neurofeedback and epilepsy. Epilepsy Behav 2002;3:214–8.
59. Sterman MB, Egner T. Foundation and practice of neurofeedback for the treatment of epilepsy. Appl Psychophysiol Biofeedback 2006;31:21–35.
60. Nijboer F, Furdea A, Gunst I, et al. An auditory brain-computer interface (BCI). J Neurosci Methods 2008;167:43–50.
61. Schaechter JD. Motor rehabilitation and brain plasticity after hemiparetic stroke. Prog Neurobiol 2004;73:61–72.
62. Tecchio F, Zappasodi F, Tombini M, et al. Brain plasticity in recovery from stroke: an MEG assessment. Neuroimage 2006;32:1326–34.
63. Jurkiewicz MT, Mikulis DJ, McIlroy WE, et al. Sensorimotor cortical plasticity during recovery following spinal cord injury: a longitudinal fMRI study. Neurorehabil Neural Repair 2007;21:527–38.
64. Celnik P, Stefan K, Hummel F, et al. Encoding a motor memory in the older adult by action observation. Neuroimage 2006;29:677–84.
65. Celnik P, Webster B, Glasser DM, et al. Effects of action observation on physical training after stroke. Stroke 2008;39:1814–20.
66. Lotze M, Cohen LG. Volition and imagery in neurorehabilitation. Cogn Behav Neurol 2006;19:135–40.
67. Stefan K, Classen J, Celnik P, et al. Concurrent action observation modulates practice-induced motor memory formation. Eur J Neurosci 2008;27:730–8.
68. Feldman DE, Brecht M. Map plasticity in somatosensory cortex. Science 2005; 310:810–5.
69. Hebb DO. Organization of behavior. New York: Wiley; 1949.

70. Buccino G, Vogt S, Ritzl A, et al. Neural circuits underlying imitation learning of hand actions: an event-related fMRI study. Neuron 2004;42:323–34.
71. Fabbri-Destro M, Rizzolatti G. Mirror neurons and mirror systems in monkeys and humans. Physiology (Bethesda) 2008;23:171–9.
72. Iacoboni M, Dapretto M. The mirror neuron system and the consequences of its dysfunction. Nat Rev Neurosci 2006;7:942–51.
73. Rizzolatti G, Sinigaglia C. Mirror neurons and motor intentionality. Funct Neurol 2007;22:205–10.
74. Iacoboni M. Neural mechanisms of imitation. Curr Opin Neurobiol 2005;15: 632–7.
75. Hari R, Forss N, Avikainen S, et al. Activation of human primary motor cortex during action observation: a neuromagnetic study. Proc Natl Acad Sci U S A 1998;95:15061–5.
76. Iacoboni M, Woods RP, Brass M, et al. Cortical mechanisms of human imitation. Science 1999;286:2526–8.
77. Caetano G, Jousmaki V, Hari R. Actor's and observer's primary motor cortices stabilize similarly after seen or heard motor actions. Proc Natl Acad Sci U S A 2007;104:9058–62.
78. Tkach D, Reimer J, Hatsopoulos NG. Congruent activity during action and action observation in motor cortex. J Neurosci 2007;27:13241–50.
79. Tkach D, Reimer J, Hatsopoulos NG. Observation-based learning for brain-machine interfaces. Curr Opin Neurobiol 2008;18:589–94.
80. Jeannerod M. Neural simulation of action: a unifying mechanism for motor cognition. Neuroimage 2001;14:S103–9.
81. Mast FW, Jancke L. Spatial processing in navigation, imagery and perception. New York: Springer; 2007.
82. Dunsky A, Dickstein R, Marcovitz E, et al. Home-based motor imagery training for gait rehabilitation of people with chronic poststroke hemiparesis. Arch Phys Med Rehabil 2008;89:1580–8.
83. Ertelt D, Small S, Solodkin A, et al. Action observation has a positive impact on rehabilitation of motor deficits after stroke. Neuroimage 2007;36(Suppl 2): T164–73.
84. Page SJ, Szaflarski JP, Eliassen JC, et al. Cortical plasticity following motor skill learning during mental practice in stroke. Neurorehabil Neural Repair 2009;23: 382–8.
85. PRWeb. World neurostimulation market to reach $5.2 billion by 2012, according to new report by global industry analysts; 2008. Available at: Bio-Medicine.org. Accessed: May 1, 2009.
86. Middlebrooks JC, Bierer JA, Snyder RL. Cochlear implants: the view from the brain. Curr Opin Neurobiol 2005;15:488–93.
87. Sharma A, Nash AA, Dorman M. Cortical development, plasticity and re-organization in children with cochlear implants. J Commun Dis 2009;42:272–9.
88. Morita I, Keith MW, Kanno T. Reconstruction of upper limb motor function using functional electrical stimulation (FES). Acta Neurochir Suppl 2007;97:403–7.
89. Moritz CT, Perlmutter SI, Fetz EE. Direct control of paralysed muscles by cortical neurons. Nature 2008;456:639–42.
90. Morrow MM, Pohlmeyer EA, Miller LE. Control of muscle synergies by cortical ensembles. Adv Exp Med Biol 2009;629:179–99.
91. Caspi A, Dorn JD, McClure KH, et al. Feasibility study of a retinal prosthesis: spatial vision with a 16-electrode implant. Arch Ophthalmol 2009;127: 398–401.

92. Cohen ED. Prosthetic interfaces with the visual system: biological issues. J Neural Eng 2007;4:R14–31.

93. Wong YT, Chen SC, Kerdraon YA, et al. Efficacy of supra-choroidal, bipolar, electrical stimulation in a vision prosthesis. Conf Proc IEEE Eng Med Biol Soc Minneapolis, MN; 2008.

94. Jackson A, Mavoori J, Fetz EE. Long-term motor cortex plasticity induced by an electronic neural implant. Nature 2006;444:56–60.

95. Kaczmarek KA, Webster JG, Bach-y-Rita P, et al. Electrotactile and vibrotactile displays for sensory substitution systems. IEEE Trans Biomed Eng 1991;38:1–16.

96. Childress DS. Closed-loop control in prosthetic systems: historical perspective. Ann Biomed Eng 1980;8:293–303.

97. Scott RN. Feedback in myoelectric prostheses. Clin Orthop Relat Res 1990;58–63.

98. Prior RE, Lyman J, Case PA, et al. Supplemental sensory feedback for the VA/NU myoelectric hand. Background and preliminary designs. Bull Prosthet Res 1976;170–91.

99. Shannon GF. A comparison of alternative means of providing sensory feedback on upper limb prostheses. Med Biol Eng 1976;14:289–94.

100. Anani A, Korner L. Discrimination of phantom hand sensations elicited by afferent electrical nerve stimulation in below-elbow amputees. Med Prog Technol 1979;6:131–5.

101. Clippinger FW. A system to provide sensation from an upper extremity amputation prosthesis. In: Fields WL, editor. Neural organization and its relevance to prosthetics. London: International Medical Book Corporation; 1973.

102. Riso RR. Strategies for providing upper extremity amputees with tactile and hand position feedback – moving closer to the bionic arm. Technol Health Care 1999;7:401–9.

103. Micera S, Navarro X, Carpaneto J, et al. On the use of longitudinal intrafascicular peripheral interfaces for the control of cybernetic hand prostheses in amputees. IEEE Trans Neural Syst Rehabil Eng 2008;16:453–72.

104. Dhillon GS, Horch KW. Direct neural sensory feedback and control of a prosthetic arm. IEEE Trans Neural Syst Rehabil Eng 2005;13:468–80.

105. Weber DJ, Stein RB, Everaert DG, et al. Limb-state feedback from ensembles of simultaneously recorded dorsal root ganglion neurons. J Neural Eng 2007;4:S168–80.

106. Waltz JM. Spinal cord stimulation: a quarter century of development and investigation. A review of its development and effectiveness in 1,336 cases. Stereotact Funct Neurosurg 1997;69:288–99.

107. Yamamoto T, Katayama Y, Obuchi T, et al. Thalamic sensory relay nucleus stimulation for the treatment of peripheral deafferentation pain. Stereotact Funct Neurosurg 2006;84:180–3.

108. Romo R, Hernandez A, Zainos A, et al. Sensing without touching: psychophysical performance based on cortical microstimulation. Neuron 2000;26:273–8.

109. Chapman A. Seeing with your fingers: a transcranial magnetic stimulation investigation of multimodal sensory perception. J Neurosci 2007;27:7081–2.

110. Blankenburg F, Ruff CC, Bestmann S, et al. Interhemispheric effect of parietal TMS on somatosensory response confirmed directly with concurrent TMS-fMRI. J Neurosci 2008;28:13202–8.

111. Antal A, Paulus W. Transcranial direct current stimulation and visual perception. Perception 2008;37:367–74.

112. Hummel FC, Cohen LG. Non-invasive brain stimulation: a new strategy to improve neurorehabilitation after stroke? Lancet Neurol 2006;5:708–12.

113. Harvey RL, Nudo RJ. Cortical brain stimulation: a potential therapeutic agent for upper limb motor recovery following stroke. Top Stroke Rehabil 2007;14:54–67.

114. Nudo RJ, Jenkins WM, Merzenich MM. Repetitive microstimulation alters the cortical representation of movements in adult rats. Somatosens Mot Res 1990;7:463–83.

115. Ziemann U, Wittenberg GF, Cohen LG. Stimulation-induced within-representation and across-representation plasticity in human motor cortex. J Neurosci 2002;22:5563–71.

116. Adkins-Muir DL, Jones TA. Cortical electrical stimulation combined with rehabilitative training: enhanced functional recovery and dendritic plasticity following focal cortical ischemia in rats. Neurol Res 2003;25:780–8.

117. NorthstarNeuroscience: safety and effectiveness of cortical stimulation in the treatment of stroke patients with upper extremity hemiparesis (EVEREST). Available at: http://clinicaltrials.gov/ct2/show/NCT00170716; 2007, Accessed May 1, 2009.

118. Plow EB, Carey JR, Nudo RJ, et al. Invasive cortical stimulation to promote recovery of function after stroke: a critical appraisal. Stroke 2009;40:1926–31.

119. Hummel F, Celnik P, Giraux P, et al. Effects of non-invasive cortical stimulation on skilled motor function in chronic stroke. Brain 2005;128:490–9.

120. Reis J, Schambra HM, Cohen LG, et al. Noninvasive cortical stimulation enhances motor skill acquisition over multiple days through an effect on consolidation. Proc Natl Acad Sci U S A 2009;106:1590–5.

121. Pascual-Leone A, Tormos JM, Keenan J, et al. Study and modulation of human cortical excitability with transcranial magnetic stimulation. J Clin Neurophysiol 1998;15:333–43.

122. Perez MA, Lungholt BK, Nielsen JB. Short-term adaptations in spinal cord circuits evoked by repetitive transcranial magnetic stimulation: possible underlying mechanisms. Exp Brain Res 2005;162:202–12.

123. Zuur AT, Christensen MS, Sinkjaer T, et al. Tibialis anterior stretch reflex in early stance is suppressed by repetitive transcranial magnetic stimulation. J Physiol 2009;587:1669–76.

124. Chen R, Classen J, Gerloff C, et al. Depression of motor cortex excitability by low-frequency transcranial magnetic stimulation. Neurology 1997;48:1398–403.

125. Huang YZ, Edwards MJ, Rounis E, et al. Theta burst stimulation of the human motor cortex. Neuron 2005;45:201–6.

126. Di Lazzaro V, Oliviero A, Mazzone P, et al. Short-term reduction of intracortical inhibition in the human motor cortex induced by repetitive transcranial magnetic stimulation. Exp Brain Res 2002;147:108–13.

127. Gilio F, Rizzo V, Siebner HR, et al. Effects on the right motor hand-area excitability produced by low-frequency rTMS over human contralateral homologous cortex. J Physiol 2003;551:563–73.

128. Kobayashi M, Hutchinson S, Theoret H, et al. Repetitive TMS of the motor cortex improves ipsilateral sequential simple finger movements. Neurology 2004;62:91–8.

129. Peinemann A, Lehner C, Mentschel C, et al. Subthreshold 5-Hz repetitive transcranial magnetic stimulation of the human primary motor cortex reduces intracortical paired-pulse inhibition. Neurosci Lett 2000;296:21–4.

130. Stefan K, Kunesch E, Benecke R, et al. Mechanisms of enhancement of human motor cortex excitability induced by interventional paired associative stimulation. J Physiol 2002;543:699–708.

131. Boroojerdi B, Battaglia F, Muellbacher W, et al. Mechanisms underlying rapid experience-dependent plasticity in the human visual cortex. Proc Natl Acad Sci U S A 2001;98:14698–701.

132. Butefisch CM, Davis BC, Wise SP, et al. Mechanisms of use-dependent plasticity in the human motor cortex. Proc Natl Acad Sci U S A 2000;97:3661–5.
133. Huang YZ, Chen RS, Rothwell JC, et al. The after-effect of human theta burst stimulation is NMDA receptor dependent. Clin Neurophysiol 2007;118:1028–32.
134. Touge T, Gerschlager W, Brown P, et al. Are the after-effects of low-frequency rTMS on motor cortex excitability due to changes in the efficacy of cortical synapses? Clin Neurophysiol 2001;112:2138–45.
135. Jankowska E. Interneuronal relay in spinal pathways from proprioceptors. Prog Neurobiol 1992;38:335–78.
136. Valero-Cabre A, Oliveri M, Gangitano M, et al. Modulation of spinal cord excitability by subthreshold repetitive transcranial magnetic stimulation of the primary motor cortex in humans. Neuroreport 2001;12:3845–8.
137. Gandiga PC, Hummel FC, Cohen LG. Transcranial DC stimulation (tDCS): a tool for double-blind sham-controlled clinical studies in brain stimulation. Clin Neurophysiol 2006;117:845–50.
138. Hummel FC, Voller B, Celnik P, et al. Effects of brain polarization on reaction times and pinch force in chronic stroke. BMC Neurosci 2006;7:73.
139. Ragert P, Vandermeeren Y, Camus M, et al. Improvement of spatial tactile acuity by transcranial direct current stimulation. Clin Neurophysiol 2008;119:805–11.

Virtual Coach Technology for Supporting Self-Care

Dan Ding, PhD[a,b,*], Hsin-Yi Liu, MS[a,b], Rosemarie Cooper, MPT, ATP[a,b,c], Rory A. Cooper, PhD[a,b], Asim Smailagic, PhD[d], Dan Siewiorek, PhD[e]

KEYWORDS

- Virtual coach • Preventive health management • Self-care
- Secondary condition • Disability • Context awareness
- Intelligent prompting • Power wheelchair seating functions

The term virtual coach appeared in the 1950s and was used to refer to an athletic coach leading the team behind the scenes or over distance. The earliest virtual coach was reported in 1997 when an electronic device (ie, a laptop) was used to guide a rare surgical procedure in an operating room.[1] Now virtual coach is used to refer to a coaching program or device aimed at guiding users through tasks for the purpose of prompting positive behavior or assisting with learning new skills.[2-7] Cognitive orthosis, virtual trainer, occupational enabler, and prompting device are some of the terms used to name the devices or programs having similar functions as a virtual coach.[8-10] Virtual coach also shares similar features as persuasive technology defined as interactive computing systems intentionally designed to change people's attitudes and behaviors.[11] Virtual coach, however, influences people by placing more emphasis on providing instructions on how to complete the target activity correctly than simply motivating them to start doing the activity if they have not done so.

[a] Department of Rehabilitation Science and Technology, University of Pittsburgh, Pittsburgh, PA 15260, USA
[b] Department of Veterans Affairs, Human Engineering Research Laboratories, VA Pittsburgh Healthcare System, 7180 Highland Drive, Building 4, 2nd Floor East, 151R1-H, Pittsburgh, PA 15206, USA
[c] Center for Assistive Technology, 200 Lothrop Street, Forbes Tower, Suite 3010, Pittsburgh, PA 15213, USA
[d] School of Computer Science, Institute for Complex Engineered Systems, Carnegie Mellon University, Hamburg Hall 1217, Pittsburgh, PA, USA
[e] School of Computer Science, Carnegie Mellon University, Newell-Simon Hall 3519, Pittsburgh, PA, USA
* Corresponding author. Human Engineering Research Laboratories, Department of Veterans Affairs, VA Pittsburgh Healthcare System, 7180 Highland Drive, Building 4, 2nd Floor East, 151R1-H, Pittsburgh, PA 15206.
E-mail address: dad5@pitt.edu (D. Ding).

Phys Med Rehabil Clin N Am 21 (2010) 179–194
doi:10.1016/j.pmr.2009.07.012
1047-9651/09/$ – see front matter

One of the greatest areas of innovation for virtual coach is to support preventative health management and self-care. Healthy People 2010 emphasizes that a primary focus of health promotion for people with disabilities is on preventing or reducing secondary conditions.[12] The Institute of Medicine also identifies the use of assistive technologies for managing and preventing secondary conditions as one of the major areas in need of future research in the field of rehabilitation.[13] The current state of practice regarding preventing or managing secondary conditions among people with disabilities is to provide patient education during the rehabilitation process or service. With increased cost containment, however, the rehabilitation process or service continues to be compressed, and limited time is available to provide such education. Information overload or feeling the information may not apply to them can interfere with retention or application of the education materials in patients' daily living environment.[14] Also forgetfulness, complexity of the regimen, and disruption of daily routines may contribute to poor adherence to clinical recommendations. Many people, especially those having cognitive deficits, rely on caregivers or family members to provide verbal reminders or instructions to complete target activities.[15] Virtual coach interventions ranging from simple time-based reminders to interactive Web-based applications have been used to address these issues.[6,16,17] Most of these interventions, however, are designed to be used in a fixed space and cannot provide assistance as needed. They also generally operate open loop or rely on self-report, and the information delivered is more generic and not suited to an individual user's context or situation.

This article focuses on virtual coach interventions that incorporate sensor technologies, context-aware computing, and adaptive coaching strategies. Such interventions are able to infer elements of a person's context and activity and reason about when, how, and what messages to deliver based on the person's performance, progress, and context. They rely on extensive pervasive sensing of the person and his or her environment and include powerful software engines that can process, mine, and send coaching messages tailored to the person's condition and context in an automated way.

This article reviews virtual coach interventions with the purpose of guiding rehabilitation researchers to comprehend the essential components of such interventions, the underlying technologies and their integration, and exemplar applications. The authors' goal is also to provide insight by addressing key challenges and opportunities in designing and implementing virtual coach interventions, and promote such interventions in rehabilitation to support self-care and prevent secondary conditions in individuals with disabilities.

COMPONENTS OF VIRTUAL COACH INTERVENTIONS

To systematically understand virtual coach interventions, the authors have identified four components that define the design space of such interventions and address when, how, and what message to deliver in an automated and intelligent way (**Fig. 1**).

Self-monitoring

Self-monitoring refers to observing and recording a target activity, such as medication usage, activity levels, and calorie intake, or an outcome of the target activity, such as weight. Self-monitoring often is achieved through self-report, which could be tedious and inaccurate. Additionally, it relies on user cooperation. With the advance of sensor technologies and wearable computing, self-monitoring in virtual coach interventions can be achieved automatically and in real time using various sensors such as heart rate monitors, accelerometers, global positioning system (GPS), and cameras. The

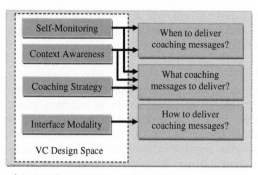

Fig. 1. Design space of a virtual coach intervention.

sensors collect, store, and share relevant data with users and make it easier for them to know how well they are performing the target activity. Psychology research has shown that self-monitoring feeds the natural human drive for self-understanding and is an important strategy to motivate desired behaviors or avoid undesired behaviors.[18] More importantly, sensor-based self-monitoring enables the system to track user performance and progress over time, and makes sure the coaching messages will be triggered only when necessary and that the message contents are more relevant to the user. Ijsselsteijn and colleagues used heart rate monitors to measure training intensity when participants cycled in a virtual environment with a stationary home exercise bike. The heart rate information was used to provide feedback to the participants via a virtual agent who could encourage participants to do better or tell them to slow down if the heart rate became too high.[19] Mihailidis and colleagues[20] developed a hand washing coach device for people with moderate-to-severe dementia, where a ceiling-mounted video camera in the washroom and computer vision algorithm were used to track hands and task objects to monitor hand washing steps and guide users through the steps as necessary.

Context Awareness

Location, time, identity, and activity have been proposed as the primary elements of context.[21] People usually take a great deal of context into account when they communicate. Previous research has shown that intervening at the right context likely will increase the chance of getting responses.[22] Studies in task interruption also have shown that responsiveness to an interruption depends crucially on what the user is doing at the time the interruption occurs, in addition to many other factors such as the emotional state of the user and the modality of the interruption.[23] Sensor technologies and machine learning algorithms could enable machines to perceive certain elements of context such as location and user activity to determine levels of user interruptibility, and deliver prompting messages at the opportune moment when users are likely to respond. For example, if the user happens to be sitting idly when the prompting messages are delivered, these messages may result in a relatively high response rate. Siewiorek and colleagues[24] designed a context-aware mobile phone that can modify its behavior such as ringer volume and vibration based on its user's state and surrounding environment using motion, light, and microphone sensors in a device worn on the body. Kaushik and colleagues evaluated a proximity-based reminder system for home medical tasks in a 10-day case study where proximity to the location where the task must be completed was used to delay the reminder until execution of the task was convenient based on location. The study showed that 96% of the proximity-triggered reminders were acted upon within 5 minutes of being acknowledged compared with only 8% of timer-triggered reminders, and 25% of the proximity-triggered messages received the most favorable rating compared with 9% of the timer-triggered ones.[15]

Interface Modality

Various modalities such as light, auditory, visual, and tactile interfaces can be used to present coaching messages to users. Within an interface modality, there are also different stimuli such as multiple sounds and text, graphics, or animation-based displays. Research has shown that different modalities/stimuli or combinations have different effects on user perception, performance, and acceptance.[23] Mayer and colleagues[25] found that participants performed better on a learning transfer test when the interface agent had a standard accent compared with foreign accent, and when the agent's voice was human rather than machine synthesized. Bickmore and colleagues[23] evaluated the impact of four different types of audio alert tones on the compliance of the target wrist rest behavior and found that compliance dropped off quickly with the very impolite alert tone. Mihailidis used the prerecorded voice of a professional male actor to prompt the correct sequence of hand washing for people with moderate-to-severe dementia.[20] Some of the subjects, however, did not like the male voice because it reminded them of "being in the Army," and one subject even became agitated by the male voice.

Animated agents recently have become one of the most popular interface modalities with the advance in graphical user interfaces (GUI) and computing technology. These agents range from animated shapes to human-like entities including cartoon-like shapes and characters, talking animals, or various other forms. A current trend is to design animated human-like agents with various features such as visual appearance, fidelity, expressiveness, and social–emotional skills. There is well documented research showing the effect of an animated agent on user performance, perception, and acceptance.[26] Atkinson suggested that the dual mode of presentation (animated agent with narrated instructions) enhanced learning outcomes.[27] King and Ohya[28] found that a dynamic three-dimensional human agent whose eyes blinked was rated more intelligent than other forms such as caricatures and geometric shapes. Walker and colleagues[29] found that people who interacted with a talking face spent more time on an online questionnaire, made fewer mistakes, and wrote more comments than those who answered a text questionnaire. Bickmore and colleagues[30] conducted a study comparing an animated health counseling agent on a mobile device with equivalent agents that had text only or text and static image representations, and found that the animated versions led to significantly better social bonding with users. The same group of scientists also researched the role of emotional and relational skills in an animated human agent to support a behavioral intervention for physical activity adoption. They found that there was no significant difference between the amount of physical activity performed by subjects working with the agent equipped with emotional and relational skills versus those working with a nonrelational agent. Subjects working with a relational agent, however, reported a significantly greater desire to continue working with the relational agent.[31] There are also negative effects reported with animated agents such as distraction and discomfort. Moreno and colleagues[32] found that visual presence of the agent was no more effective than a voice-only condition. Given the mixed results, it appears that a virtual coach intervention should consider the combined elements of physical characteristics of the user (such as personality, gender, background knowledge, and capability), attributes of the agent (such as appearance, fidelity, speech quality, or expressiveness), and the type of target task (such as intent, difficulty, or complexity).

Coaching Strategy

Coaching strategies determine what content is presented to the user, such as general versus specific messages, and incorporating different effects such as positive or emotional effects into the messages. Steege and colleagues evaluated two prompt strategies for teaching common household tasks to students with severe disabilities. One of the strategies used the least-to-most restrictive sequence, where students received instructional prompts in the order of nonspecific verbal prompt, specific verbal prompt, gesture and verbal prompt, partial physical and verbal prompt, and total physical and verbal prompt if they failed to initiate a response to the prompt with 5 seconds. The other prescriptive strategy was based on user progress, where the prompt was given at a level just above the prompt that had induced a correct response in the previous trial. The results showed both strategies were equally effective in increasing independent task acquisitions; however, the prescriptive strategy was more efficient.[33] Most-to-least restrictive sequence is another coaching strategy where the most specific message is provided at the beginning and the message specificity gradually decreases.[34] This strategy holds the most control over the user's behavior, but has a risk of message dependency. Usually the most-to-least restrictive sequence is used to help establish the confidence in performing the target activity when a user just starts to learn the new task. When the error rate decreases, the least-to-most restrictive strategy can take over to help retain the learning outcome by gradually removing message dependency. Ideally, a coaching strategy dynamically adapts to the need, performance, and progress made by the user through self-monitoring and context awareness, which will help avoid a nagging effect and enable a trustworthy relationship between the user and the system. The hand washing coach for older adults with dementia developed by Mihailidis and colleagues[20] used coaching messages with three levels of assistance including low-guidance verbal prompt, high-guidance verbal prompt, and verbal prompt with a video demonstration of the action. The level of assistance was determined based on factors such as the error committed, sensory and cognitive status of the user, and past responsiveness to the previous coaching messages. This strategy gave the coach the adaptive ability to select the most appropriate support for each individual's stage of dementia and overall responsiveness.

Coaching strategies also involve adding different affects to the messages. Coaching messages can be designed to minimize affect, or adopt a positive or negative effect. Positive messages may help reinforce the desired performance and increase comfort and interest in using the system. A study found that people who received computer praise after they played an experimental game felt the interaction was more engaging and were more willing to work with the system again.[35] Also, coaching messages that respond empathetically and encouragingly to users rather than state cold hard facts may appeal to the emotion of reaching a goal and help promote a trustworthy relationship between the user and the system.[36] Negative messages, on the other hand, should be used with caution and are generally not appropriate even when the purpose is to decrease the instances of errors or undesired behaviors.

EXAMPLES OF VIRTUAL COACH INTERVENTIONS

The use of technologies to coach activities for supporting preventive health management and self-care has been an active domain for research. **Table 1** summarizes some typical virtual coach interventions including those mentioned in previous sections. The authors also discuss their preliminary work in developing a wheelchair seating virtual coach in this section.

Table 1
Summary of some typical virtual coach interventions

Reference	Target Activity	Portability	Interface Modality	Coaching Strategy	Evaluation	Outcome
The coach prompting system to assist older adults with dementia through hand washing: an efficacy study[20]	Hand washing	Fixed station with a video camera to monitor hand washing performance	Prerecorded male voice, video demonstration	Three levels of instructions determined based on the error committed, user conditions, and past responsiveness	Pilot test with six older adults with dementia using single-subject design	More steps completed independently, fewer interactions with caregivers, 23% false alarm or miss detection
Virtual fitness: stimulating exercise behavior through media technology[19]	Physical exercise	Fixed bicycle station with virtual environment and heart rate was monitored	Female virtual agent with prerecorded voice and synchronized lip movements, text in a cartoon-like text balloon	Feedback based on heart rate	Test with 24 subjects who do not exercise regularly using within-subject design	Significantly lowered the perceived control and pressure, but did not affect enjoyment
Bringing mobile guides and fitness activities together: a solution based on an embodied virtual trainer[8]	Physical exercise	PocketPC with GPS that monitors the trial and user speed	Annotated trail map with prerecorded voice to support navigation, and embodied virtual trainer to provide motivation support and exercise demonstration	Positive feedback based on user speed on the trail; location aware exercise demonstration	Test with 12 users using within subject design	More useful for navigation than trail maps and more effective to teach how to correctly perform exercise

Lifelogging memory appliance for people with episodic memory impairment (EMI)[45]	Memory	Wearable camera, audio recorder, and GPS logger to record personal experiences	Visual and audio cues in a slideshow narrative on a Tablet PC	Self-guided review based on automated heuristics to exact meaningful memory cues	Pilot test with three subjects with EMI and their caregivers, compared with two other strategies	Support the memory of people with EMI better and reduce the burden placed on their caregivers
Context awareness in a handheld exercise agent[30]	Walk	PDA with an integrated two-dimensional accelerometer to detect if walking at a moderate intensity	Animated agent in a close-up shot with a range of nonverbal behaviors such as head nod or eyebrow raise and text display (no speech)	Positive feedback based on accelerometer readings	Pilot test with eight subjects using within-subject design (sensor-based feedback on and off)	More perceived awareness and closer relationship with the agent, but less walking when feedback based on accelerometer

Wheelchair Seating Virtual Coach

Power seating functions (PSFs), including tilt-in-space, backrest recline, and elevating leg rests (**Fig. 2**), usually are prescribed for power wheelchair users who are often unable to adjust their body positions independently, and therefore predisposed to secondary conditions related to prolonged sitting such as pressure ulcers, spasticity, edema, orthostatic hypotension, and chronic pain.[37,38] Power wheelchair users who have these seating functions may not use them as prescribed, however, and frequently come back to clinics for problems such as fatigue, pain, or pressure sores that could be improved or solved by changing seating positions. Although client education on proper use of PSFs is part of the clinical evaluation process in assistive technology clinics, these clinics have limited time and resources to devote to extended periods of client training. Users may know that using PSFs is good for their conditions, but simply may not remember when they should use them, and how to operate them. In a previous survey study, most individuals used the PSFs for comfort rather than the specific medical reasons for which they are provided.[39] The authors also have tracked actual PSFs use of 11 subjects with a suite of sensors and a datalogger for 2 weeks. They found that subjects did not adjust seating positions frequently and seldom used large tilt angles (greater than 30°), which was found to provide sufficient weight shift in previous laboratory studies.[40] Given the fact that a full complement of PSFs can double the cost of a power wheelchair, and many wheelchair users are not using the technology in an appropriate and effective way, it is important to develop interventions that address this problem. The authors are currently developing a wheelchair seating virtual coach (**Fig. 3**). **Fig. 4** shows the system diagram of the seating coach, which is comprised of

- A suite of sensors that monitor the actual PSF use and elements of a user's context such as location and activity
- A single board computer that synthesizes sensor information to determine the appropriate coaching protocol to assist wheelchair users to use PSFs for effective pressure relief and other activities of daily living such as transfers
- A touch screen that delivers the coaching messages to the user via a multi-modal interface.

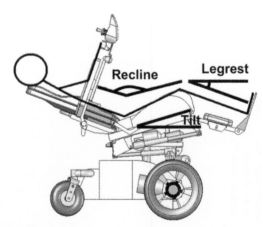

Fig. 2. Power seat functions.

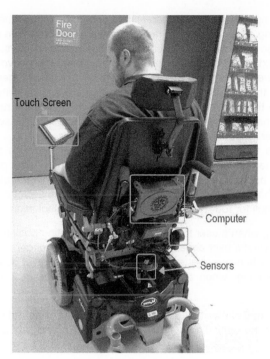

Fig. 3. Virtual seating coach.

The seating coach also can transfer actual PSF use and compliance information to clinicians to assist further client education and decision making with PSF prescription.[41]

The authors instrumented a Permobil C500 power wheelchair with a suite of sensors to monitor the actual PSF use (Permobil Corp., Lenanon, Tennessee). User access to PSF is detected by three encoders coupled to the shafts of three actuators for tilt-in-space, backrest recline, and elevating leg rests, respectively. Nine pressure sensors underneath the cushion are used to detect wheelchair occupancy and activate the seating coach and other sensors. All sensor data are processed by a single-board computer attached behind the backrest to track actual PSF use such as duration of maintaining the same seating position, frequency and duration of accessing pressure relief positions, and sequence of using three PSFs. The actual PSF use also is compared with clinician recommendations to determine user compliance status.

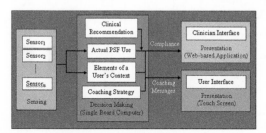

Fig. 4. System diagram of the virtual seating coach.

The sensors, computer, and touch screen are powered by the wheelchair battery, making the seating coach available when the power wheelchair is in use.

The authors also plan to add more sensors such as accelerometers, light, and audio sensors for context detection to determine opportune moments or avoid inappropriate moments for delivering coaching messages. As prior research suggested, time-shifting interruptions that coincide with changes in posture and mobility, or happen in a location where the task is likely to be completed might reduce reminder burden. Locations and changes in mobility state will be detected in the seating coach to help increase user responsiveness to coaching messages.

As appropriate feedback features can be varied according to the intervention purpose and the target audience, the authors are conducting a user preference study to determine the appropriate interface modalities and coaching strategies. A survey program (**Fig. 5**) has been created that allows participants to select different interface modalities or stimuli for four types of coaching scenarios, including

> Reminding (eg, when a user forgets to change the seating position for an hour)
> Warning (eg, when a user accesses PSF in a wrong sequence)
> Guidance (eg, when a user attempts to access pressure relief positions)
> Encouragement (eg, when a user responds to the message with appropriate actions).

For example, **Fig. 5** shows that a participant is to select preferred interface modalities or stimuli for the reminding scenario on page A. Page B lists a combination of

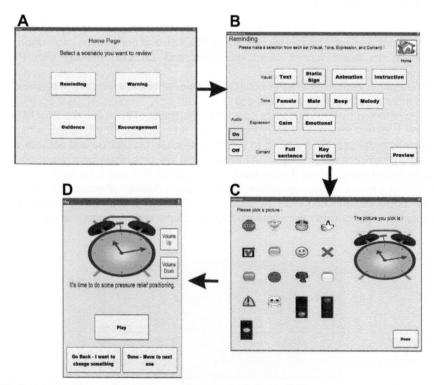

Fig. 5. Survey program for the user preference study (A, B, C, D).

modalities or stimuli for the reminding scenario. Page C shows several icons if the participant selects Static Sign as the preferred visual modality on page B. Page D displays the combination of selected modalities or stimuli and allows the participant to review the final interface for the reminding scenario. Participants can go back to page B to choose a different set of modalities or stimuli, or go back to page A to repeat the selection process for another scenario. **Fig. 6** shows four animation characters if the participant selects Animation as the preferred visual modality on page B. Genie and Merlin are from Microsoft Agent Animations (Microsoft Corp., Seattle, Washington), and the female and male faces represent an average face developed by Braun and colleagues. **Fig. 7** shows the final interface for the warning scenario if the participant selects Instruction as preferred visual modality on page B. An animated power wheelchair figure is used to illustrate the instruction.

The authors' preliminary data with six participants who used power wheelchairs equipped with PSFs showed that participants preferred to have the cartoon animation to inform them of the task they need to do, as they are funny and entertaining. They also preferred to have the animated power wheelchair figure to illustrate the instructions for the specific task, which not only conveys the essential point of a message, but makes them feel it is important to follow the instructions. The participants did not show specific interest in either one of the human agents. This is partly because of the static faces instead of animated faces being used in the study. The participants also commented that they would like to work with a human agent whose face is someone they knew or someone who was significant to them.

Currently the virtual seating coach provides specific coaching messages when detecting conditions when a user forgets changing seating positions or uses the seating function inappropriately. The messages, however, remain the same no matter how many times the same condition occurs. The authors intend to implement an adaptive coaching strategy, where the content specificity, frequency, and effect of coaching messages will change dynamically based on user compliance, responsiveness, and context.

One of the unique components of the virtual seating coach is the clinician interface. Feedback on user compliance to clinicians should be easy to understand. Traditionally, feedback is provided in the form of daily, weekly, or monthly graphs, which may be difficult to comprehend at a glance. The authors use Kiviat Graphs (often used in computer system performance analysis), which summarize high dimensional data and indicate user compliance.[42,43]

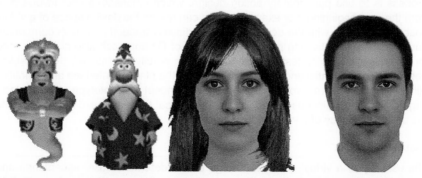

Fig. 6. Four animated characters (from left: Genie, Merlin, average female face, and average male face).

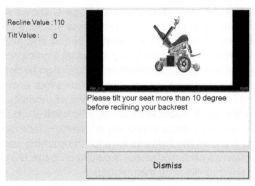

Fig. 7. An example interface for the warning scenario.

OPPORTUNITIES AND CHALLENGES

Although virtual coach technology has shown promising results, the authors identified some key challenges and opportunities that need to be addressed as the technology matures and help shape future directions.

Evaluation

Evaluating a virtual coach intervention can be complicated. Few user studies are available that have looked at the long-term acceptance and effectiveness of virtual coach interventions. All the studies presented in this article are pilot projects involving a short period of time with a small number of subjects. Given the complex nature of designing a virtual coach intervention, it seems reasonable and necessary to use iterative pilot testing to refine the design until the intervention is field-ready for large-scale long-term evaluation. Mihailidis and colleagues[20] developed three versions of their hand washing coach for older adults with dementia over 10 years.[9,10] Each version was tested with a small number of subjects (less than or equal to 10) and had significant advances in the sophistication and versatility compared with those in the previous version. For example, the first version of their coach used an accelerometer-based wristband to track user performance and only used audio prompts, with one prompt for each step of hand washing. The third version used a camera and computer vision algorithms to detect performance and dynamically determine the level of assistance with audio and audio–video prompts. Perhaps one way to speed up the evaluation process is to use participatory action design, which emphasizes user involvement from the very beginning. For example, users can review the design space of a virtual coach intervention with the design team and discuss tradeoffs for each component during the project planning phase. The Wizard of Oz approach also could be used for preliminary usability testing before a system is fully operational, thus enabling observation of potential end users' responses to the planned interface and functionalities as the system evolves from proof-of-concept to prototype. Nonetheless, large-scale longitudinal user studies such as clinical trials are needed to determine the ultimate efficacy of a virtual coach intervention.

Usability

The usability of a virtual coach to a large extent determines user acceptance and possibly performance. Self-monitoring and context-awareness are important to improve the usability by delivering relevant just-in-time messages. This benefit, however, is crucially dependent on the quality and relevance of the machine sensing and inference algorithms. As the physical world and human behavior are both highly complex and ambiguous, reliable activity inference is a difficult problem. It is important to understand how tolerant will the target audience be to incorrect inferences, improper feedback, and bad timing, and strike a balance between the level of intelligence and reliability of a virtual coach.

Few existing virtual coach interventions incorporate adaptive effect into their coaching strategies. The hand washing coach is the only study the authors found that can adapt the level of prompting assistance to each subject's performance, cognitive status, and overall responsiveness.[20] Ideally, a virtual coach intervention should reduce the number of and level of detail in the cues it provides as a user learns and his/her ability changes, which could enable a trustworthy relationship between the user and the system, leading to better usability and coaching effectiveness.

Virtual Coach on a Mobile Device

With mobile devices such as smart phones and personal digital assistant (PDA)s becoming more plentiful and powerful, and the fact that they become an integral part of everyday life, one of the further directions is to use mobile devices to deliver virtual coach interventions.[44] Mobile devices are always with their users and stay on most of the time, which enables a virtual coach to be consulted whenever and wherever a user needs his or her help and proactively intervene in real time. The time and frequency of contact with a mobile device could also help build greater social bonding between the user and the virtual coach. Context awareness is essential in mobile applications to avoid annoying users and maximize coaching effectiveness. The ability to actively interrupt and help a user in a situation that is automatically sensed by a virtual coach could lead to increased perception of trust and caring by the user.

SUMMARY

Prevention and self-care play increasingly important roles in the overall health of an individual. Virtual coach technology potentially can enable a new class of intelligent devices and applications that facilitate self-management and improve compliance to clinical regimens. The ability to provide coaching messages in a way that is tailored both to the user and the situation likely will enable a trustworthy relationship between the technology and the user, improving technology acceptance and effectiveness. Future work should focus on improving technology reliability, usability, and portability, and conducting large-scale longitudinal evaluations.

ACKNOWLEDGEMENTS

Funding for this study was provided by the National Science Foundation, Engineering Research Center (EEC0540865), and the US Department of Veterans Affairs Rehabilitation Research and Development Service Center of Excellence for Wheelchairs and Associated Rehabilitation Engineering (B3142C).

REFERENCES

1. Virtual coach: disk offers expert guidance. CD-ROM saves man's only leg: a Sarasota surgeon would have had to amputate without the disk to guide him through a rare procedure. Sarasota Herald-Tribune. 1997.
2. Plan and schedule your season. TRAININGPEAKS. The ultimate training & nutrition software. 2009.

3. Pondera virtual coach sports program. In: Virtual Coach Sports LLC, 2007, volume 2009.

4. Virtual coach program. Business development services. In: Big Time Business, 2005.

5. Virtual coach/basic training combo. In: Financial Strategies, Incorporated, 2007, volume 2009.

6. Andrade AS, McGruder HF, Wu AW, et al. A programmable prompting device improves adherence to highly active antiretroviral therapy in HIV-infected subjects with memory impairment. Clin Infect Dis 2005;41:875.

7. Richardson M, Frank AO. Electric powered wheelchairs for those with muscular dystrophy: problems of posture, pain, and deformity. Disabil Rehabil Assist Technol 2009;4:181.

8. Buttussi F, Chittaro L, Nadalutti D. Bringing mobile guides and fitness activities together: a solution based on an embodied virtual trainer. In: MobileHCI, Helsinki, Finland.

9. Mihailidis A, Barbenel JC, Fernie G. The efficacy if an intelligent cognitive orthosis to facilitate handwashing by persons with moderate-to-severe dementia. Neuropsychol Rehabil 2004;14:134.

10. Mihailidis A, Davis J. The potential of intelligent technology as an occupational enabler. Occupational Therapist Now 2005;22–3.

11. Fogg BJ. Persuasive technology: using computers to change what we think and do. San Francisco (CA): Morgan Kaufmann; 2003.

12. U.S. Department of Health and Human Services. Healthy people 2010: understanding an improving health. 2nd edition. Washington, DC: US Government Printing Office; 2000.

13. Field MJ, Jette AM. The future of disability in America. Washington, DC: National Academics Press; 2007.

14. White GW, Gutierrez RT, Seekins T, et al. Preventing and managing secondary conditions: a proposed role for independent living centers. J Rehabil 1996;62.

15. Kaushik P, Intille SS, Larson K. Observations from a case study on user adapative reminders for medication adherence. Second international conference on pervasive computing technologies for healthcare. Tampere, Finland, January 30–February 1, 2008.

16. Chang JS, Lee DA, Petursson G, et al. The effect of a glaucoma medication reminder cap on patient compliance and intraocular pressure. JOP 1999;7: 117.

17. Riva A, Smigelski C, Friendman R. WebDietAID: an interactive Web-based nutritional counselor. Proceedings of the American Medical Informatics Association Annual Symposium. Los Angeles, California, November 4–8, 2000.

18. Clark NM, Zimmerman BJ. A social cognitive view of self-regulated learning about health. Health Educ Res 1990;5:371.

19. IJsselsteijn WA, de Kort YAW, Westerink J, et al. Virtual fitness: stimulating exercise behavior through media technology. Presence 2006;15:688.

20. Mihailidis A, Boger JN, Craig T, et al. The coach prompting system to assist older adults with dementia through handwashing: an efficacy study. BMC Geriatr 2008;8(28).

21. Dey A, Abowd G. Towards a better understanding of context and context awareness. Presented at the CHI 2000 Workshop on the What, Who, Where, When, and How of Context Awareness. The Hague, Netherlands, April 3, 2000.

22. McBride CM, Emmons KM, Lipkus IM. Understanding the potential of teachable moments: the case of smoking cessation. Health Educ Res 2003;18:156–70.

23. Bickmore T, Mauer D, Crespo F, et al. Persuasion, task interruption, and health regimen adherence. Presented at the Second International Conference on Persuasive Technology. Palo Alto, California, April 26–27, 2007.

24. Siewiorek D, Smailagic A, Furukawa J, et al. Sensay: a context-aware mobile phone. Presented at the IEEE International Symposium on Wearable Computers. White Plains, New York, October 21–23, 2003. p. 248–9.

25. Mayer RE, Sobko K, Mautone PD. Social cues in multimedia learning: role of speaker's voice. J Educ Psychol 2003;95:419.

26. Mohamad Y, Hammer S, Haverkamp F, et al. Evaluation study: training with animated pedagogical agents. Computer helping people with special needs. Linz, Austria, July 15–20, 2002. p. 3–25.

27. Atkinson RK. Optimizing learning from examples using animated pedagogical agents. J Educ Psychol 2002;94(2):416–27.

28. King WJ, Ohya J. The representation of agents: anthropomorphism, agency, and intelligence. Conference on Human Factors in Computing Systems. Vancouver, British Columbia, April 13–18, 1996. p. 289–90.

29. Walker JH, Sproull L, Subramani R. Using a human face in an interface. In: Proceedings of the SIGCHI conference on human factors in computing systems: celebrating interdependence. Boston, Massachusetts, 1994. p. 85–91.

30. Bickmore T, Mauer D, Brown T. Context awareness in a handheld exercise agent. PMC 2009;5(3):226–35.

31. Bickmore TW, Picard RW. Establishing and maintaining long-term human–computer relationships. ACM Trans Comput Hum Interact 2005;12(2):293–327.

32. Moreno R, Mayer RE, Spires HA, et al. The case for social agency in computer-based teaching: do students learn more deeply when they interact with animated pedagogical agents? Cognit Instruct 2001;19(2):177–213.

33. Steege MW, Wacker DP, McMahon CM. Evaluation of the effectiveness and efficiency of two stimulus prompt strategies with severely handicapped students. J Appl Behav Anal 1987;20(3):293–9.

34. McDonnell J, Ferguson B. A comparison of time delay and decreasing prompt hierarchy strategies in teaching banking skills to students with moderate handicaps. J Appl Behav Anal 1989;22(1):85–91.

35. Andrew A, Borriello G, Fogarty J. Toward a systematic understanding of suggestion tactics in persuasive technologies. Presented at the Second International Conference on Persuasive Technology. Palo Alto, California, April 26–27, 2007. p. 259–70.

36. Bickmore T, Schulman D. Practical approaches to comforting users with relational agents, Presented at the Conference on Human Factors in Computing Systems. San Jose, California, April 28–May 3, 2007. p. 2291–6.

37. Dicianno BE, Margaria E, Arva J, et al. RESNA position on the application of tilt, recline, and elevating legrests for wheelchairs. RESNA, Arlington, Virginia, 2008.

38. Klingbeil H, Baer HR, Wilson PE. Aging with a disability. Arch Phys Med Rehabil 2004;85:68.

39. Lacoste M, Weiss-Lambrou R, Allard M, et al. Powered tilt/recline systems: why and how are they used? Assist Technol 2003;15:58.

40. Ding D, Leister L, Cooper RA, et al. Usage of tilt-in-space, recline, and elevation seating functions in natural environment of wheelchair users. J Rehabil R D 2008; 45:973.

41. Cooper R. Virtual Coach to monitor powered seat functions (PSF) usage. RESNA: Washington DC, June 26–30, 2008.

42. Elliott RW. Kiviat-graphs as a means for displaying performance data for on-line retrieval systems. Am Soc Info Sci 2007;27(3):178–82.

43. Saary MJ. Radar plots: a useful way for presenting multivariate health care data. J Clin Epidemiol 2008;60:311.
44. Chatterjee S, Price A. Healthy living with persuasive technologies: framework, issues, and challenges. J Am Med Inform Assoc 2009;16:171.
45. Lee ML, Dey AK. Lifelogging memory appliance for people with episodic memory impairment. In: 10th International Conference on Ubiquitous Computing. Seoul (Korea). p. 44.

Enhancing Quality of Life through Telerehabilitation

Michael McCue, PhD[a,b,*], Andrea Fairman, OTR[a],
Michael Pramuka, PhD[c]

KEYWORDS

- Telerehabilitation • Telehealth • Telepractice
- Telemedicine • Remote

Telerehabilitation is an emerging method of delivering rehabilitation services that uses technology to serve clients, clinicians, and systems by minimizing the barriers of distance, time, and cost. More specifically, "telerehabilitation can be defined as the application of telecommunication, remote sensing and operation technologies, and computing technologies to assist with the provision of medical rehabilitation services at a distance."[1] Much attention has been paid to the efficacy of telerehabilitation in efforts to decrease time and cost in the delivery of rehabilitation services. Some studies have also compared telerehabilitation services to face-to-face interventions to discover whether these approaches are "as good as" traditional rehabilitation approaches. However, telerehabilitation may in fact provide new opportunities that are more effective by increasing accessibility and creating the least restrictive environment.

Telerehabilitation was first documented in 1959, when interactive video was first used at Nebraska Psychiatric Institute in the delivery of mental health services. Over the past 50 years, technologists and clinicians have investigated the use of bridging the gap between individuals with specialized medical needs living in remote areas and the source of specialty care.[2] Closely related to the emergence and use of telerehabilitation are solutions to problems associated with technological, functional,

---

This work was supported by The Rehabilitation Engineering Research Center (RERC) on Telerehabilitation, funded by NIDRR, US Department of Education, Washington DC, Grant #: H133E040012.

[a] Department of Rehabilitation Science and Technology, University of Pittsburgh, 5040 Forbes Tower, 3600 Forbes Avenue, Pittsburgh, PA 15260, USA
[b] University of Pittsburgh's Rehabilitation Engineering Research centre (RERC) on Telerehabilitation, 5040 Forbes Tower, 3600 Forbes Avenue, Pittsburgh, PA 15260, USA
[c] School of Health and Rehabilitation Science, University of Pittsburgh, 5040 Forbes Tower, 3600 Forbes Avenue, Pittsburgh, PA 15260, USA
* Corresponding author.
E-mail address: mmccue@pitt.edu (M. McCue).

economic, political, and geographic convergence. Technologies that enable telereha-bilitation services, such as increased computer power and availability of high-speed data transmission lines, have become more prominent in recent years.[3]

Winters provides a comprehensive review of the conceptual models of telerehabili-tation.[4] He explains that telerehabilitation falls under a broader category of services that use telecommunication to provide health information and care across distance, termed telehealth. Telehealth is broken into 3 subcategories: telemedicine, telehealth-care, and e-health/education. Telerehabilitation is classified into the category of tele-healthcare along with telehomecare, telenursing, and telecoaching. Not clearly defined, these terms are often used interchangeably throughout the research litera-ture. There is an existing need for consensus of the terminology used in this field to allow for a clear description of services. It has been proposed that telerehabilitation warrants a separate and parallel identity alongside telehealthcare and telemedicine.[5]

AN ALTERNATIVE MODEL OF TELEREHABILITATION TO PROMOTE QUALITY OF LIFE

Much of the research literature on telerehabilitation has focused on the outcome measure of decreasing costs, saving travel time, and improving access to specialty services and expert practitioners.[6] The rationale proposed to support the exploration and implementation of telerehabilitation has been essentially based on the use of various technologies to address geographic and economic barriers, and potentially enhance cost effectiveness. An alternative perspective is that the potential benefit of telerehabilitation technologies is that effective rehabilitation services can be imple-mented in the individual's environment (home, community, workplace, and so forth).

Examples are found in the behavior therapy literature, in which there is substantial evidence that interventions delivered in vivo, or in the patient's natural environment, have been more effective than the same therapy delivered in the clinic. This benefit has been demonstrated with treatment of agoraphobia,[7,8] panic,[9] pain,[10,11] fear of reinjury in patients with back pain,[12] and social phobia.[13,14]

There is also significant impetus to support the value of medical rehabilitation services delivered in the home. Although much of this literature seems to be motivated by providing a rationale for expeditious discharge from the inpatient setting for cost-saving purposes, the research supports that the delivery of some home-based reha-bilitation services is at least as effective as the delivery of those services in hospitals, and in some cases adds contextual factors that enhance rehabilitation and outcomes. These findings support the development and implementation of telerehabilitation approaches to facilitate naturalistic rehabilitation treatment in the home.

In a study by Von Koch and colleagues,[15] a comparison between therapy following stroke delivered in the home versus in the clinic revealed that patients treated in the home took greater initiative and were more likely to express goals than patients treated in the hospital. In a similar randomized clinical control study of poststroke patients, Holmqvist and colleagues[16] determined a systematic positive effect for those treated in the home in levels of social activity, activities of daily living, motor capacity, manual dexterity, and walking. Significant differences were also noted in rate of read-mission and in patient satisfaction in favor of the home treatment group. Legg and Langhorne[17] completed a systematic review of randomized clinical trials of rehabilita-tion therapy provided at home, and found that therapy at home resulted in improved ability to undertake personal activities of daily living and reduce risk of deterioration in ability. In-home treatment was found to reduce the incidence of delirium, reduce the duration of rehabilitation, and reduce rehabilitation costs in a frail elderly population.[18]

Telerehabilitation approaches have been recommended to facilitate in-home intervention approaches with persons with traumatic brain injury[19] and the elderly.[20]

Attention to contextual factors in rehabilitation is reinforced by the World Health Organization framework that emphasizes an individual's functioning within the context of their environment.[21,22] Recognizing that the social and physical environment can be facilitative (or inhibitory), rehabilitation that can occur within the patient's own home and community has greater relevance to the patient. Ylvisaker[23] states that for individuals with brain injury, cognitive rehabilitation that occurs in the natural setting and within the context of everyday interaction and demand domains is more relevant to the individual. Willer and Corrigan[24] cite that the issue of generalization can be a major obstacle to achieving a successful rehabilitation outcome. What is learned or accomplished in one setting (eg, a clinic) does not necessarily generalize to other settings. Willer and Corrigan[24] assert that the problem of failure of generalizability can be successfully addressed by conducting rehabilitation in the environment in which the skills must be applied.

The literature on supported employment, a demonstrated effective vocational rehabilitation strategy for enabling persons with severe disabilities to achieve competitive employment outcomes, stresses 2 naturalistic features. The model is built on the "place and train" premise, which states that individuals with disabilities should be placed in the real workplace as soon as possible, and that "pretraining" in clinical or simulated environments is less effective. The second feature is that supports and interventions (including cognitive rehabilitation, assistive technology, and adjustment counseling) can be delivered in the natural environment, through a job coach.[25] Job coaching can be delivered by a live job coach, on-site, or through the use of telerehabilitation technologies to monitor and intervene remotely.[26]

In summary, there is considerable evidence to support the value of conducting some aspects of rehabilitation within the natural environment. The literature suggests that such naturalistic treatment increases functional outcomes, addresses problems with generalizability, and enhances patient satisfaction and self-direction. These factors have also been related to quality of life issues. Therefore, telerehabilitation can play a key role in the accessibility and implementation of naturalistic and in vivo treatment.

As of April 2009, 63% of adult Americans reported broadband usage within their homes, up from 55% in May 2008.[27] Given that the availability of Internet access is increasing extensively, and that wireless access is projected to become much more universally available,[28] the potential to integrate treatment and monitoring into the environments where people live and work through in vivo telerehabilitation applications can become a viable option.

TELEREHABILITATION TECHNOLOGIES

Traditional models of telemedicine began with videoconference interactions between a service provider, such as a physician or nurse, directly to a patient at the remote site. In recent years the model has been broadened, and the technologies supporting the remote service provision have diversified dramatically. This section briefly addresses models and then provides an overview of telerehabilitation technologies.

Models for providing telerehabilitation may provide services either synchronously (in real time) or asynchronously, in which data are collected and then later forwarded via email, bluetooth technology, or other electronic format for review by a clinician. Asynchronous applications are therefore often referred to as a "store and forward" approach. The exchange may occur directly between provider and patient, but more frequently includes a paraprofessional or facilitating staff person at the remote site who may be tasked simply with technology management, or may play a significant role in engaging the patient in interview or physical tasks. Telerehabilitation may alternatively follow a consultative model, in which the telerehabilitation provider participates in an assessment with the patient and his or her primary clinician at the remote site. Technology may also be developed in Web-based, robotic, or virtual reality-based formats and used autonomously by patients remotely, with the clinician observing patient responses and modifying the tasks accordingly. Here a variety of commonly used technologies for telerehabilitation are briefly reviewed, including telephones and videophones, video-conferencing, sensors, personal digital assistants (PDAs) and smart phones, virtual reality, and robotics.

Plain old telephone service (POTS) technologies use a real-time, standard analog voice-grade telephone service that remains the basic form of residential and small business service connection to the telephone network in most parts of the world. POTS is available in 97% of United States households.[4] Despite the growing availability of high-speed Internet availability in individuals' homes throughout the United States, the use of the POTS is still the most widely used mechanism for providing home tele-services.[5] This situation may be in part due to the fact that prevalence and acceptance of technologies depend largely on ease of use and keeping implementation costs low.[26] One step further is the *videophone* that is basically a telephone with a video screen, and is capable of full bidirectional video and audio transmissions for communication between people in real time. Videophones can especially be useful to persons who are deaf or who have hearing impairments, and can use them with sign language or for lip reading. *Video-conferencing* differs from the videophone in that it is designed to serve multiple participants through a conference rather than individuals. Video-conferencing is a set of interactive telecommunication technologies that allow 2 or more locations to interact via 2-way video and audio transmissions simultaneously. These interactive systems consist of some version of a video monitor, video camera, speakers, microphone, and a CODEC. The CODEC (stands for COder-DECoder) uses hardware or software to simultaneously code and decode (compress and decompress) digital video and audio information, and sends it to another CODEC where the same process is also occurring.[29]

Real-time access may also be provided through *wireless technologies* that transfer information over a distance without the use of electrical conductors or "wires." The distances involved may be short (a few meters as in television remote control) or long (thousands of miles for radio communications). When the context is clear, this term is often shortened to "wireless." Technology that is able to be provided wirelessly allows increased freedom to be used within various environments and unrestricted movement.

PDAs and cell phones are some of the most common and widely used wireless devices. PDAs are handheld computers, also known as palmtop computers or handheld mobile computing. Newer PDAs also have both color screens and audio capabilities, enabling them to be used as mobile phones (smart phones), web browsers, or portable media players. Many of today's PDAs or smart phones can access the Internet, intranets, or extranets wirelessly. Wireless, interactive, Web-based interventions are particularly suited to providing rehabilitation intervention and monitoring in the home and community environments. Gentry has completed studies in the use of PDAs as cognitive supports for persons with traumatic brain injury and multiple sclerosis. Positive outcomes were found with the use of PDAs as an intervention to improve performance of everyday life tasks for both of these populations.[30,31] Technology is quickly converging with the development of smart phones, which combine PDAs with Internet access and cellphone technology as the convention of today.

Likewise, newer technologies include software applications that allow the user to make a voice or video call over the Internet, such as in the popular application called

Skype.[32] However, clinicians must consider the need for security and ensure that all precautions are taken to maintain patient confidentiality in accordance with *Health Insurance Portability and Accountability Act* regulations. Other technologies, including remote desktop control by the therapist (or desktop "push"), are examples of how rehabilitation services, such as job coaching and career development counseling, can be applied remotely.[33]

Many *motion sensors* and technology involving *body monitoring* are now available wirelessly. A motion sensor is a device that contains a physical mechanism or electronic sensor that quantifies motion, which can be integrated with or connected to other devices that alert the user of the presence of a moving object (or person). Some examples of these devices include accelerometers for determining position in space and rate of movement, physiologic monitoring sensors that can track or check blood pressure or body temperature, electrocardiogram for heart rate, contactless sensors fatigue electromyogram for monitoring muscle activity, or electroencephalogram for monitoring brain electrical activity.[34]

A newer technology that is being used with increasing frequency is *Virtual Reality* (VR). VR technology allows a user to interact with a 3-dimensional computer-simulated environment, whether that environment is a simulation of the real world or an imaginary world. VR systems provide sensory feedback to the user and whereas most systems use visual feedback, some simulations include additional sensory information, such as sound through speakers or headphones. Although VR is not geared toward the natural environment, it approximates or recreates it. For example, the popular game called The Sims encourages players to make choices while fully engaged in an interactive environment. This characteristic has helped the game successfully attract casual gamers.[35] The Sims does not have the person engage in their natural environment to practice social skills, but creates a quasi-realistic setting to safely practice skills, with consequences but without long-term detrimental effects.

Other advanced systems called haptic systems now include tactile information, known as force feedback in applications. *Haptic technology* interfaces with the user through the sense of touch by applying forces, vibrations, or motions to the user. The user can "feel" objects in the virtual environment, and with practice can become skilled at subconsciously using an object as if it were an extension of their own body (ie, a pen for writing).[4] Rehabilitation robotics is a growing area in which haptic technology is being used to aid and augment the traditional therapy intended for patients with motor disabilities to improve motor performance, shorten the rehabilitation time, and provide objective parameters for patient evaluation.[36]

TELEREHABILITATION APPROACHES TO ENHANCE QUALITY OF LIFE

Rehabilitation services often comprise a scope of services, beginning with assessment, moving on to intervention, and then assure patient success and outcome via follow-up services. Telerehabilitation strategies and applications provide additional venues to allow for provision of rehabilitation services at a distance where persons live, work, and play. Not only has home and community-based rehabilitation been found to be preferred by persons with disabilities,[37] provision of services within the naturalistic and least restrictive settings has also been found to be more effective in several ways, as noted earlier. In particular, skills are more likely to generalize if taught in the environment(s) in which they will eventually be used in the person's daily life. Although it is not possible to provide a description of every possible clinical application of telerehabilitation in an article of this brevity, reviews of several venues for telerehabilitation focused on home and community-based rehabilitation efforts are included to exemplify the variety of clinical applications and the magnitude of potential to improve quality of life.

Remote assessment of rehabilitation needs has been described for neuropsycholog-ical status,[38] apraxia,[39] motor speech disorders,[40] wheeled mobility and seating,[5] and gait,[41] among numerous other applications. A particularly time-consuming assessment critical to everyday function has been the evaluation of a patient's home environment for accessibility and potential home modification. As part of the University of Pittsburgh's Rehabilitation Engineering Research Center on Telerehabilitation, a protocol with sup-porting software has been developed to allow accessibility assessment of a home without the need for on-site assessment via data (photos), which can then be sent elec-tronically back to the University. The software can produce a detailed 3-dimensional visual layout of the home with adequate specificity to render architectural drawing, and to make recommendations to the patient and family about potential interventions without the professional making a time-consuming trip to distant locations.[42]

Intervention in the home or work environment has been provided remotely for numerous needs, including cognitive rehabilitation using the Internet,[43] constraint-induced movement therapy using a computer and sensors to guide the patient through exercises,[44] and speech pathology for children with autism.[45] In recent years, there has been a trend toward self-management programs as a long-term intervention tool for individuals with chronic medical conditions. Although these programs were initially pre-sented in face-toface, usually group-based formats, they have now moved to Internet-based modalities.[46] Whereas the original interventions were focused on a few medical conditions such as asthma and diabetes, they have now expanded to a wider variety of chronic conditions such as epilepsy,[47] and have incorporated a variety of self-assess-ment tools, education, goal-setting, and discussion board modalities to support increased self-management. These Internet-based interventions can be conducted without requiring the patient to travel to a central site, allowing them to learn and be provided feedback on daily functions specific to their progress, and also engage with others, with the relatively simple technology of a computer and the Internet.

Another area for intervention and monitoring in rehabilitation is falls. Falls are one of the most commonly occurring problems within the aging population, often resulting in prolonged periods of or permanent disability, and typically require rehabilitation inter-ventions. In a recent study conducted by the University of California at Los Angeles (UCLA), "falls were responsible for 70% of accidental deaths in persons age 75 or older."[48] Several new devices have recently been created to reduce the incidence of falls, or at least decrease the severity of injury and impact on the individual. The SmartCane was developed by researchers at UCLA to prevent falls. Equipped with contact pressure sensors in its handle and base, this device can predict risk for falling and communicate this information wirelessly to the individual, caregivers, or medical providers. This information reveals whether the person is using the cane properly. If improper use of the SmartCane is identified, the person can then receive additional training in the proper use of the device. The lightweight SmartShoe similarly is able to determine fall risk by analyzing walking behavior patterns. Also, training can take place to improve safety and proper ambulation with use of a mobility device such as a walker.[48]

The need for ongoing case management, follow-up, or monitoring in the home envi-ronment has also found varied support in telerehabilitation, ranging from videophone support of families caring for individuals in a minimally conscious state[49] to monitoring of the number of steps taken in patients with Parkinson disease at home via a wearable sensor.[50] A more complex and well-developed system of case management and monitoring in rehabilitation was developed for veterans with polytrauma.[51] In this project, the Low Activities of Daily Living Monitoring System (LAMP) used therapists as care coordinators to provide assistive technology (AT), hands-on and remote training on AT, as well as computer and Internet access for daily completion of LAMP questionnaires on functional status, ongoing remote support for self-care, and home modifications.

OBSTACLES AND OPPORTUNITIES

There are multiple challenges and potential barriers to the implementation of telerehabilitation services in everyday clinical practice. Primary among them are concerns held by clinicians, policy issues with reimbursement and licensure, privacy, and confidentiality, and the limited scope of current research on telerehabilitation.

Schopp and colleagues[52] identified several reasons for the decreased satisfaction of clinicians that is relevant to many applications of telerehabilitation. Of note, it is the patient, not the health care provider, who is inconvenienced by the need to travel to an appointment at a distant location to see a specialist, and is therefore most likely to appreciate the opportunities afforded by telerehabilitation. For persons with disabilities or illness, traveling is often very difficult. In addition, most health care providers are accustomed to practicing in an environment over which they have full control, rather than introducing an external environment into clinical service. Many health care providers are also uneasy about use of any technological mediation between them and their clients, and believe that it may hinder therapeutic rapport. Finally, remote service provision is perceived as initially time-consuming for clinicians to learn and to implement.

Policy issues have recently been reviewed in detail, with the finding that there is a paucity of published literature that addresses policy in telerehabilitation; few policy papers have adequate empirical data, and typically only comprise a small part of a larger research article.[53] In terms of licensure issues, licensure restricts the practice of most clinicians to the state in which they are licensed. Telerehabilitation services provided across state lines may jeopardize the clinician's status and render their services as practice without a license. Physicians and other licensed rehabilitation professionals in the federal government are typically allowed to practice anywhere in the country as long as they are legitimately licensed in one state, which has allowed the Veterans Healthcare system and the American military to move quickly to implement telemedicine and telerehabilitation. Policy issues for reimbursement of clinical services are typically led by Medicare, which has implemented funding for telemedicine services (ie, teledermatology, telepathology, telepsychiatry, and so forth) in many states, but has had very limited funding for telerehabilitation.[54]

Due to the electronic nature of data transmission associated with telerehabilitation, there are differing challenges to privacy of clinical service and confidentiality of data and records compared with traditional face-to-face services with written or typed documentation. Conducting services in vivo does increase the requirement to explore who might be in the remote environment, and to carefully explain and disclose risks and benefits of telerehabilitation services to prospective patients. Transmission of data electronically affords numerous opportunities for breach of confidentiality, but as with finance and other industries, there are numerous opportunities to enhance security through encryption, networks, and so forth. In addition, many medical systems have migrated to paperless, electronic health records, negotiating many of the challenges to secure electronic communication ahead of time.

The current research literature on telerehabilitation is burgeoning in number of studies, but remains limited to clinical observations and equivalence trials, or is restricted in generalizability by small sample size. There are few large-scale clinical trials, and research in rehabilitation has traditionally been underfunded.[53] This limited empirical support for specific telerehabilitation practices negatively impacts the ability to convince prospective payers of the viability of telerehabilitation, and suggests that the field would benefit from clinicians and research activity working in tandem to document the appropriate uses of telerehabilitation for improving the quality of life.

RESOURCES

Much of the clinical work and research being done in telerehabilitation is not described in common rehabilitation journals or resources, but a familiarity with professional resources in telemedicine will provide a venue to explore applications that may have direct relevance to rehabilitation. Journals include *Telemedicine and e-health*, *Cyberpsychology and Behavior*, and the *Journal of Telemedicine and Telecare*. Given the emphasis on telemedicine in the military and the Veterans Healthcare system, journals oriented to serving those populations are also more likely to include specific clinical applications or research on telerehabilitation, such as the *Journal of Rehabilitation Research and Development* (JRRD) or *Military Medicine*.

The predominant professional organization in telemedicine is the American Telemedicine Association (ATA) (www.americantelemed.org). The ATA has a Special Interest Group in Telerehabilitation currently finalizing standards for provision of Telerehabilitation services, based in part on the nearly completed standards for Telementalhealth (http://www.americantelemed.org/i4a/pages/index.cfm?pageid=3311). Several professional organizations of rehabilitation therapies have produced position papers on the use of telerehabilitation, including AOTA,[55] ASHA,[56] and APTA.[57] Policy and advocacy issues for telemedicine and telerehabilitation are supported by the Center for Telemedicine and e-Health Law at www.telehealthlawcenter.org/.

SUMMARY

Telerehabilitation is an emerging method of delivering rehabilitation services that uses technology to serve clients, clinicians, and systems by minimizing the barriers of distance, time, and cost. The driving force for telerehabilitation has been as an alternative to face-to-face rehabilitation approaches to reduce costs, increase geographic accessibility, or act as a mechanism to extend limited resources. Most of the literature on telerehabilitation targets these needs, and justifies the use of telerehabilitation by attempts to empirically equate remote services delivered via telerehabilitation to face-to-face services. Another rationale for telerehabilitation is the potential to enhance outcomes beyond what may result from face-to-face interventions by enabling naturalistic, in vivo interventions. There is considerable support for the value of interventions delivered in the natural environment, ranging from addressing efficacy concerns by addressing problems of generalization, to increasing patient participation, including environmental context in rehabilitation, and increasing patient satisfaction. These potential outcomes are consistent with promoting quality of life. Further clinical and research exploration should explore telerehabilitation as a tool for the delivery of rehabilitation services in vivo.

REFERENCES

1. Cooper R, Fitzgerald S, Boninger M, et al. Telerehabilitation: expanding access to rehabilitation expertise. Proceedings of the IEEE 2001;89(8):1174–91.

2. Ricker J, Rosenthal M, Garay E, et al. Telerehabilitation needs a survey of persons with acquired brain injury. J Head Trauma Rehabil 2002;17(3):242–50.
3. Diamond BJ, Shreve GM, Bonilla JM, et al. Telerehabilitation, cognition and user-accessibility. NeuroRehabilitation 2003;18(2):171–7.
4. Winters JM. Telerehabilitation research: emerging opportunities. Annu Rev Biomed Eng 2002;4:287–320.
5. Schmeler MR, Schein RM, McCue M, et al. Telerehabilitation clinical and vocational applications for assistive technology: research, opportunities, and challenges. International Journal of telerehabilitation. Available at: http://telerehab. pitt.edu/ojs/index.php/Telerehab/article/viewFile/701/950. Accessed May 2, 2009.
6. Bashshur R. Telemedicine and health care. Telemed J E Health 2002;8(1):5–12.
7. Zitrin CM, Klein DF, Woerner MG. Treatment of agoraphobia with group exposure in vivo and imipramine. Arch Gen Psychiatry 1980;37(1):63–72.
8. de Beurs E, van Balkom AJ, Lange A, et al. Treatment of panic disorder with agoraphobia: comparison of fluvoxamine, placebo, and psychological panic management combined with exposure and of exposure in vivo alone. Am J Psychiatry 1995;152:683–91.
9. Ost LG, Thulin U, Ramnero J. Cognitive behavior therapy vs exposure in vivo in the treatment of panic disorder with agoraphobia: comparison of fluvoxamine, placebo, and psychological panic management combined with exposure and of exposure in vivo alone. Am J Psychiatry 1995;152:683–91.
10. Vlaeyen JW, de Jong JR, Geilen M, et al. Graded exposure in vivo in the treatment of pain-related fear: a replicated single-case experimental design in four patients with chronic low back pain. Behav Res Ther 2001;39(2):151–66.
11. Vlaeyen JW, De Jong JR, Onghena P, et al. Can pain-related fear be reduced? The application of cognitive-behavioural exposure in vivo. Pain Res Manag 2002;7(3):144–53.
12. Vlaeyen JW, de Jong JM, Geilen MP, et al. The treatment of fear of movement/(re)-injury in chronic low back pain: further evidence on the effectiveness of exposure in vivo. Clin J Pain 2002;18(4):251–61.
13. Mersch P. The treatment of social phobia: the differential effectiveness of exposure in vivo and an integration of exposure in vivo, rational emotive therapy and social skills training. Behav Res Ther 1995;33(3):259–69.
14. Salaberria P, Echeburua P. Long-term outcome of cognitive therapy's contribution to self-exposure in vivo to the treatment of generalized social phobia. Behav Modif 1998;22(3):262–84.
15. Von Koch L, Wottrich AW, Holmqvist LW. Rehabilitation in the home versus the hospital: the importance of context. Disabil Rehabil 1998;20(10):367–72.
16. Holmqvist WH, von Koch L, Kostulas V, et al. A randomized clinical control of rehabilitation at home after stroke in Southwest Stockholm. Stroke 1998;29(3):591–7.
17. Legg L, Langhorne P. Rehabilitation therapy services for stroke patients living at home: a systematic review of clinical trials. Lancet 2004;363(9406):352–6.
18. Caplan GA, Coconic J, Board N, et al. Does home treatment affect delirium? A randomized controlled trial of rehabilitation of elderly and care at home or unusual treatment. Age Ageing 2006;35(1):53–60.
19. Warden DL, Salazar AM, Martin EM, et al. A home program for rehabilitation of moderately severe brain injury patients. J Head Trauma Rehabil 2000;15(5):1092–102.
20. Hoenig HH, Sanford JA, Butterfield T, et al. Development of a technology protocol for in-home rehabilitation. J Rehabil R D 2006;43(2):287–98.

21. World Health Organization. International classification of functioning, disability and health (ICF). Geneva: WHO; 2001.
22. Kuipers P, Foster M, Smith S, et al. Using ICF-environment factors to enhance the continuum of outpatient ABI rehabilitation: an exploratory study. Disabil Rehabil 2009;31(2):144–51.
23. Ylvisaker M. Context-sensitive cognitive rehabilitation after brain injury: theory and practice. Brain Impair 2003;4(1):1–16.
24. Willer B, Corrigan JD. Whatever it takes: a model for community-based services. Brain Inj 1994;8(7):647–59.
25. Wehman PH, Kreutzer JS, West MD, et al. Return to work for persons with traumatic brain injury: a supported employment approach. Arch Phys Med Rehabil 1990;71(13):1047–52.
26. Tran BQ, Krainak DM, Winters JM. Performance evaluation of commercial POTs-based videoconferencing systems. Technical report HCTR-11-v1.0. Available at: http://faculty.cua.edu/tran/cprl/Abstract/TR-HCTR-11-v1.pdf. Accessed May 4, 2009.
27. Horrigan J. Home broadband adoption. PewInternet & American life project. Pew Research Center Publications. 2009. Available at: http://pewresearch.org/pubs/1254/home-broadband-adoption-2009. Accessed July 6, 2009.
28. Della LJ, Eroglu D, Bernhardt JM, et al. Looking to the future of new media in health marketing: deriving propositions based on traditional theories. Health Mark Q 2008;25(1&2):147–74.
29. Said A, Pearlman WA. A new, fast, and efficient image codec based on set partitioning in hierarchical trees. IEEE Trans Circuits Syst Video Technol 1996;6(3):243–50.
30. Gentry T, Wallace J, Kvarford C, et al. Personal digital assistants as cognitive aids for individuals with severe traumatic brain injury: a community-based trial. Brain Inj 2008;22(1):19–24.
31. Gentry T. PDAs as cognitive aids for people with multiple sclerosis. Am J Occup Ther 2008;62(1):18–27.
32. Skype™. Available at: http://www.skype.com/. Accessed July 6, 2009.
33. Pramuka M, Chase SL, Danilko N, et al. Telerehabilitation and Vocational Rehabilitation: Supported Self-Employment using Web-based Applications. Proceedings of the RESNA Annual Conference. Atlanta, GA: June; 2006.
34. Jovanov E, Milenkovic A, Otto C, et al. A wireless body area network of intelligent motion sensors for computer assisted physical rehabilitation. J Neuroeng Rehabil 2005;2:6.
35. Maxi™ Electronic Arts Inc. Redwood City (CA):2005. The Sims™. Available at: http://thesims.ea.com/us. Accessed May 1, 2009.
36. Brewer BR, McDowell SK, Worthen-Chaudhari LC. Poststroke upper extremity rehabilitation: a review of robotic systems and clinical results. Top Stroke Rehabil 2007;14(6):22–44.
37. Vladek BC, Miller NA, Clausen SB. The changing face of long-term care. Health Care Financ Rev 1993;14(4):5–23.
38. Girard P. Military and VA telemedicine systems for patients with traumatic brain injury. J Rehabil R D 2007;44(7):1017–26.
39. Hill A, Theodoros D, Russell T, et al. Using telerehabilitation to assess apraxia of speech in adults. Int J Lang Commun Disord, iFirst 2008;99999(1):1–17.
40. Hill AJ, Theodoros DG, Russell TG, et al. The effects of severity of aphasia upon the ability to assess language disorders via telerehabilitation. Aphasiology, iFirst 2008;23(5):627–42.
41. Russell TG, Jull GA, Wootton R. The diagnostic reliability of internet-based observational kinematic gait analysis. J Telemed Telecare 2003;9(Suppl 2):548–51.

42. Kim JB, Brienza DM, Lynch RD, et al. Effectiveness evaluation of a remote accessibility assessment for wheelchair users using virtual reality. Arch Phys Med Rehabil 2008;89(3):470–9.

43. Bergquist T, Gehl C, Lepore S, et al. Internet-based cognitive rehabilitation in individuals with acquired brain injury: a pilot feasibility study. Brain Inj 2008;22(11): 891–7.

44. Lum PS, Uswatte G, Taub E, et al. A telerehabilitation approach to delivery of constraint-induced movement therapy. J Rehabil R D 2006;43(3):391–400.

45. Parmanto B, Saptano A, Murthi R, et al. Secure telemonitoring system for delivering telerehabilitation therapy to enhance children's communication function to home. Telemed J E Health 2008;14(9):905–11.

46. Lorig KR, Ritter PL, Laurent DD, et al. Internet-based chronic disease self-management: a randomized trial. Med Care 2006;44(11):964–71.

47. DiIorio C, Escoffery C, McCart F, et al. Evaluation of WebEase: an epilepsy self-management web site. Health Educ Res 2009;24(2):185–97.

48. Naditz A. Still standing: telemedicine devices and fall prevention. Telemed J E Health 2009;15(2):137–41.

49. Hauber RP, Jones ML. Telerehabilitation support for families at home caring for individuals in prolonged states of reduced consciousness. J Head Trauma Rehabil 2002;17(6):535–41.

50. Giasanti D, Macellari V, Maccioni G. Telemonitoring and telerehabilitation of patients with Parkinson's disease: health technology assessment of a novel wearable step counter. Telemed J E Health 2008;14(1):76–83.

51. Bendixen RM, Levy C, Lutz BJ, et al. A telerehabilitation model for victims of polytrauma. Rehabil Nurs 2008;33(5):215–20.

52. Schopp LH, Johnstone BR, Merveille OC. Multidimensional telecare strategies for rural residents with brain injury. J Telemed Telecare 2000;6(1):146–9.

53. Seelman K, Hartman L. Telerehabilitation: policy issues and research tools. International Journal of telerehabilitation. Available at: http://telerehab.pitt.edu/ojs/index.php/Telerehab/article/viewFile/704/954. Accessed May 2, 2009.

54. Palsbo SE. Medicaid payment for telerehabilitation. Arch Phys Med Rehabil 2004; 85:1191–8.

55. Wakeford L, Whitman P, White MW, et al. Telerehabilitation position paper. Am J Occup Ther 2005;59(6):656–60.

56. American Speech-Language-Hearing Association. Speech-language pathologists providing clinical services via telepractice: position statement. Available at: http://www.asha.org/docs/html/PS2005-00116.html. Accessed July 6, 2009.

57. American Physical Therapy Association Government Affairs. Telehealth—definitions and guidelines BOD G03-06-06-19 (Program 19) [retitled: telehealth; amended BOD G03-03-07-12; initial BOD 11-01-28-70]. Alexandria (VA): American Physical Therapy Association.

Using Architecture and Technology to Promote Improved Quality of Life for Military Service Members with Traumatic Brain Injury

Paul F. Pasquina, MD[a],*, Lavinia Fici Pasquina, MArch[b],
Victoria C. Anderson-Barnes, BA[c], Jeffrey S. Giuggio, MArch[d,e],
Rory A. Cooper, PhD[d,e]

KEYWORDS

- Architecture • Traumatic brain injury • Quality of life
- Universal design • Assistive technology

The US Census Bureau reports that more than 41.2 million individuals older than 5 years live with some type of disability. Of this population, more than 11 million persons older than 6 years require personal assistance with every day activities.[1] Each year, approximately 1.5 million Americans sustain a traumatic brain injury (TBI), with direct medical costs and indirect costs (such as lost productivity) totaling to an estimated

[a] Department of Orthopaedics & Rehabilitation, Walter Reed National Military Medical Center, 6900 Georgia Avenue, Washington, DC 20307, USA
[b] School of Architecture and Planning, The Catholic University of America, Crough Center, 620 Michigan Ave, Washington, DC 20307, USA
[c] Center for Neuroscience and Regenerative Medicine, Uniformed Services University, 4301 Jones Bridge Road, Bethesda, MD 20814, USA
[d] Human Engineering Research Laboratories, Department of Veterans Affairs, Rehabilitation Research and Development Service, VA Pittsburgh Healthcare System, 7180 Highland Drive, Building 4, 2nd Floor East, 151R-1 Pittsburgh, PA 15206, USA
[e] Department of Rehabilitation Science & Technology, University of Pittsburgh, Pittsburgh, PA, USA
* Corresponding author.
E-mail address: paul.pasquna@u.s.army.mil (P.F. Pasquina).

Phys Med Rehabil Clin N Am 21 (2010) 207–220
doi:10.1016/j.pmr.2009.08.001
1047-9651/09/$ – see front matter © 2010 Elsevier Inc. All rights reserved.

$60 billion in the United States in 2000.[2] More than 5 million Americans are estimated to be living with long-standing disability from TBI, including cognitive, physical, behavioral, and emotional difficulties.[3–5] For veterans with service-connected disabilities in the fiscal year 2007, more than $28.2 billion was spent in compensation.[6] This number can only be expected to increase as military operations continue in support of the Global War on Terrorism.

Since military operations began in Iraq and Afghanistan, more than 1.6 million US service members have been deployed.[7] Improvements in protective body armor, medical evacuation techniques, and forward area surgical resuscitation have dramatically improved battlefield survival rates.[8] Today, injured service members are surviving wounds that would have been fatal in the previous wars. A recent RAND Corporation report estimates that approximately 320,000 service members may have experienced a TBI during deployment.[9] Because of the mechanism of the injury, which is most commonly from a blast, it is not uncommon for a soldier to sustain multiple associated injuries in addition to the TBI, including limb loss, paralysis, sensory loss, and psychological damage. As a result, many military service members and their families face significant challenges returning to a high quality of independent life.

Military reports suggest that more than 850 service members have sustained a major limb loss as a result of military service since 2001, with more than 20% of them losing more than one limb and greater than 50% also sustaining a TBI.[10] Many of these individuals have also sustained vision loss in one or both eyes, hearing deficits, pain syndromes, and difficulty with balance and orientation.[11–13] Related cognitive difficulties, such as poor memory, decreased concentration, impaired executive functioning, and emotional lability, which are manifested by irritability, anger, and depressed mood, make it difficult for many individuals to live alone or even with others.[13,14] Further complicating the problem is the young age of many of the individuals who are challenged to live with their acquired disabilities for the rest of their lives.

Current paradigms in medical rehabilitation primarily focus on teaching individuals the strategies to adapt and reintegrate into existing environments. Architecture, however, focuses more on how to adapt the environment to the individual. Architects are skilled at integrating new materials, construction methods, and design to customize an environment for an individual client. By listening to a client's needs, the architect attempts to optimize a living and work environment to improve productivity and efficiency, and also influence the mood of those who enter the space. By manipulating interior and exterior spaces through the use of volumes, light, and materials, it is the hope of architects to improve the quality of life for those who encounter their design. Just as there is a symbiosis between nature and animal life, one also exists between humans and the built environment around them. It seems only fitting, therefore, that architects work with medical and rehabilitation professionals to embrace the current challenges faced by many severely injured service members to create new environments for those with significant disabilities.

Since the signing of the Americans with Disabilities Act (ADA) of 1990, building codes have provided minimum standards to help reduce the architectural barriers experienced by individuals with disabilities.[15] Unfortunately, architecture and its role in improving the lives of individuals with disabilities have been relatively stagnant over the past 2 decades. Although advocates for "universal design" (UD) and organizations such as the Paralyzed Veterans of America (PVA) continue to promote "barrier-free environments," the field remains lacking in high-end design quality and options for individuals with disabilities.[16–18]

The concept of UD was developed in the 1990s for the purpose of creating new products that are usable by all consumers, including those with disabilities and the elderly.[19] UD involves the creation of new environments, devices, materials, and tools that provide accessibility, adaptability, ease of use, and safety to all users.[20] The concept emphasizes the importance of designing buildings, appliances, and tools that are easy to use for all individuals of all ages and abilities.[21]

Since the introduction of UD, research universities and organizations involved with disabled veterans have made efforts to spread the concept of UD to product designers and marketing firms. North Carolina State University was involved in this process, and subsequently developed 7 principles of UD. The principles include (1) equitable use, (2) flexibility in use, (3) simple and intuitive use (ie, single color pictograms), (4) perceptible information (ie, cell phones with speed dial), (5) tolerance for error (ie, temperature limiter on a shower to prevent burning), (6) low physical effort, and (7) size and space for approach and use (ie, sliding doors than hinging doors).[22] The implementation of UD in hospitals, in and around the city, and at home can have many benefits for people with disabilities. When universally designed products are integrated into everyday living, individuals with disabilities can have more control over their environment, ultimately leading to more independence and a better quality of life.

"Evidence-based design" (EBD) has gained interest by architects, builders, and clients. EBD involves applying the use of sound research to make decisions on a project to achieve the best outcome. EBD is frequently used by architects and others involved in the design and construction of commercial buildings. An evidence-based designer works with an informed client, or group of clients, to determine the best solution that will meet the needs of the clients. By implementing EBD, needs of the clients can be met through a collaborative effort between architects, interior designers, facility managers, and anyone else closely involved with the project.

The Center for Health Design, created in 1993, is an advocacy and research organization that seeks to promote the implementation of EBD within the health care system. The mission of the Center is to "transform healthcare environments for a healthier, safer world through design research, education, and advocacy."[22] The organization seeks to promote forward thinking within the health care discipline, and it supports the implementation of personalized architecture or design. The Center for Health Design is involved in several research projects throughout the United States that are associated with the implementation of EBD.[23] The Pebble Project is one initiative that has received growing attention throughout the past several years.

Founded in 2000, the Pebble Project is a nationwide research effort designed to provide evidence to health care professionals regarding the importance of a health care facility's design.[24] The goal of the initiative was to establish that the design and layout of a room or building has a significant impact on patient and staff outcomes. The Pebble Project has research initiatives throughout the United States, and preliminary data have been gathered from several research sites. The PeaceHealth Organization in Eugene, Oregon, for example, installed ceiling lifts and booms in the intensive care unit and neurology department to see what the effect would be on patient handling injuries.[25] The results were encouraging; patient handling injuries decreased by 99%. Another medical center in Boise, Idaho, Saint Alphonsus Regional Medical Center, discovered that after renovations were made to a nursing unit (including larger rooms within the ward, carpet in the hallways, and acoustic tiles on walls and ceilings), noise levels had dropped significantly and quality of sleep improved from 4.9 to 7.3 (on a 10-point scale).[26] Hospitals and clinics throughout the nation that are involved with the Pebble Project have experienced similar positive changes associated with patient outcomes, and staff morale has increased in hospitals where EBD has been implemented.

Health care organizations have begun to take notice of EBD principles. Schweitzer and colleagues[26] conducted a review of optimal healing environments within the health care setting, emphasizing the need for designing healing spaces that contribute to making improvements in patient satisfaction and well-being. Schweitzer's group discussed a variety of stimuli that have an effect on patient recovery and overall well-being. Examples include personal space, sensory environment (including smells and sound or noise), environmental complexity, fresh air and ventilation, light, color, viewing and experiencing nature, art esthetics and entertainment, and positive distractions (including humor entertainment). The complexity of the environment was reported to positively influence elderly cognitive function.

EBD supports the principle of using design to promote patient comfort and reduce any detrimental effects on the patients' physical or psychological well-being. The use of EBD becomes particularly challenging, however, when given the unique considerations for each patient. Many health care settings treat patients of multiple different injuries and illnesses with varied social and cultural backgrounds. Regardless of the widespread patient diversity, EBD advocates that a patient's physical, mental, emotional, and spiritual healing must be considered in the design of a health care facility.

The literature highlights several approaches that hospitals and clinics may take for better incorporation of patient needs. To begin with, research conducted on geriatric patients suggested that the arrangement of furniture within hospital lounges and even individual rooms has an effect on social interactions and communication.[27] As a result, proper placement of furniture can lead to increased social interactions and increased communication between patients, family members, and staff. In addition to furniture arrangements, location and number of nursing stations can also affect patient and staff relationships. Increasing the number of nursing stations within a ward may be valuable for patients, because this may allow for increased confidentiality and more privacy between patients and staff. Likewise, increased visiting hours for family and friends can have a positive effect on patient well-being, because contact with caring individuals during the recovery process has been shown to reduce stress and is a positive contributor to health.[28] Furthermore, widening doors to patient bathrooms may reduce patient falls, and single-bed hospital rooms have been reported to lead to fewer medication errors and improved comfort for the family and friends of the patient.[29] Patients with depression may experience a reduction or relief from symptoms when their environment encourages physical activity.[30] Finally, various images and symbols located within the hospital bedroom or hallways may influence the behavior of patients.[31]

Improved environments within health care organizations may also positively influence the medical staff. For example, relationships among hospital staff members may be improved by designing an environment that encourages positive interactions among staff members, such as gardens and staff-only lounges. In addition, redesigning nursing stations to allow for more opportunities for patient and staff interactions may improve staff satisfaction and patient outcomes.[27] It is well known that stress, anxiety, depression, and loss of control are detrimental to health.[26,32,33] The opposite is also true: optimism, self-efficacy, and a sense of control are associated with positive outcomes and good health.[26,34,35] Proponents of EBD believe that this can and should be influenced by architecture.

In addition to the initiatives taking place in advanced design, rehabilitation engineers and scientists continue to apply emerging technologies and materials to advance assistive technology (AT) to improve the lives of individuals with disabilities. AT devices, such as ultralight wheelchairs, robotic systems, and microprocessor prostheses, allow individuals with impaired mobility to be much more independent than they were even a decade ago.[19] Current adaptive equipment will allow a person with tetraplegia, limb loss, or visual impairment to ski down a mountain, sail across a lake, or return to activities such as hunting, fishing, or even scuba diving. Cognitive aids, including a personal digital assistant (PDA), are frequently used to help individuals with memory problems to remember names, phone numbers, appointments, or medication regimens. Improved personal computers and new software applications are able to turn text into Braille, operate various entertainment systems from a single platform, interpret voice commands, and automatically activate emergency support systems as needed in cases of home fires or burglary. Despite these fascinating advances, there has been little effort in how to best incorporate these AT devices into modern architecture and design practice.[36]

The concept of "smart homes" has also emerged as a way to bridge advanced technology, especially AT, into the home environment of individuals with disabilities. Over the past few years, the media have started reporting on the concept of a "smart home." According to a CNN report by Julie Clothier,[36] eNeo Labs, a company in Barcelona, Spain, has created an environment-friendly "smart home." Clothier reported that eNeo Labs has designed and developed a home that is controlled by the click of a button: all household appliances are connected and controlled by a single remote control; settings can be personalized for different family members; and the house can accept, respond to, and send text messages to its owner, notifying him, for example, that there is a water leak. Although seemingly unreal, this concept is being tested on a family of 4 living outside Barcelona. The CNN report and another report featured in LiveScience highlighted the unique abilities of the house, stating that it would be "security-conscious and aware of its inhabitants at all times," noting when a person enters and exits a room, and eventually being able to respond to voice commands.[19]

The General Manager of eNeoLabs, Javier Zamora, stated that there are 2 main components to a smart home: the "information network" and the "brain." The "information network" serves to connect all of the household appliances within the home, and the "brain" coordinates the activities of the appliances and connects them to the outside world. Although "smart home" technology is in its infancy in the United States, it seems promising that the technology will be obtainable in the coming years.

Of particular interest of many civilian, military, and veterans groups is what can be done to help service members with TBI and associated comorbidities reintegrate successfully into society. The authors believe that the importance of one's environment during recovery and rehabilitation, whether in a hospital setting or at home, is underemphasized and that through collaborative efforts between architects, designers, engineers, and clinicians, better solutions can be achieved to improve the quality of life for many severely injured service members.

The authors' team recently explored the role that architecture could play in helping injured service members with TBI. Through a collaborative effort between the Catholic University of America; University of Pittsburgh, the US Department of Veterans Affairs, the Rehabilitation Research and Development Service, and the Walter Reed Army Medical Center (WRAMC), a team of architects and students met clinical experts and also individuals with TBI and their family members to better understand their needs. Focus groups conducted structured and nonstructured interviews with medical staff, patients, and families. In addition, as part of his architectural master's thesis, Jeffrey Giuggio immersed himself at WRAMC, where he directly observed patients and families, and also interviewed members of the TBI clinical teams to best understand their unique needs.

It was clear that existing environments, whether in hospitals, commercial buildings, or private residences were not optimal for individuals who had difficulty with orientation, irritability, light sensitivity, or emotional lability, even though all these environments met ADA standards. More troubling, however, was the patient's and family's report of the difficulty in returning home. Fundamental in the rehabilitation and recovery of individuals with severe injury is their return home and reintegration in society. In fact the World Health Organization places great emphasis on "participation" as a meaningful measure of outcomes from a disability.[37,38] "Participation" may involve activities such as work, education, parenting, or volunteerism, but at its core seeks to improve the lives of individuals with disabilities by having them be active participants in the world and in the lives of people around them. Many individuals with TBI continue to have significant difficulty in living independently. Some injured service members, who were once high-functioning soldiers responsible for operating million-dollar equipment and who were models of self-reliance and independence, due to their acquired disability are now forced to move back in with their parents, relying on them for basic functions such as feeding, bathing, and toileting. This loss of independence only exacerbates their state of mind and may often cause the development of serious negative mental health.

Hearing these concerns, the authors' team sought to concentrate its efforts by trying to improve the home environment for this challenging patient population. The authors offer the following thesis, which was developed by Mr Giuggio and his advisors, as an example of how architecture, design, and technology may be applied to help mitigate the effect of disabilities on a military population with TBI, at the same time hoping that it will be only the first step in further studies for bringing professionals together from various disciplines to improve the lives of all persons with disabilities.

The thesis was to design a contemporary living environment for service members with TBI and its associated disabilities. While emphasis was placed on incorporating the latest technology in AT, equal importance was also given to the functionality of the environment and to the esthetics. To avoid the "sterile" atmosphere created in most medical facilities, this project sought to create a unique, clean, and modern space, commiserate with a young population of individuals with disabilities, with the belief that this would also be more conducive to healing. Because of the complexities of associated injuries and resultant disabilities, it was decided that such an intervention would need to be modular, so that it could be customized for each individual and family.

During the early stages of development, it was clear that a new "vocabulary" of design features needed to be formulated to meet the unique needs of this patient population. To this end, a legend of design graphics was created that could be translated into architectural drawings to denote specific needs (**Fig. 1**). Patients with TBI may have multiple cognitive impairments, accompanied by loss of vision or the use of one or more limbs. A suitable environment, therefore, must address issues such as privacy, pathfinding, acoustics, orientation, mobility, access, comfort, and mood control. In architectural terms, these must be displayed in graphic form to facilitate the design process. The conceptual diagrams in **Fig. 1** were derived to designate UD features that would accommodate a multitude of impairments in association with TBI. The conceptual diagrams serve as guidelines in the design to accommodate both patient and caregiver needs.

On reviewing the existing literature and technologic capabilities available in UD, EBD, smart homes, and AT, the authors' research revealed multiple interventions that could be used to help meet the needs of patients and their families with complex injuries. For example, colors and textures could be used to aid with pathfinding. New lighting systems could be used to assist in orientation to time and space. The use of chromatherapy or ambient noises may help with mood adjustments or pain management, and the use of radiofrequency identification devices may be used to trigger smart devices to turn switches on and off throughout the environment to fully

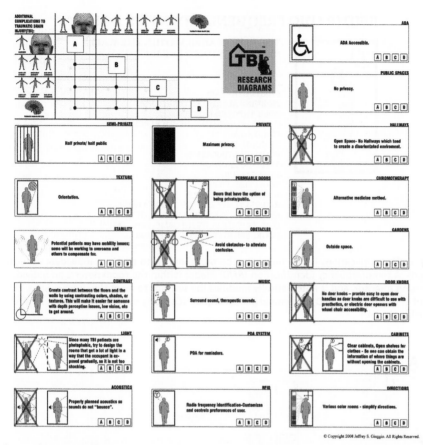

Fig. 1. The upper left-hand corner presents various combinations of possible TBI complications, labeled with letters A to D. The surrounding diagrams represent architectural and personal elements beneficial to all injury types. (*Courtesy of* Jeffrey S. Giuggio, MArch., Pittsburgh, PA.)

customize to an individual's needs (**Fig. 2**). As the authors' study continued, however, it was clear that many of these features were contradictory, which created unforeseen challenges. For example, while it is important to enhance orientation to make the bathroom readily visible and accessible for an individual with cognitive or visual impairments, this space must also become private once the users find their destination. Likewise, natural light often enhances mood and time orientation, but may need to be "turned off" suddenly for a patient who develops a migraine headache, which may be exacerbated by light exposure. It was therefore important for the design to be able to address these challenges graphically at first, before establishing possible solutions.

At the core of this thesis was the development of a modular wall system that could be applied to either new construction or retrofit into an existing home. Each wall panel could be constructed to address the unique needs of each individual. Within the wall systems, various devices could be incorporated into the vertical sections of each wall to add or subtract features as needed (**Fig. 3**). These wall panels could then be placed in a modular sequence to create a room or home (**Fig. 4**). The wall systems should be

RFID (RADIO FREQUENCY IDENTIFICATION)

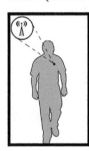

THE RFID READER WITHIN THE WALL SYSTEM CUSTOMIZES BASED ON USER:

-MUSIC
-LIGHTING
-CHROMOTHERAPY
-MORNING ALARM(LED LIGHTING)
-DIRECTION(LED LIGHTING)
-CONTRAST/LIGHTING(DEPTH PERCEPTION)
-PDA SYSTEM
-REMINDERS
-ROOM IDENTIFICATION
-APPLIANCES(ON/OFF)
-TEMPERATURE
-ROOM TEMPERATURE
-WATER TEMPERATURE
-RAILING TEMPERATURE(ORIENTATION)
-SPD WALL SYSTEM(PUBLIC/PRIVATE)
-LOUVER WALL SYSTEM(PUBLIC/PRIVATE)
-DOORS SPD SYSTEM(PUBLIC/PRIVATE)

Fig. 2. The applications in the figure can be programmed to meet an individual's specific needs. A radiofrequency identification (*RFID*) reader within the room detects an individual wearing a sensor, and it automatically modifies the settings to meet the user's desires. LED, light-emitting diode; SPD, suspended partial display. (*Courtesy of* Jeffrey S. Giuggio, MArch., Pittsburgh, PA.)

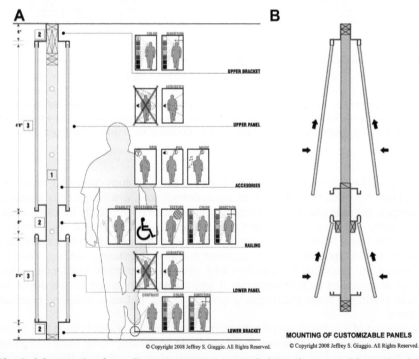

Fig. 3. (*A*) Example of a wall system containing LED lighting (*upper and lower brackets*), a hand railing, acoustic panels (*upper and lower panels*), and accessories including an RFID reader, a PDA, and speakers. (*B*) The wall system contains panels that can clip in and out to customize design. (*Courtesy of* Jeffrey S. Giuggio, MArch., Pittsburgh, PA.)

3D ASSEMBLY

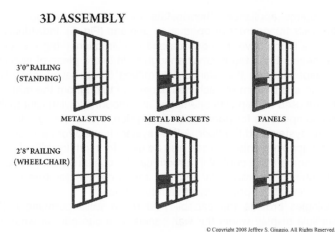

Fig. 4. The assembly process. The wall can be customized to standing and wheelchair height. The device can be retrofitted into an existing home by attaching brackets to studs and clipping desired panels. This 3-dimensional plan depicts all of the technologies and design cues throughout the apartment or living space. (*Courtesy of* Jeffrey S. Giuggio, MArch., Pittsburgh, PA.)

made of durable acoustic panels that can modify sound transmission and resist damage caused by wheelchair or prosthetic collision. In addition, the wall panels should be easily removable to service or install new technology as it is developed. A handrail is added to enhance stability and facilitate orientation, but is built "in," or subtracted from the panel volume, instead of built "out," for practical and esthetic reasons. Within each wall, a radiofrequency identification (RFID) reader is installed to create a smart environment that interacts with the user, whether it is with the injured patient or the patient's family member. The RFID reader is able to customize music,

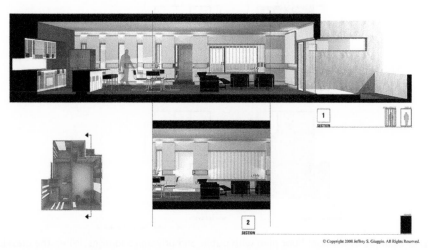

Fig. 5. The wall system has the capability of being public or private by using suspended particle display. Section 1 shows the translucent walls (*public*) and section 2 shows the opaque walls (*private*). (*Courtesy of* Jeffrey S. Giuggio, MArch., Pittsburgh, PA.)

lighting, PDA systems, appliances, thermostats, window and door opening systems, and can make walls transparent or opaque on demand (**Fig. 5**). Individuals entering or living within the home have an individualized radiofrequency tag that designates their particular needs. Each tag is small enough to fit into a piece of jewelry or into a wheelchair, depending on the user. Light-emitting diode–based (LED) lighting is emitted at the top and bottom of each wall panel and throughout the railing system; various colors are used to help with orientation and mood. Allowing light to illuminate the floor helps compensate for poor depth perception, thus creating a firm contrast between the wall system and the floor. A PDA system is used for reminders such as medications and appointments, and can also be used for room identification for blind individuals. The temperature control in a room can be customized for the comfort of the individual entering the room. In addition, the water temperature can also be programmed to prevent the possibility of harmful burns.

New technologies provide the capability to make walls permeable. By using suspended particle display within the wall panels, one can control what is private

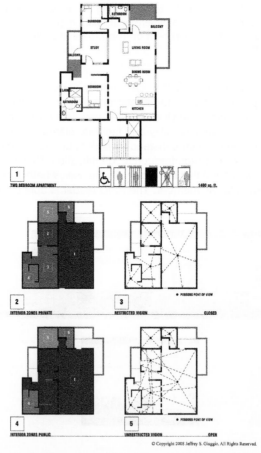

© Copyright 2008 Jeffrey S. Giuggio. All Rights Reserved.

Fig. 6. Example of a model floor plan with public and private conditions. When the glass is translucent (public), visual obstructions are alleviated. When the glass is opaque (private), vision is constrained to each individual room. (*Courtesy of* Jeffrey S. Giuggio, MArch., Pittsburgh, PA.)

and what is public by passing an electric current through glass panels that alter the view between transparent/clear and opaque, thus providing a means of better privacy instantaneously. Allowing the walls to open, however, eases orientation and the burden of tracking individuals by a caregiver or video surveillance system. This same concept can be used for glass panels within the kitchen cabinets. When a person is in the kitchen the cabinets become transparent, making it easier to obtain information, and when they leave the kitchen the cabinet panels become opaque.

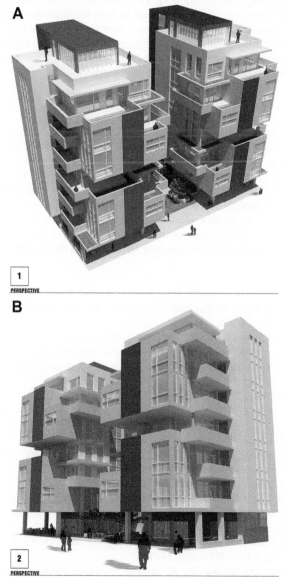

Fig. 7. Front (A) and rear (B) perspectives of the building rendering. (*Courtesy of* Jeffrey S. Giuggio, MArch., Pittsburgh, PA.)

Laying each panel in series allows endless possibilities of creating various floor plans. **Fig. 6** depicts a possible layout of an apartment of 1400 square feet, which was influenced by several factors. It was important to create a plan that removed visual obstructions or hallways where someone suffering from TBI could become easily disoriented or confused. While entering a house, furniture is all that separates the living room, dining room, and kitchen. This setting allows the person to obtain all the desired information within a single room. The floor plan layout also allowed the stacking of these apartments into a contemporary apartment or residential building to achieve a living community (**Fig. 7**). These residential buildings ideally would be constructed within an urban landscape to help facilitate reintegration into society, to obtain access to public transportation, restaurants, museums, theaters, vocational rehabilitation programs; and to be in proximity to medical facilities. Each complex was also designed to have available commercial space for retail shops, a café, and a courtyard to help further enhance socialization.

SUMMARY

The possibilities that exist to integrate the latest technologies into today's architecture design are limitless, but they are in need of active study. Collaboration between experts in clinical care, rehabilitation engineering, AT, and architecture will lead to improved solutions and, hopefully, improved long-term outcomes for individuals with disabilities, and further mitigate the negative effect of these disabilities on the health care system and the public. Investment in these strategies now may have significant long-term dividends for society. Moreover, helping individuals and families who have sacrificed so much in the service of their country merit the full intent of those countries to use all possibilities to optimize their recovery and reintegration.

REFERENCES

1. U.S. Census Bureau Facts for Features: Americans with Disabilities Act: July 26. U.S. Newswire 26 May, 2009.
2. Vanderploeg RD, Schwab K, Walker WC, et al. Rehabilitation of traumatic brain injury in active duty military personnel and veterans: defense and veterans brain injury center randomized controlled trail of two rehabilitation approaches. Arch Phys Med Rehabil 2008;89:2227–38.
3. Thurman DJ, Alverson C, Dunn KA, et al. Traumatic brain injury in the United States: a public health perspective. J Head Trauma Rehabil 1999;14:602–15.
4. Rimel RW, Giordani B, Barth JT, et al. Disability caused by minor head injury. Neurosurgery 1981;9:221–8.
5. Thornhill S, Teasdale GM, Murray GD, et al. Disability in young people and adults one year after head injury: prospective cohort study. BMJ 2000;320:1631–5.
6. Available at: http://www.census.gov/compendia/statab.
7. Tanielian T, Jaycox LH. Invisible wounds of war: psychological and cognitive injuries, their consequences, and services to assist recovery. Santa Monica (CA): RAND Corporation; 2008.
8. Gawande A. Causualties of war – military care for the wounded from Iraq and Afghanistan. N Engl J Med 2004;351:2471–5.
9. Tanielian T, Jaycox LH, Schell TL, et al. The Invisible Wounds Study Team. Invisible wounds of war: summary and recommendations for addressing psychological and cognitive injuries. Santa Monica (CA): RAND Corporation; 2008. MG-720/1-CCF, p. 64. Available at: http://veterans.rand.org.

10. Data obtained from the Proceedings of the Armed Forces Amputee Program, Walter Reed Army Medical Center, July 2009.
11. Sayer NA, Chiros CE, Sigford B, et al. Characteristics and rehabilitation outcomes among patients with blast and other injuries sustained during the Global War on Terror. Arch Phys Med Rehabil 2008;89(1):163–70.
12. Radfar-Baublitz LS, Pickett TC, McDonald SD, et al. (2006, March). Objectively assessing balance deficits after TBI: the role of computerized posturography. Association of Academic Physiatrists 2006 Annual Meeting. Daytona, Florida, March 2, 2006.
13. Walker WC, Seel RT, Curtiss G, et al. Headache after moderate and severe traumatic brain injury: a longitudinal analysis. Arch Phys Med Rehabil 2005;86:1793–800.
14. Vanderploeg RD, Curtiss G, Luis CA, et al. Long-term morbidities following self-reported mild traumatic brain injuries. J Clin Exp Neuropsychol 2007;29(6): 585–98.
15. Americans with Disabilities Act Law & Legal definition. Available at: http://definitions.uslegal.com/a/americans-with-disabilities-act.
16. Breaking down barriers: after 10 years, Marc Mendelsohn's efforts to promote universal design are finally paying off. Reeves Journal 2002.
17. The Center for Universal Design home page. Available at: http://www.design.ncsu.edu/cud/index.htm.
18. Lichter M. Architecture. (PVA in Action). Paraplegia News Paralyzed Veterans of America 2002.
19. Cooper RA, Ohnabe H, Hobson D, editors. An introduction to rehabilitation engineering. New York: Taylor and Francis Group LLC; 2006. p. 1–18, 129–55, 239–59.
20. Universal design and occupational therapy. The Canadian J of OT. June 2003. Pangrazio P. Universal design: the right fit. (Around the House).
21. Pangrazio P. Universal design: the right fit. (Around the House). Paraplegia News, Sep 2002.
22. The Center for Health Design. Available at: http://www.healthdesign.org/aboutus/index.php.
23. The Center for Health Design. Available at: http://www.healthdesign.org/research.
24. The Center for Health Design. Available at: http://www.healthdesign.org/research/pebble.
25. The Center for Health Design. Available at: http://www.healthdesign.org/research/pebble/data.php.
26. Schweitzer M, Gilpin L, Frampton S. Healing spaces: elements of environmental design that make an impact on health. J Altern Complement Med 2004; 10(Suppl 1):S71–83.
27. Melin L, Gotestam KG. The effects of rearranging ward routines on communication and eating behaviors of psychogeriatric patients. J Appl Behav Anal 1981; 14:47–51.
28. Lepore S, Mata AK, Evans G. Social support lowers cardiovascular reactivity in an acute stressor. Psychosom Med 1993;55:518–24.
29. Page A. Keeping patients safe: transforming the work environment of nurses. Washington, DC: National Academy of Sciences; 2004.
30. Jackson RJ. Physical spaces, physical health. AIA J Arch 2003;1:1–2.
31. Astorino LD. Enhancing the design process through visual metaphor. Healthcare Des 2003;3:12–7.
32. Lindheim R, Syme L. Environments, people and health. Annu Rev Public Health 1983;4:335–59.

33. Taylor S, Repetti R, Seeman T. Health psychology: what is an unhealthy environment and how does it get under the skin? Annu Rev Psychol 1997;48:411–7.
34. Lorig KR, Sobel DS, Steward AL, et al. Evidence suggesting that a chronic disease self-management program can improve health status while reducing hospitalization: a randomized trial. Med Care 1999;37:5–14.
35. Sobel D. Rethinking medicine: improving health outcomes with cost effective psychosocial interventions. Psychosom Med 1995;57:234–44.
36. Clothier J. 'Smart' homes not far away. CNN.com. May 31, 2005.
37. Parry J, Wright J. Community participation in health impact assessments: intuitively appealing but practically difficult. Bull World Health Organ 2003; 81(6):388.
38. Smith LK. Community participation in health: a case study of world health organization's healthy cities project in Barcelona and Sheffield. Community Dev J 1991;26:112–7.

Current State of Mobility Technology Provision in Less-Resourced Countries

Alexandra N. Jefferds, BS[a], Nahom M. Beyene, MS[a],
Nekram Upadhyay, MS[c], Puneet Shoker, BPT[c],
Jonathan L. Pearlman, PhD[a],*, Rory A. Cooper, PhD[a],
Joy Wee, MSc, MD, FRCPC[b]

KEYWORDS

- Wheelchairs • Mobility • Quality of life • Provision
- Less-resourced countries • International

Many rehabilitation specialists understand that in lower-income countries, the need for assistive technology (AT) outweighs availability; research and development are called for. Since the publication of the earliest papers, appropriate technology for people with disabilities (PWD) has, to a limited extent, become more available and of better quality. International convention has recognized the need for progress toward the inclusion of PWD in their communities through a social model of disability.[1,2] Although there remains a great deal of work to meet the needs of millions worldwide, better tools and technologies are in development. This paper provides an overview of the work that has been done thus far in low- and middle-income countries, including recent research carried out by the authors' laboratory in collaboration with the Indian Spinal Injuries Centre in New Delhi.

This work was supported by the National Science Foundation under a supplement to REU Grant No. EEC 0552351. This material is the result of work supported with resources and the use of facilities at the Human Engineering Research Laboratories, VA Pittsburgh Healthcare System.
[a] Department of Veterans Affairs, VA Pittsburgh Healthcare System, 7180 Highland Drive, Building 4, 2nd Floor, 151R1-H, University of Pittsburgh, Pittsburgh, PA 15206, USA
[b] Providence Care, St Mary's of the Lake Hospital Site, Queen's University, Postal Bag 3600, Kingston, Ontario, K7L 5A2, Canada
[c] Indian Spinal Injuries Centre, Sector C, Vasant Kunj, New Delhi, 110070, India
* Corresponding author. VA Pittsburgh Healthcare System, 7180 Highland Drive, Building 4, 2nd Floor, 151R1-H, Pittsburgh, PA 15206.
E-mail address: jlp46@pitt.edu (J.L. Pearlman).

Phys Med Rehabil Clin N Am 21 (2010) 221–242
doi:10.1016/j.pmr.2009.07.011
1047-9651/09/$ – see front matter. Published by Elsevier Inc.

SNAPSHOTS

Although appropriate technology is scarce throughout much of the world, varying political stability, national resources, and societal attitudes affect the lives of PWD. Although rehabilitation specialists often talk in terms of "technology for less-resourced environments," the situation in each country is different and may need to be evaluated on its own terms. This section gives examples of several countries in various stages of progress for PWD.

Afghanistan

In recent decades, Afghanistan has experienced political upheaval and violence. Years of civil war have left the country littered with landmines, and consequently with a large number of amputees. Historically, some provision of AT was given to men with amputations, although this service was not rendered to women or individuals with other types of orthopedic disabilities.[3] Taliban rule forbade employment of women, which compromised the quality of health services. Traditional societal views and isolation from international convention have contributed to a lack of social progress with respect to disability.[4] War wounds frequently disable men, and the deterioration of infrastructure and services has taken its toll on the physical and mental well-being of women and children.[5] An effort was made to include women in a study to evaluate a wheelchair designed for Afghanistan[6]; however, among those recruited, women were still a minority.

There have been several internal and international efforts to bring relief to this situation. The Physical Therapy Institute in Kabul trains therapists, although employment of these approximately 200 individuals is concentrated in urban areas. The Rehabilitation of Afghans with Disability (RAD) program trains physical therapy assistants to work in rural areas and implements several rehabilitation programs. Even with these efforts, the physical therapy needs of the Afghan people are not well met.[5]

India

India is an emerging economic power where poverty, accessibility barriers, and repair resources present challenges to wheelchair use.[7] However, the Indian government is concerned with promoting the welfare of its citizens with disabilities. The Persons with Disabilities Act of 1995 was passed to protect PWD in education, employment, and other situations in which they encounter discrimination.[8] Implementation of this act is difficult, as is the enforcement of much of India's human rights legislation. However, the Ministry of Social Justice and Empowerment's Assistance to Disabled Persons for Purchase (ADIP) Scheme is intended to assist PWD with acquiring AT,[9] and parts of India's infrastructure, such as the buses in New Delhi, are slowly being made wheelchair accessible.[10]

Kosovo

One of the world's newest nations faces the challenge of rebuilding a health care system after decades of soviet bureaucracy and war. When the country was part of Yugoslavia, the health care system was hierarchical and inefficient. Since Kosovo gained its independence from Serbia, it has begun to develop its own health care system.[11] Kosovo still struggles to care for the health needs of all its citizens, and consequently support for PWD is limited.

Because Kosovo is focused on its survival and stability, the government has few resources to devote to service provision. The nongovernmental organization Handi-KOS (Association of Paraplegics and Paralysed Children of Kosovo) attempts to fill this void by distributing AT, educating PWD and their communities, and encouraging networking among families concerned with similar disabilities. However, the effectiveness of HandiKOS is dependent on the support of charitable foundations and the availability of other resources for PWD in Kosovo. HandiKOS continues to lobby the government for public services.[12]

Zimbabwe

Before the recent collapse of Zimbabwe's economy, the country had one of the more advanced and progressive rehabilitation systems in the developing world. Two parallel sectors existed: the informal sector of traditional medicine and rehabilitation techniques, and the formal, Western-oriented sector that had remained in Zimbabwe since British colonial rule. Each sector eyed the other with suspicion and lack of respect, and referrals between the 2 were limited. However, PWD enjoyed a level of acceptance within their families and communities. Disability was not viewed as inherently isolating. Although access to disability services was in part determined by socioeconomic status and in particular living location (urban vs rural), Zimbabweans overall enjoyed some presence of services.[13]

Recent political upheaval and economic turmoil in Zimbabwe have made necessities such as food and sanitation scarce, and it is uncertain if much rehabilitation is being conducted. Zimbabwe's history of social inclusion of PWD may facilitate recovery of the rehabilitation system, if the country stabilizes enough that its people can focus on more than basic survival. However, "health in Zimbabwe is presently largely unavailable, unacceptable, inaccessible and of poor quality."[14]

PROVISION EFFORTS
Provision Models

Several approaches have been taken to providing wheelchairs in less-resourced countries. These include the "charitable model," "workshop model," "manufacturing model," "globalization model," and a fifth model that integrates aspects of the other 4 according to the needs of local people.[15]

In the charitable model, organizations donate wheelchairs in mass numbers to people in lower-income countries. Some charities provide used wheelchairs with or without custom fitting and local repair efforts. The Free Wheelchair Mission (FWM) donates a proprietary wheelchair model that is mass produced in China and shipped throughout the world. The wheelchair, which can be distributed for about $52 USD, has a seat made from a plastic lawn chair. In recent years, a thin foam seat cushion has been included, although concerns about complications such as pressure ulcers remain. One study reported modest benefits to participation, pain, and skin health among recipients of FWM wheelchairs in India and Peru; however, this study was retrospective rather than longitudinal (surveys were not conducted before the wheelchair was received). The study found that only 11.7% of individuals used their wheelchair more than 8 h/d.[16] This is in contrast to wheelchair users in the United States, who spend an average of more than 12 h/d in their wheelchairs.[15]

Charitable donations of used wheelchairs have been criticized for providing technology that cannot be maintained locally, undercutting efforts to develop sustainable sources of wheelchair provision.[17] Donated wheelchairs are quickly abandoned or rarely used because of poor fit and comfort, rapid breakdown of chairs, and inaccessibility of the local environment.[7]

Workshop and manufacturing model enterprises involve the establishment of local wheelchair fabrication facilities. They have the potential to be sustainable, produce wheelchairs that are less expensive than imported equipment, and provide employment for local wheelchair users.[15,17] However, they are subject to local economic influences, including competition from charitable wheelchair donations. Individuals assisting with the establishment of these shops must be prepared to teach wheelchair building and seating skills using methods that convey knowledge effectively to members of the local community.[17]

In the globalization model, an established wheelchair manufacturer builds or imports wheelchairs in an emerging market. This model can be sustainable and effective provided the product and sale cost are appropriate for the local community.[15] A "multimodal" model combines various strategies according to what works in a particular region, and allows efforts to be scaled depending on what is feasible. In this model, the need for wheelchairs in a region may be addressed by several different providers using diverse approaches.[15]

Design Efforts

There have been numerous efforts by researchers to design mobility technology appropriate for less-resourced environments. It is unknown how many have been successful. The most familiar organizations and technologies are those that have a large presence in rehabilitation literature or on the Internet. These include a ground-level mobility device,[16–19] a manual wheelchair,[18] a pediatric tilt-in-space wheelchair,[19] and a low-cost electric-powered wheelchair,[20] which were all designed with a focus on India. The ground-level mobility device was given to local developers after the initial research (Susan J. Mulholland, personal communication, 7 June 2009). Freely available designs have made it obtainable in India and other countries such as Nepal, where it is produced (Joy Wee, personal communication, 27 June 2009). Several wheelchair designs appear in the book *Disabled Village Children*[21] and can be built with simple materials and techniques (**Fig. 1**). Hope Haven's KidsChair wheelchair incorporates seating supports for individuals with varying postural needs.[22]

Whirlwind Wheelchair International has established itself as a network of independent wheelchair shops around the globe. Whirlwind's staff serve to integrate design concepts gathered from innovators throughout the network. The result has been a series of wheelchair designs intended for regions in Latin America, Africa, and Asia.[23] A study to evaluate a wheelchair specifically designed for people in Afghanistan found that users ranked the study wheelchair significantly higher than their original wheelchair in ease of propulsion, stability, transportability, seating

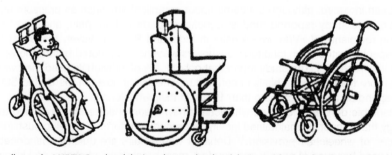

Fig. 1. (l to r) AHRTAG wheelchair, plywood wheelchair, and metal tube (a Whirlwind design). (*From* Werner D. Disabled village children: a guide for health workers, rehabilitation workers, and families. Palo Alto (CA): Hesperian Foundation; 1987, with permission from the Hesperian Foundation, 1919 Addison Street, Suite 304, Berkeley, CA 94704, USA.)

comfort, and appearance.[6] For many years, Whirlwind has offered a wheelchair construction class at San Francisco State University.[24] Similarly, a class at Massachusetts Institute of Technology, "Wheelchair Design in Developing Countries" (SP.784), addresses the improvement of appropriate wheelchairs and mobility tricycles.

Motivation Charitable Trust, from the United Kingdom, contributes in mobility technology, advocacy, community employment programs, and training.[25] Motivation has created the Worldmade brand, a wheelchair-provision process that combines mass production, flat packing, and on-site fitting. These chairs, although mass produced, are designed such that their configuration can be customized upon assembly. The Worldmade 3-wheel wheelchair, which was designed with rural areas in mind, has customizable seat width, seat depth, backrest height, footrest height, footrest position, and drive wheel axle position.

Freedom Technology, a wheelchair and tricycle shop based in the Philippines, offers a comprehensive line of everyday, sport, geriatric, and pediatric wheelchairs and tricycles. The company values quality and appropriateness of its technology and has conducted user research to assess its products.[26] This research concluded that a tricycle may best benefit someone with limited walking or crawling ability, that the tricycle should be able to be used easily over rough terrain, that it should support the user and be ergonomic, that it should be configurable to be used with significant cargo, and that repair frequency and costs should be comparable to a standard bicycle.[27]

In Nicaragua, Mobility Builders focuses particularly on children with complex seating needs, many of whom come from the poorest of families. They use a combination of clinical evaluation, computer-aided design, and local wheelchair fabrication to bring mobility to these children. Mobility Builders is an offshoot of The Wheelchair Project, a broader organization that raises funds to buy wheelchairs for those in need, trains therapists, and advocates for children's medical care.[28]

RECENT RESEARCH IN INDIA
Introduction

Many similarities exist between the needs of wheelchair users worldwide, such as the need for access, appropriate seating and mobility, and employment opportunities. However, the specifics are not universal. Infrastructure accessibility and employment opportunities vary widely, and the appropriateness of technology depends on the environment and aspects of local culture (eg, where cooking is done). Thus, to serve PWD properly in a given location, it is important to understand the specific needs of individuals.

Although proponents of the various provision models believe in the effectiveness of their own efforts, there exists little reliable evidence to indicate that one strategy is superior to another. There has been praise for one type of wheelchair and complaints about another, but these are anecdotes and may not represent the totality of wheelchair-provision outcomes. Stronger evidence would come in quantitative data that evaluates many outcomes in a region during a period of time. Ideally, this evidence would be collected using a standard survey tool appropriate for widespread use, so that results could be compared across regions and service-delivery techniques.

Some of the technology development in the authors' laboratory[18-20] has focused on India, as has the research presented in this article. Community participation, life satisfaction, wheelchair skills, and technology satisfaction were studied among clients of the Indian Spinal Injuries Centre (ISIC) who received new AT.

ISIC is one of a few locations in India where wheelchairs are clinically prescribed. The Department of Assistive Technology (DAT) has collaborated with the authors' laboratories for several purposes: (1) to assess the impact of AT in India, (2) to improve clinical provision at the ISIC DAT by evaluating the effectiveness of its practices, and (3) to pilot the collection of such data in less-resourced environments. The authors hypothesized that the provision of new AT to clients of the hospital would increase their community participation and life satisfaction, and also that the provision of clinician-evaluated wheelchairs would immediately increase wheelchair skill proficiency and technology satisfaction.

The authors aim to improve the level of evidence available to support appropriate mobility technology. With this evidence, providers such as the ISIC DAT should be able to improve their quality of care and inform donors, providers, and designers about which AT makes the most impact on the people who use it.

PART survey: participation and life satisfaction of Indian wheelchair users
The World Health Organization (WHO) has taken a lead in promoting a holistic approach toward disability. WHO's International Classification of Functioning, Disability and Health (ICF) considers disability to be a result of the interaction between a person's body and the environment. Body functions, body structure, activity, and participation are taken into account. Because "an individual's functioning and disability occurs in a context,"[2] a person with a particular impairment will live a unique life depending on socioeconomic status, educational work opportunities available, perception of the impairment by others, and any number of other factors. Furthermore, the ICF recognizes the concept of parity, in which the repercussions of an impairment are largely independent of the cause of that impairment (eg, limb losses caused by landmines and illness have similar consequences).[29] The ICF was designed to complement the International Classification of Diseases (ICD) system, which classifies health conditions without addressing the repercussions of those conditions.

Recently WHO, in collaboration with other international agencies, published a best practices guidebook for manual-wheelchair provision.[30] The book emphasizes the effects of appropriate technology on the health and happiness of wheelchair users, supplementing provision information with profiles of individuals who have benefited from wheelchairs. The message of many of these anecdotes is that appropriate technology benefits participation in the community.

In addition to the best practice evidence, substantial research has been carried out in the area of participation. Vissers and colleagues[31] investigated barriers to physical activity after spinal cord injury (SCI). This study found evidence that the logistical needs of individuals with SCI dominate immediately following injury, whereas social, economic, and health maintenance issues dominate in the long term. In other words, depending on the time since disability onset, different issues may predominantly influence physical activity. After self-care challenges become routine, physical and social public barriers seem most limiting. Similarly, Chaves and colleagues[32] found that wheelchair users with SCI in 2 US cities identified mobility technology as the most limiting factor to overall participation, even compared with the physical impairment. Participants in this study were an average 14 ± 9 years post injury. Chaves and colleagues' findings agree with those of Vissers and colleagues, in that individuals accepted their physical impairments in time and became more frustrated with the inadequacies of available technology (the wheelchair) and infrastructure (concerning environmental accessibility, or that which the wheelchair cannot traverse). Other studies[33,34] have also identified AT and adaptations as facilitators to participation. Shoulder pain has been shown to correlate with decreased participation among men with SCI[35] and standard practice guidelines recommend a customizable wheelchair that is as lightweight as possible to reduce the risk of pain and injury in the upper extremities.[30,36] Thus, there is an established influence of pain and barriers on participation, with technology as a known mediating factor.

To benefit the Indian population, with and for whom the authors have developed several wheelchairs, it is important to understand the influence of such technology on their lives. Though appropriate technology may have similar effects worldwide, factors such as the wheelchair user's physical environment, and the social role of the person with the disability, will likely influence what defines "appropriate" technology. A first step in gathering this information is to assess whether current AT provision practices in India have a positive benefit on the lives of consumers. Few data of this type have been collected because of the nascent state of clinical provision in India, though even if provision were commonplace, the data would not necessarily exist. Rehabilitation specialists working to establish quality-care practices and technologies can improve their effectiveness by assessing their current strengths and weaknesses.

The Participant Assessment (PART) questionnaire, used in this study, is an update to the Craig Handicap Assessment and Reporting Technique (CHART).[37] The objective section collects information such as the frequency that the individual does certain activities (such as childrearing and involvement in community religious activities), and the subjective section asks people to rank the importance of and their satisfaction with certain aspects of their life (such as family relationships). The PART is currently being developed. The developers are exploring multiple scoring methods (Marcel Dijkers, personal communication, 15 May 2009).

Wheelchair Skills Test/Quebec User Evaluation of Satisfaction with assistive Technology: wheelchair skills and satisfaction of Indian wheelchair users

The prescription of customized wheelchairs has become a practice, albeit uncommon, in India in the last 5 to 10 years. Most wheelchairs in India are acquired through vendors or government agencies without clinician input. They tend to be heavy, poorly designed, prone to mechanical failure, and do not allow their users to be independent or to move about efficiently with assistance.[7,38] Such wheelchairs are often inappropriate for the terrains within India. Many are manufactured locally, but chairs of similarly poor quality are also donated.[7] Because the built environment of India is more challenging to wheelchair users than in Western countries, durability and stability are much more important than some charities and manufacturers realize. In a recent study of Indian home accessibility by Pearlman and colleagues[39] unstable surfaces, narrow doorways, steps, steep ramps, and inaccessible bathrooms were found to be some of the most frequent and challenging obstacles. Several of these correspond with "community" skills described by developers of the Wheelchair Skills Test (WST).[40] Wheelchair skills performance[41] and mobility level[42] have been shown to increase participation, possibly because of individuals' increased ability to traverse physical barriers within the home and community. Though accessibility in India may be slowly improving, a more immediate impact on participation could come through the provision of wheelchairs that allow the user to exercise better skills. Given the documented failings of poor-quality wheelchairs, the authors hypothesized that individuals would demonstrate better proficiency using clinician-evaluated wheelchairs than they did using hospital-style wheelchairs. In this project, wheelchairs were categorized as either "old/heavy/hospital" (about 50 lb [22 kg], not fitted by a clinician, frequently inappropriate for user) or "active/fitted" (<35 lb [15.5 kg], fitted by a clinician, an educated guess at appropriate technology provision). Pictures of these 2 types of wheelchairs can be seen in **Fig. 2**. If results support the hypothesis that custom-fitted wheelchairs provide users with increased independent mobility and technology

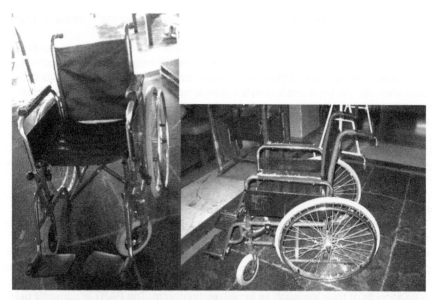

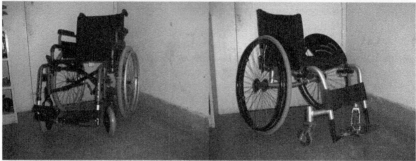

Fig. 2. (*Top*) A hospital-style wheelchair. (*Bottom*) Two types of wheelchairs available through the ISIC DAT.

satisfaction, this will provide evidence in favor of wheelchair distribution models that incorporate fitted chairs.

The WST was developed to fill a need for a standardized wheelchair proficiency instrument in research and rehabilitation.[43] Version 4.1 consists of 32 skills ranging in difficulty from rolling the wheelchair and applying the brakes to ascending stairs. Participants are spotted on all skills. A rater judges whether the participant has passed or failed each skill, and whether failures occur safely or unsafely. It is not possible to pass a skill unsafely. According to the manual,[40] several different percentage scores can be calculated. The Total Performance Score (TPS) measures how many skills out of the total were passed, the Total Attempted Score (TAS) measures how many skills out of the total were attempted, and the Total Safety Score (TSS) measures how many skills out of the total attempted were awarded a safe score. Higher scores indicate more success at completing skills, attempting skills, and safely attempting skills, respectively. Formulas for these calculations can be seen in the Equations. Additionally, the WST can be evaluated in the context of skills that a therapist believes are particularly relevant to an individual participant's rehabilitation goals.

The Quebec User Evaluation of Satisfaction with assistive Technology (QUEST) 2.0 consists of 12 questions that are scored on a scale of 1 to 5, where 5 indicates highest satisfaction. There are 2 principal subsections: device, which contains 8 questions and addresses user satisfaction with the physical properties and utility of the wheelchair; and services, which contains 4 questions and addresses user satisfaction with the sale, information, and maintenance of the wheelchair. In addition, there is a third section that asks users to select from a list the 3 wheelchair characteristics that they consider most important. The contents of the list correspond to topics of questions in the device and satisfaction subsections.

A selection of the literature suggests there are multiple strategies for scoring the QUEST. In a validation of the QUEST with a population of adults with multiple sclerosis, mean subscores for satisfaction with the device and for its services were calculated.[44] Other studies[45–47] used this technique. Alternatively, several studies[45,46,48] calculated the mean score for each individual question (the line-by-line score).

Methods

PART survey

A longitudinal repeated measures survey study was conducted through the analysis of medical records of clients of ISIC who were new recipients of AT. The authors assisted with an ISIC project to assess the quality of its AT provision services, and records from this project were ultimately transferred to the University of Pittsburgh as de-identified existing medical data. Hospital clients were enrolled in the project as they used the DAT's services (typically wheelchair evaluation), although if they did not have time to complete the measures or were suspected not to understand the questions, they were not included in the transferred dataset.

DAT clients were asked to complete intake forms on demographic data (sex, age, diagnosis/injury level, inpatient/outpatient status, and AT currently owned). Contact information was collected directly into ISIC records as part of the standard hospital intake. Upon completion of these documents, the clients provided responses to questions in the PART questionnaire. Follow-up interviews (repeated PART questionnaires) were conducted by ISIC staff at 6 and 12 months after the baseline. The purpose of these follow-ups was to determine whether community participation and life satisfaction had changed in the year since technology was received from the DAT.

The PART scoring method used involved assigning a numerical value to each response using a scoring key, and then taking a numerical average of the objective and subjective sections. Linear regression was used to evaluate the influence of gender and rural/urban location on responses. Data normality was verified using Q-Q plots of the baseline, 6-month, and 12-month objective and subjective scores. These plots allowed for assessment of data normality with a low sample size. Regression models were built, controlling for gender, semi-urban versus rural (S-R), and urban versus rural (U-R).

WST/QUEST

The WST and QUEST were administered to clients of ISIC receiving new wheelchairs from the DAT. In addition to the client, 3 personnel were involved in each test: an evaluator, a spotter, and a translator (English and Hindi). After the WST was completed, the QUEST survey was conducted. If an individual was unable to respond to a question, it was left blank. The WST and QUEST were administered to clients in their old personal (outpatients) or hospital-provided (inpatients) wheelchair. These measures were then repeated in the new wheelchair. No specific wheelchair training was given to the clients in the interim, although it was provided afterward if a client's schedule permitted.

WST evaluation and course setup were conducted as outlined in the WST manual.[40] The obstacle course was set throughout the physiotherapy department, hospital hallways, and on the ISIC grounds. Obstacles such as ramps, cross slopes, and thresholds were identified in existing hospital terrain features. Others (such as steep ramp and pothole) consisted of wheelchair skills training equipment already at the hospital. Some, such as maneuvering paths (**Fig. 3**), were constructed temporarily using small traffic cones placed on the floor.

Several different WST scores were calculated: (1) TPS, documenting how many skills out of the total were passed; (2) the TAS, indicating how many skills out of those attempted were passed; and (3) TSS, indicating how many skills out of the total attempted were awarded a safe score.[40] The subsection[47–50] and line-by-line[45,46,48] methods were used to score the QUEST. The first scoring method was used to compare pre- and posttest scores, whereas the second method was used to identify the individual factors that contributed to the overall differences between time points. These approaches were taken based on an understanding of the purposes of each scoring method; the subsection method allows for general comparisons of technology satisfaction between time points or groups, whereas the line-by-line method can be used to examine responses in individual domains such as safety and wheelchair effectiveness.

Results

PART survey
Data were transferred for 24 clients who completed the baseline questionnaire, 14 who completed the 6-month follow-up, and 13 who completed the 12-month follow-up. This decrease in available data points was caused by ISIC's lack of contact information to contact some individuals for follow-up. All but one of the included clients had received a new wheelchair close to the time of the baseline survey. The

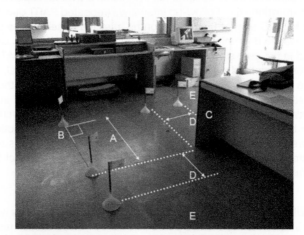

A. 1.2 m wide, smooth surface (marble tile)

B. 90 degree turns

C. Solid barrier

D. Start and finish line 0.5 m from corner

E. 1.5 m space before/after start and finish lines

Fig. 3. The 90 degree corner turning obstacle, set up using cones on the floor.

remaining client had recently acquired an accessible vehicle. Seventeen (71%) clients were male. Their ages ranged between 19 and 67 years (mean 36.4±14.8). Twelve (50%) had paraplegia as a result of SCI, 5 (21%) had tetraplegia as a result of SCI, and 7 (29%) had other conditions such as poliomyelitis and syringomyelia. The majority (92%) were outpatients, although some had been recently discharged from the hospital. Demographic information can be seen in **Table 1**. Scores for the objective and subjective sections at the baseline, 6 months, and 12 months are presented in **Table 2**.

R^2 values were higher (≈ 0.50) for the objective regression models than for the subjective models (≈ 0.27). The best significance (values <0.1) could be found in the objective U-R comparison coefficient (**Table 3**). For this calculation, there were 10 urban dwellers, 1 semi-urban dweller, and 2 rural dwellers.

Information about AT owned was collected at the baseline and the 6-month follow-up, but not at the 12-month. On average (mean and median), individuals owned more AT at 6 months than they had at the baseline. At the baseline, there was a trend toward higher objective scores with greater numbers of AT devices, and a marked higher subjective score with the individual who owned more than 10 devices. At 6 months, there were slightly higher objective scores for individuals who owned more than 10 devices, and a trend toward higher subjective scores with greater number of devices (**Table 4**).

WST/QUEST

Thirteen clients completed at least one set of WST and QUEST. Eight (62%) clients were male. Their ages ranged between 21 and 60 years (mean 33.0±12.2). Eight (62%) had paraplegia as a result of SCI, 2 (15%) had tetraplegia as a result of SCI, and 3 (23%) had other conditions such as a combination of SCI and traumatic brain injury (TBI). The majority (69%) were inpatients. Client demographics can be seen in **Table 5**.

At the time data were transferred, 7 clients had successfully completed a full set of pre- and posttests. Of these 7 individuals, 5 (71%) were male. Their ages ranged between 21 and 60 years (mean 35.1±14.5). Five (71%) had paraplegia as a result of SCI, one (14%) had tetraplegia as a result of SCI, and 1 (14%) had paraplegia as

Table 1
ISIC client demographic information

		Number	Percentage
All		24	
Sex	M	17	71
	F	7	29
Age	18–29	12	50
	30–39	6	25
	40–49	1	4
	50–59	4	17
	60+	2	8
Diagnosis	SCI (paraplegia)	12	50
	SCI (tetraplegia)	5	21
	Other	7	29
Status at baseline	Inpatient	2	8
	Outpatient	22	92

Table 2
Mean PART scores at the baseline and follow-ups

	n	Objective	Subjective
Baseline	24	1.91 (0.62)	6.99 (1.91)
6-month	14	2.38 (0.66)	6.52 (1.46)
12-month	13	2.45 (0.58)	7.07 (1.07)

a result of SCI and a TBI. Most (5, 71%) were inpatients. Demographics of these clients can be seen in **Table 6**.

Interval time between the initial and final data collection was determined by client schedule and date of wheelchair receipt, and ranged from 7 to 19 days (mean 12). Data from the 7 clients with complete data formed the basis for the direct pre/post comparison. Clients with less than the complete set of data were analyzed according to the category of wheelchair used (old/heavy/hospital or active/fitted).

TPS, TAS, and TSS averages for the 7 pre/post clients can be seen in **Table 7** and **Fig. 4**. TPS scores increased in all cases, as did TAS scores. TSS scores increased on average but decreased in 2 individuals.

The scored results of the posttest wheelchair skills as clinical goals can be seen in **Fig. 5**. Successful completion of these participation-relevant skills became less frequent as the skills increased in difficulty. All individuals were able to roll across a soft surface. Most could traverse a door, a threshold, and a cross slope, and perform a level transfer. Some could descend a 5-cm level change and a pothole. None was able to traverse a 15-cm level change or ascend a 5-cm level change.

Respective device and service subsection scores for the QUEST can be seen in **Table 8**. Pretest scores averaged approximately 2.7 (out of 5) for the device and services subsections, although other users of hospital-style wheelchairs rated them higher. Posttest scores averaged 3.44 in the device domain and 2.93 in the services domain; other users of fitted wheelchairs provided higher scores. In addition, the line-by-line scores of the pre- and postprescription QUEST surveys can be seen in **Table 9**. Fewer service-related questions were completed, although this trend was diminished in the posttest. There seemed to be little correlation between the line-by-line scores and wheelchair characteristics that the clients identified as most important (**Table 10**).

Discussion

PART survey
Statistical analysis of the PART data indicates that U-R location partially accounted for variation in scores. In the objective section, those living in rural environments had

Table 3
Analysis of regression models for B-6 (baseline to 6-month) and B-12 (baseline to 12-month) scores

		R^2	Gender Significance	Semi-Urban-Urban Significance	Urban-Rural Significance
Objective	B-6	0.449	0.475	0.961	0.079
	B-12	0.520	0.875	0.881	0.032
Subjective	B-6	0.271	0.719	0.175	0.366
	B-12	0.275	0.208	0.887	0.197

Table 4
Number of AT devices owned, relative to PART scores

		Baseline			6-month	
Number of devices	n	Objective	Subjective	n	Objective	Subjective
<6	7	1.72	6.04	7	2.29	6.10
6 to 10	6	2.17	6.51	6	2.28	6.25
>10	1	2.65	9.25	2	2.93	7.70

higher participation scores. It is possible that some feature of rural environments, such as housing structure or availability of social supports, may be more conducive to participation. However, this apparent rural favor may also be due to participation bias; the 2 rural dwellers with whom the DAT staff were able to follow-up may have a social or economic advantage that others lack. The U-R distribution present in this study was not representative of India as a whole, where the majority live in rural areas (a limitation of this study).[49] However, the male majority was consistent with existing statistics on people with locomotor disabilities in India.[50,51]

Modest increases in the objective scores indicated a trend that community participation increased. On the other hand, subjective scores decreased at 6 months and then returned approximately to baseline. Because the vast majority of clients were outpatients at the baseline, this cannot be attributed to the influence of a hospital stay. Objective and subjective scores improved during the course of 12 months, suggesting that the intervention of new AT may have improved their participation and life satisfaction. An analysis of the PART data suggests a population size of 32 would be required to achieve 90% power. The effect size at 6 months was calculated to be 0.6. Given that data for only 13 individuals were available at 12 months, the need for further quality assurance study of ISIC clients by DAT staff is indicated.

At baseline, most clients were outpatients who had been living in a community setting before their interactions with the DAT for this intervention. Some were outpatients recently discharged from ISIC and may still have been primarily concerned with self-care, as discussed by Vissers and colleagues[31] By the 12-month follow-up,

Table 5
WST/QUEST demographics

		Number	Percentage (%)
All		13	
Sex	M	8	62
	F	5	38
Age	18–29	7	54
	30–39	3	23
	40–49	2	15
	50–59	0	0
	60+	1	8
Diagnosis	SCI (paraplegia)	8	62
	SCI (tetraplegia)	2	15
	Other	3	23
Status	Inpatient	9	69
	Outpatient	4	31

Table 6
WST/QUEST demographics for complete client data

		Number	Percentage
Complete		7	
Sex	M	5	71
	F	2	29
Age (years)	18–29	4	57
	30–39	1	14
	40–49	2	29
	50–59	0	0
	60+	0	0
Diagnosis	SCI (paraplegia)	5	71
	SCI (tetraplegia)	1	14
	Other	1	14
Status	Inpatient	5	71
	Outpatient	2	29

however, all had experience living in the community rather than the hospital. Average participation scores may have increased because of this shift of environment and client acclimation to life with a disability. Future research should record and explore the influence of time since disability onset on PART survey results.

A comparison of the number of AT devices owned with PART scores yielded several trends. There seems to be a correlation between higher scores and owning more AT, an effect which is most apparent when more than 10 devices are owned. AT ownership appears to correlate more strongly with subjective scores (life satisfaction) than with objective scores (participation). Overall, these relationships may be due to a positive impact that the AT has on the lives of those who own it (an influence indicated by existing literature). It may also be that individuals on a stronger financial footing may enjoy higher life satisfaction because of their economic status while simultaneously having the capability of purchasing more equipment.

The PART questionnaire used in this study is a measure currently in development, and use of an established survey such as the CHART would have better facilitated comparisons to existing data. However, communications with Dr Marcel Dijkers indicate that the PART has been formulated after careful analysis of the advantages and

Table 7
TPS, TAS, and TSS averages for the WST

	TPS Pretest	TPS Posttest	TAS Pretest	TAS Posttest	TSS Pretest	TSS Posttest
1	50.00	59.38	53.13	65.63	53.13	62.50
2	68.75	62.50	71.88	75.00	71.88	65.63
3	68.75	71.88	75.00	81.25	75.00	78.13
4	34.38	53.13	46.88	62.50	43.75	53.13
5	59.38	62.50	71.88	68.75	68.75	65.63
6	18.75	25.00	46.88	53.13	46.88	53.13
7	65.63	78.13	75.00	84.38	75.00	81.25
Mean	52.23 (19.24)	58.93 (17.06)	62.95 (13.31)	70.09 (10.95)	62.05 (13.67)	65.63 (10.97)

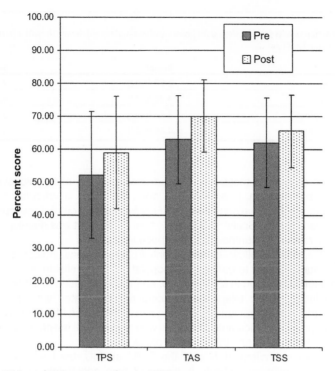

Fig. 4. TPS, TAS, and TSS averages for the WST.

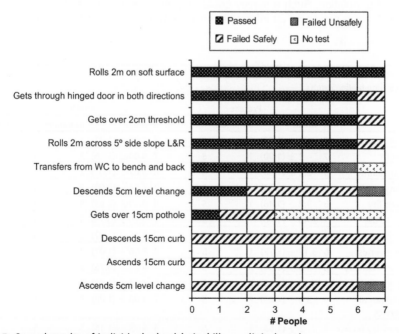

Fig. 5. Scored results of individual wheelchair skills, as clinical goals.

Table 8
QUEST subsection results for complete data points and incomplete old/heavy/hospital (O/H/H) and active/fitted (A/F) points

	Device	Services
Pretest (O/H/H)	2.72 (1.02)	2.69 (0.63)
Posttest (A/F)	3.95 (0.77)	4.21 (0.83)
O/H/H (incomplete)	3.44 (0.92)	2.93 (1.59)
A/F (incomplete)	4.44 (0.44)	4.00 (0.45)

disadvantages of existing measures, and an understanding of the biopsychosocial influences on participation. It is likely that when the PART is validated and documented in literature, it will be considered an improvement on current measures. Alternatively, the Participation Scale[52] could have been used, as it was developed in India and other low-resource countries, and has been validated.

Clients unavailable for follow-up were mainly from rural areas, indicating that it was more difficult for ISIC staff to contact this population. Some clients were reported to have no contact information in ISIC records, and the information of others may have changed. In India, mobile telephone numbers are associated with the SIM card purchased, and a lapse in minute purchasing can result in loss of the number. If there were a way to provide participants of studies with prepaid cell telephones guaranteed to last the duration of a study, this could improve retention.

Since the original implementation of the PART at ISIC, the DAT staff have not continued its use with new clients because of time constraints in the provision process, but staff are exploring alternate methods of deploying a participation survey (perhaps online) that would allow data to be collected efficiently among India's disabled population. Such a survey could be publicized using the SCI-India Yahoo group,[53] which serves as an information and networking site for individuals in India

Table 9
QUEST line-by-line results

	Pretest				Posttest			
	n	Mean	Minimum	Maximum	n	Mean	Minimum	Maximum
Dimensions	7	2.71 ± (1.70)	1	5	7	4.00 ± (1.41)	1	5
Weight	7	2 ± (1.00)	1	3	7	4.00 ± (1.15)	2	5
Adjustability	5	2.2 ± (1.30)	1	4	6	3.67 ± (1.03)	2	5
Safety	7	3.29 ± (1.25)	2	5	7	4.14 ± (0.90)	3	5
Durability	5	3.2 ± (1.48)	1	5	6	4.00 ± (0.63)	3	5
Easy to use	7	2.43 ± (1.40)	1	5	7	4.29 ± (0.76)	3	5
Comfort	7	2.71 ± (1.25)	1	5	7	3.86 ± (1.07)	2	5
Effectiveness	6	3.17 ± (1.72)	1	5	7	3.86 ± (1.07)	3	5
Service delivery	5	3.6 ± (1.34)	2	5	7	4.23 ± (0.79)	3	5
Repairs/servicing	4	3.25 ± (1.50)	2	5	6	4.33 ± (1.03)	3	5
Professional service	4	3.5 ± (1.29)	2	5	7	4.00 ± (1.00)	3	5
Follow-up service	4	3 ± (1.63)	1	5	3	4.33 ± (1.15)	3	5

Table 10
Reported frequency of preferred wheelchair properties, and the mean scores
of the corresponding questions

	Frequency (Pretest)	Mean (Pretest)	Frequency (Pos-test)	Mean (Posttest)
Easy to use	22	2.43	6	4.29
Comfort	15	2.71	6	3.86
Safety	14	3.29	3	4.14
Effectiveness	10	3.17	2	3.86
Weight	8	2.00	1	4.00
Dimensions	7	2.71	2	4.00
Adjustments	2	2.20	1	3.67
Durability	2	3.20	0	4.00
Follow-up services	1	3.00	0	4.33
Service delivery	0	3.60	0	4.23
Repairs/servicing	0	3.25	0	4.33
Professional service	0	3.50	0	4.00

with SCI. The use of online methods would introduce a socioeconomic bias to the data, but it would reach individuals who could not be reached in person and reduce the administrative load on ISIC DAT staff. Until the PART survey is validated, the CHART may be a better instrument with which to collect the needed data. CHART data could be directly compared with existing literature and provide a clearer picture of the impact of AT on the lives of users.

WST/QUEST
Though the results were not significant, there was a trend toward better scores on the WST after the wheelchair prescription. On average, clients successfully completed more skills in the posttest, as demonstrated by the 6.7% increased mean TPS.[d] In addition, individuals attempted more skills in their new wheelchairs (7.1%). That individuals were willing to attempt more skills suggests the immediate benefits of a fitted wheelchair. Safety scores increased overall by 3.6%, although the scores of some individuals decreased. Skills that most commonly became unsafe in the posttest were those that involved ascending ramps and curbs (rear tipping). This is not unexpected because fitted wheelchairs are often less stable than hospital wheelchairs because of a more forward axle position that shifts the user center of gravity further back. The lightweight wheelchairs provided by ISIC typically come with antitippers, but the ultralight models do not. Larger safety increases might have been observed if the posttests had been conducted later, after clients had become accustomed to their new wheelchairs. An examination of the construct validity of the WST indicated that wheelchair users with more than 21 days' experience performed significantly better than those with less than this amount.[54] ISIC clients who fell within this 21-day period might demonstrate a learning effect between pre- and posttests in addition to the effect of the wheelchair, whereas long-term wheelchair users would probably demonstrate an effect only because of differences in wheelchair characteristics.

A wheelchair training program for hospital clients would allow a user to make the most use of the maneuverability benefits of the fitted wheelchair while optimizing

---

[d] Percentages reported are absolute and refer to values calculated using Eqs. 1–3.

safety. Such a program exists and was trialed at ISIC before this study[55]; infrequent training sessions continue to occur. However, the authors observed that clients did not remain in the hospital with their fitted wheelchairs long enough to attend many training sessions. If wheelchair training was given to clients, it usually occurred only after they had received their new wheelchairs. Frequently, however, clients were discharged from the hospital shortly after fitting of the new wheelchair. In general, ISIC inpatients might benefit from receiving their own wheelchairs earlier rather than later, though such a modification of practice would have to be considered in the context of other factors such as changing user needs during the rehabilitation process.

The accessibility-related skills (**Fig. 5**) were scored using the posttests, because these were indicative of the skills that the clients went home with (and were therefore relevant to individuals' interactions with the home environment). An analysis of these skills suggests that clients were more competent wheeling on flat ground than they were on level changes (eg, thresholds, curbs, and steps). Most could traverse soft ground, a 2-cm threshold, and a side slope, but successful completion of skills such as curb ascent and descent was much less common. Transfer skills might allow for the use of Western-style toilets, whereas skills in traversing tight spaces might allow more use of available environments. However, Indian-style floor toilets remain challenging or impossible for wheelchair users, and doors are often simply too narrow for the wheelchair to fit through.

The QUEST results show a trend toward increased satisfaction with new wheelchairs. Each line-by-line score was higher in the posttest than in the pretest, and posttest scores were in similar ranges to scores reported in existing literature for European populations. These increases indicate that clients were more satisfied with the technology and corresponding services associated with their new, fitted wheelchairs.

In addition, response frequency increased with the new wheelchairs, especially in the services subsection, possibly reflecting optimism and confidence in the services that would be provided for their own wheelchairs. Clients rated the service-related skills no higher in importance than they had in the pretest, perhaps reflecting the reality that little wheelchair service is available throughout India. Use of the QUEST with community-based Indian populations might yield low service subsection responses such as the ones observed in the pretests presented in this article.

The wheelchair characteristics most frequently preferred by clients were "easy to use," "comfort," and "safety," followed by "effectiveness," "weight," and "dimensions." There appears to be a slight de-emphasis on wheelchair utility, as effectiveness was fourth in the list. This list may reflect that the majority of inpatient clients completed the QUEST before discharge from the hospital (where accessibility is not an issue, and assistance is available from hospital employees). Thus, clients did not anticipate that "repairs/servicing" or "durability" would be high priorities, although these attributes were considered highly important by content experts.[56] If a follow-up QUEST were conducted after individuals had lived with their wheelchair at home for some time, rankings might differ. A change in social role because of the acquired disability, or an improved understanding of accessibility and the need for wheelchair repair, could adjust an individual's preferences. Needs may become apparent as consumers become more familiar with the benefits and drawbacks of different types of wheelchairs. In addition, peer counseling and exposure of users to various types of wheelchairs could influence preferences.

An analysis of the WST data suggests a population size of 33 would be required to achieve 90% power, whereas the QUEST data suggest a population of 13 would be necessary to achieve 90% power. Because of the small sample size in this study, it was not possible to account for the numerous confounding factors that may have influenced the results of the PART and WST/QUEST studies: gender, rural/urban location, follow-up losses, time lived in the community, and types of AT acquired at ISIC.

The results of this study suggest that the use of an individually fitted wheelchair may immediately improve the skills and satisfaction of Indian users. If evidence such as this were collected and applied across India toward more widespread availability of active/fitted wheelchairs, users might gain improved skills, satisfaction, and potentially, community participation.

Evidence collected at ISIC may already have benefited the people of India. The Ministry of Social Justice and Empowerment's ADIP Scheme has granted ISIC funds to distribute clinician-evaluated wheelchairs to PWD. Each individual is allocated the equivalent of approximately $125 USD for a wheelchair, orthosis, or other piece of AT, and there is some leeway to justify shifting funds from one person's less expensive item to pay for another's more expensive one. ISIC has begun holding 3-day distribution camps each month, and will try to extend the ADIP scheme's support when the current 6-month term expires. Upon ISIC's recommendations (supported by the authors' research findings), wheelchair recipients under this program will receive foreign-purchased wheelchairs rather than the ones currently manufactured by the government agency Artificial Limbs Manufacturing Corporation of India (ALIMCO), which cannot be custom-fitted. The Ministry of Social Justice and Empowerment appears to regard ISIC as an expert resource for rehabilitation and is receptive of the hospital's advice with regard to its disability policies (Nekram Upadhyay, personal communication, 1 July 2009). This positive relationship could serve as an important channel for implementing future research findings in India, and thus improving the lives of PWD there.

SUMMARY

Numerous AT provision efforts have occurred and continue to occur throughout the world. In low- and middle-income countries, provision strategies include charitable donation of wheelchairs, local manufacture on a small or large scale, and global manufacture using international resources. Regardless of the method used, the technology provided must be appropriate for a local population to increase user function. User research can improve the chance that a developed technology will succeed in this way. At ISIC, the authors assisted with the collection of PART, WST, and QUEST data in a program intended to assess the DAT's effectiveness and pilot the collection of similar data in India and other countries. Evidence was found that wheelchairs provided by the DAT improve wheelchair skill scores and technology satisfaction, although the impact of the department's AT provision needs to be explored further to control for the influences of living environment and socioeconomic factors. Logistical experiences during the implementation of this study suggest that work is needed to reach more individuals and efficiently collect data. Electronic methods of communication (telephones, Internet) may prove useful in contacting populations difficult to reach in person.

APPENDIX

Eq. (1). Calculation of the TPS.

$$\text{Total performance score} = \frac{\text{Total skills passed}}{\text{Total skills}} \times 100 \tag{1}$$

Eq. (2). Calculation of the TAS.

$$\text{Total attempted score} = \frac{\text{Total skills attempted}}{\text{Total skills}} \times 100 \tag{2}$$

Eq. (3). Calculation of the TSS.

$$\text{Total safety score} = \frac{\text{Total skills safe}}{\text{Total skills attempted}} \times 100 \tag{3}$$

REFERENCES

1. UN Enable - Frequently Asked Questions. Available at: http://www.un.org/disabilities/default.asp?navid=12&pid=25; 2007. Accessed March 16, 2009.
2. International Classification of Functioning, Disability and Health (ICF). Available at: http://www.who.int/classifications/icf/en/; 2008. Accessed April 9, 2009.
3. François I, Lambert M-L, Salort C, et al. Causes of locomotor disability and need for orthopaedic devices in a heavily mined Taliban-controlled province of Afghanistan: issues and challenges for public health managers. Trop Med Int Health 1998;3(5):391–6.
4. Armstrong J, Ager A. Perspectives on disability in Afghanistan and their implications for rehabilitation services. Int J Rehabil Res 2005;28(1):87–92.
5. Wickford J, Hultberg J, Rosberg S. Physiotherapy in Afghanistan - needs and challenges for development. Disabil Rehabil 2008;30(4):305–13.
6. Armstrong W, Reisinger KD, Smith WK. Evaluation of CIR-Whirlwind Wheelchair and service provision in Afghanistan. Disabil Rehabil 2007;29(11):935–48.
7. Mukherjee G, Samanta A. Wheelchair charity: a useless benevolence in community-based rehabilitation. Disabil Rehabil 2005;27(10):591–6.
8. The Persons with Disabilities Act, India (1995).
9. Scheme of assistance to disabled persons for purchase/fitting of aids/appliances (ADIP scheme). Available at: http://socialjustice.nic.in/adipmain.htm. Accessed September 2, 2009.
10. Staff. Thumbs up sign for new DTC low floor buses. Available at: http://www.thehindu.com/2005/11/05/stories/2005110512530400.htm. Accessed June 16, 2009.
11. Buwa D, Vuori H. Rebuilding a health care system: war, reconstruction and health care reforms in Kosovo. Eur J Public Health 2006;17(2):226–30.
12. HandiKOS. Available at: http://www.aifo.it/english/resources/online/books/cbr/reviewofcbr/CBR-Kosova.pdf. Accessed May 21, 2009.
13. Mpofu E. Rehabilitation an international perspective: a Zimbabwean experience. Disabil Rehabil 2001;23(11):481–9.
14. ZADHR. Cholera in a time of health system collapse: violations of health rights and the cholera outbreak. Harare, Zimbabwe: Zimbabwe Association of Doctors for Human Rights; 2009.
15. Pearlman J, Cooper RA, Zipfel E, et al. Towards the development of an effective technology transfer model of wheelchairs to developing countries. Disabil Rehabil Assist Technol 2006;1(1):103–10.
16. Shore SL. Use of an economical wheelchair in India and Peru: Impact on health and function. Med Sci Monit 2008;14(12):PH71–9.
17. Kim J, Mulholland SJ. Seating/wheelchair technology in the developing world: need for a closer look. Tech Disabil 1999;11:21–7.

18. Zipfel E, Cooper RA, Pearlman J, et al. New design and development of a manual wheelchair for India. Disabil Rehabil 2007;29(11):949–62.
19. Zipfel E. Design and development of a pediatric wheelchair with tilt-in-space seating. Pittsburgh (PA): School of Health and Rehabilitation Sciences, University of Pittsburgh; 2007.
20. Pearlman J. Research and development of an appropriate electric powered wheelchair for India. Pittsburgh (PA): School of Rehabilitation Science & Technology, University of Pittsburgh; 2007.
21. Werner D. Disabled village children: a guide for health workers, rehabilitation workers, and families. Palo Alto (CA): Hesperian Foundation; 1987.
22. Wheelchairs designed to fit each individual need. Available at: http://www.rocwheels.org/wheelchairs.htm. 2007. Accessed July 1, 2009.
23. About Whirlwind: Mission Statement. Available at: http://www.whirlwindwheelchair.org/about.htm. 2004. Accessed March 30, 2009.
24. Engineering 699: wheelchair design & development. Available at: http://design.sfsu.edu/node/148. 2006. Accessed June. 30, 2009.
25. Our work. Available at: http://www.motivation.org.uk/_our_work/index.html. 2009. Accessed March 30, 2009.
26. Freedom Technology. Available at: http://www.freedomtechnology.com.ph. 2008. Accessed April 30, 2009.
27. Mellin J. Tricycle research: Available at: http://www.YouTube.com. Accessed April 30, 2009.
28. Mobility Builders. Available at: http://www.mobilitybuilders.org. 2009. Accessed June 5, 2009.
29. Üstün TB, Chatterji S, Kostansjek N, et al. Information in health records. Health Care Financ Rev 2003;24(3):77–88.
30. Armstrong W, Borg J, Krizack M, et al. Guidelines on the provision of manual wheelchairs in less-resourced settings. Geneva, Switzerland: World Health Organization; 2008.
31. Vissers M, van den Berg-Emons R, Sluis T, et al. Barriers to and facilitators of everyday physical activity in persons with a spinal cord injury after discharge from the rehabilitation centre. J Rehabil Med 2008;40:461–7.
32. Chaves ES, Boninger ML, Cooper R, et al. Assessing the influence of wheelchair technology on perception of participation in spinal cord injury. Arch Phys Med Rehabil 2004;85(11):1854–8.
33. Chan SC, Chan AP. User satisfaction, community participation and quality of life among Chinese wheelchair users with spinal cord injury: a preliminary study. Occup Ther Int 2007;14(3):123–43.
34. Meyers AR, Anderson JJ, Miller DR, et al. Barriers, facilitators, and access for wheelchair users: substantive and methodologic lessons from a pilot study of environmental effects. Soc Sci Med 2002;55:1435–46.
35. Ballinger DA, Rintala DH, Hart KA. The relation of shoulder pain and range-of-motion problems to functional limitations, disability, and perceived health of men with spinal cord injury: a multifaceted longitudinal study. Arch Phys Med Rehabil 2000;81:1575–81.
36. Boninger ML, Waters RL, Chase T, et al. Preservation of upper limb function following spinal cord injury: a clinical practice guideline for health-care professionals. Washington, DC: Consortium for Spinal Cord Medicine; 2005.
37. Whiteneck GG, Charlifue SW, Gerhart KA, et al. Quantifying handicap: a new measure of long-term rehabilitation outcomes. Arch Phys Med Rehabil 1992;73(6):519–26.

38. Saha R, Dey AK, Hatoj M, et al. Study of wheelchair operations in rural areas covered under the district rehabilitation centre (DRC) scheme. Indian J Disabil Rehabil 1990;75–87.

39. Pearlman J, Jefferds A, Nagai I, et al. Designing assistive technology for less-resourced environments: an online method to gauge accessibility barriers and collect design advice. Paper presented at: Annual Conference of Rehabilitation Engineering and Assistive Technology Society of North America. Atlanta, Georgia, June 22–26, 2006.

40. Kirby RL. Wheelchair skills test (WST) manual. Halifax (NS): Dalhousie University; 2008.

41. Kilkens OJ, Post MW, Dallmeijer AJ, et al. Relationship between manual wheelchair skill performance and participation of persons with spinal cord injuries 1 year after discharge from inpatient rehabilitation. J Rehabil R D 2005;42(8):65–74.

42. Dijkers MPJM, Yavuzer G, Ergin S, et al. A tale of two countries: Environmental impacts on social participation after spinal cord injury. Spinal Cord 2002;40: 351–62.

43. Kirby RL, Swuste J, Dupuis DJ, et al. The wheelchair skills test: a pilot study of a new outcome measure. Arch Phys Med Rehabil 2002;83:10–8.

44. Demers L, Monette M, Lapierre Y, et al. Reliability, validity, and applicability of the Quebec User Evaluation of Satisfaction with assistive Technology (QUEST 2.0) for adults with multiple sclerosis. Disabil Rehabil 2002;24(1):21–30.

45. Bergstrom AL, Samuelsson K. Evaluation of manual wheelchairs by individuals with spinal cord injuries. Disabil Rehabil Assist Technol 2006;1(3):175–82.

46. Goodacre L, Turner G. An investigation of the effectiveness of the Quebec user evaluation of satisfaction with assistive technology via a postal survey. Br J Occup Ther 2005;68(2):93–6.

47. Wessels RD, De Witte LP. Reliability and validity of the Dutch version of QUEST 2.0 with users of various types of assistive devices. Disabil Rehabil 2003;25(6): 267–72.

48. Wressle E, Samuelsson K. User satisfaction with mobility assistive devices. Scand J Occup Ther 2004;11:143–50.

49. India Statistics (Demographics). Available at: http://www.unicef.org/infobycountry/india_india_statistics.html. 2005. Accessed June 30, 2009.

50. Patel SK. An empirical study of causes of disability in India. Int J Epidemiol 2009;6:2.

51. Sarvekshana. 47th rounds, National Sample Survey Organization, Department Of Statistics: Ministry of Planning & Program Implementation, Government of India [census results]; 1991.

52. van Brakel WH, Anderson AM, Mutatkar RK, et al. The participation scale: measuring a key concept in public health. Disabil Rehabil 2006;28(4):193–203.

53. SCI India - SCI Info Forum. Available at: http://health.dir.groups.yahoo.com/group/SCI-India/?v=1&t=directory&ch=web&pub=groups&sec=dir&slk=3. 2009. Accessed July 1, 2009.

54. Kirby RL, Dupuis DJ, MacPhee AH, et al. The wheelchair skills test (version 2.4): measurement properties. Arch Phys Med Rehabil 2004;85:794–804.

55. Kirby RL, Cooper RA. Applicability of the wheelchair skills program to the Indian context. Disabil Rehabil 2007;29(11–12):969–72.

56. Demers L, Wessels RD, Weiss-Lambrou R, et al. An international content validation of the Quebec User Evaluation of Satisfaction with assistive Technology (QUEST). Occup Ther Int 1999;6(3):159–75.

Index

Note: Page numbers of article titles are in **boldface** type.

A

AAC. See *Augmentative and alternative communication (AAC).*
AAOS. See *American Association of Orthopedic Surgeons (AAOS).*
ADA. See *Americans with Disabilities Act (ADA).*
Adaptive cruise control, in motor vehicles, 119–120
ADIP Scheme. See *Assistance to Disabled Persons for Purchase (ADIP) Scheme.*
Afghanistan, assistive technology for people with disabilities in, 222
ALSFRS-R. See *Revised ALS Functional Rating Scale (ALSFRS-R).*
American Association of Orthopedic Surgeons (AAOS), 89
Americans with Disabilities Act (ADA), 111, 208
Amputation surgery, 89
ARM, 61–62, 64–66
Assessment tools, CAT, 18–21
Assistance to Disabled Persons for Purchase (ADIP) Scheme, of Ministry of Social Justice
    and Empowerment, 222
Assistive robotic manipulation devices, **59–77**
    advances in, future directions in, 73–74
    CATOR taxonomy on, 60
    described, 59–60
    effectiveness of, definitions of, in accordance with priorities of users of, 72–73
    evaluation of, 70–72
        gaps in, 73
    externally mounted manipulators, 60–66
        control of, 62–64
        evaluation of, trends in, 64–66
        future research on, 66
        overview of, 60–61
    prosthetic devices, 66–70
        alternative control techniques, 69
        future research on, 70
        overview of, 66–67
        pattern recognition, 68–69
        sensory feedback, 69–70
        targeted muscle reinnervation, 67–68
    users of, priorities of, definitions of effectiveness in accordance with, 72–73
Assistive technology, for people with disabilities, provision of, in less-resourced countries,
    221–242
    Afghanistan, 222
    described, 221
    design efforts, 224–225

Phys Med Rehabil Clin N Am 21 (2010) 243–252
doi:10.1016/S1047-9651(09)00086-2
1047-9651/09/$ – see front matter © 2010 Elsevier Inc. All rights reserved.

pmr.theclinics.com

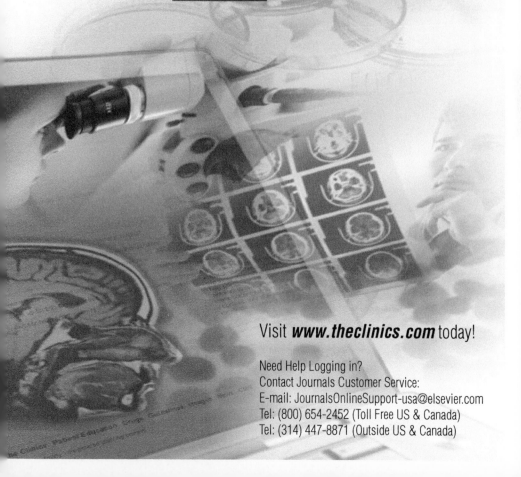

Printed and bound by CPI Group (UK) Ltd, Croydon, CR0 4YY

03/10/2024

01040464-0003